Molecular Mechanisms in Demyelinating Disorders of the Central Nervous System

Molecular Mechanisms in Demyelinating Disorders of the Central Nervous System

Guest Editor

Paschalis Theotokis

MDPI

Basel • Beijing • Wuhan • Barcelona • Belgrade • Novi Sad • Cluj • Manchester

Guest Editor
Paschalis Theotokis
Laboratory of Histology
and Embryology
Aristotle University of Thessaloniki
Thessaloniki
Greece

Editorial Office
MDPI AG
Grosspeteranlage 5
4052 Basel, Switzerland

This is a reprint of the Special Issue, published open access by the journal *Current Issues in Molecular Biology* (ISSN 1467-3045), freely accessible at: https://www.mdpi.com/journal/cimb/special_issues/58S56E5316.

For citation purposes, cite each article independently as indicated on the article page online and as indicated below:

Lastname, A.A.; Lastname, B.B. Article Title. *Journal Name* **Year**, *Volume Number*, Page Range.

ISBN 978-3-7258-4275-9 (Hbk)
ISBN 978-3-7258-4276-6 (PDF)
https://doi.org/10.3390/books978-3-7258-4276-6

Cover image courtesy of Paschalis Theotokis
White matter area from mouse lumbar spinal cord. Magnification: 6000×

Contents

About the Editor

Paschalis Theotokis

Dr. Paschalis Theotokis is a Reader in Histology and Embryology at the School of Medicine, Aristotle University of Thessaloniki, and a Researcher at the Laboratory of Experimental Neurology and Neuroimmunology at the AHEPA University Hospital, Greece. He holds an MSc and a PhD with distinction in Neuroscience. His scientific interests lie in neurodevelopment, neurodegeneration, glial biology, and regenerative medicine, with a particular focus on myelin pathology. Dr. Theotokis has extensive expertise in advanced microscopy techniques, including immunofluorescence, confocal imaging, and, notably, transmission electron microscopy (TEM), which he applies to both experimental and translational neuroscience. His academic trajectory has been distinguished by honors for teaching excellence, formal recognition from his institution, and consistently outstanding evaluations from students. His research training includes fellowships at Yale School of Medicine (USA), INSERM (France), and Monash University (Australia), supported by national and international research grants. Currently, he maintains active research collaborations with leading neuroscience laboratories at Monash University and institutions in Israel. He has published more than 60 peer-reviewed articles and regularly presents his work at international neuroscience conferences, including invited talks in Paris, Montreal, New York and Honolulu. His current work integrates molecular neurobiology with high-resolution imaging to investigate mechanisms of demyelination and repair in central nervous system disorders.

Preface

This Special Issue reprint, curated under the theme "Myelin Dynamics and Demyelinating Disorders", brings together recent advances exploring the molecular, cellular, and developmental underpinnings of myelin biology within the central nervous system. The aim of this collection is to deepen our understanding of how oligodendrocyte lineage cells contribute to both healthy myelination and disease-associated demyelination, particularly in disorders such as multiple sclerosis. As a Guest Editor, I was motivated to compile this focused issue in light of emerging technologies and model systems that can now allow us to dissect myelin-associated mechanisms with unprecedented resolution. The contributions herein—from basic research to translational applications—are intended to support both early-career and established researchers, clinicians, and neurobiologists working in the intersecting fields of glial biology, neuroinflammation, and CNS repair. I extend my sincere appreciation to the contributing authors for their high-quality submissions, to the peer reviewers for their valuable input, and to the editorial staff at *Current Issues in Molecular Biology* for their professional support throughout the process.

Paschalis Theotokis
Guest Editor

current issues in molecular biology

MDPI

Editorial

Exploring Myelin Dynamics in Demyelinating Disorders at the Molecular Level

Paschalis Theotokis [1,2]

[1] Laboratory of Experimental Neurology and Neuroimmunology, 2nd Department of Neurology, AHEPA University Hospital, 54636 Thessaloniki, Greece; ptheotokis@auth.gr

[2] Laboratory of Histology and Embryology, Medical School, Aristotle University of Thessaloniki, 54124 Thessaloniki, Greece

Investigating the subtle molecular mechanisms underlying demyelinating disorders of the central nervous system (CNS) is pivotal in advancing therapeutic strategies and improving patient outcomes. This Editorial summarizes the dynamic landscape of myelin biology and demyelination, around three key themes extracted from a selection of ten seminal papers. Beginning with myelin origin and oligodendrocyte dynamics, the discussion progresses to inflammation, encompassing multiple sclerosis (MS) and the paramount role of microglia, before exploring systemic–therapeutic approaches. Through this structured approach, the aim is to unravel the molecular nuances of demyelinating disorders, offering insights for novel therapeutic interventions.

Primordial components of the myelin sheath at the embryological level are fundamental for illuminating the mechanisms driving myelinogenesis in adult life, particularly under both normal conditions and scenarios requiring repair [1]. Dermitzakis et al. explore the role of early life developmental cues and molecular drivers in myelinogenesis. The key contributors to this process include oligodendrocyte lineage cells, extensively investigated in animal models such as zebrafish [2] and mammalian CNS [3,4]. Whilst there is a myriad of molecular cues involved, Fahim et al. have identified OLIG2 and MYT1L transcription factors as essential catalysts for enhancing the differentiation potential of human mesenchymal stem cells into oligodendrocytes, thus offering promising avenues in advancing therapeutic strategies for demyelinating disorders.

Among the demyelinating disorders, the most prevalent one is MS, affecting 2.8 million people worldwide [5]. Experimental autoimmune encephalomyelitis (EAE), an animal model of MS, recapitulates the immunological aspects of the disease [6], serving as a substrate for cell therapy [7] and drug testing. With regards to the latter, Haghmorad et al. investigate the oral administration of myelin oligodendrocyte glycoprotein as an immunomodulatory agent, revealing its ability to induce Th2/Treg cells while suppressing Th1/Th17 immune responses, thereby offering an elegant strategy to attenuate EAE. Building upon this, Papiri et al. comprehensively explore the inflammatory and neuroglial aspects of MS, shedding light on the complex molecular interactions driving disease progression. Further delving into the specific manifestations of MS, Ciapă et al. meticulously examine the molecular mechanisms underlying optic neuritis, enhancing our understanding of the challenges posed by optic nerve involvement in MS.

Transitioning to the role of glial cells in inflammatory-based CNS demyelination, Dermitzakis et al. present a historical account of microglia origins, unraveling its eccentric journey within the CNS and contributing to a holistic perspective on neuroinflammation. Microglial fluctuations are intricately linked to key neurodevelopmental hallmarks and play a crucial role in regulating CNS myelin growth and integrity [8–10]. Microglia play a tremendous role in the healthy brain [11,12], MS-related diseased conditions [13,14] and aged CNS [15]. Notably, Piper et al. investigates the pro-inflammatory and pro-apoptotic effects of l-azetidine-2-carboxylic acid in BV2 microglial cells, offering valuable insights into potential neuroprotective strategies amidst microglial responses.

The focus shifts to diagnostic markers and therapeutic approaches addressing immune-mediated demyelinating disorders. Tonev et al. underscore the impact of plasma exchange in MS on circulatory factors, nerve growth factor and sphingosine-1-phosphate plasma levels, shedding light on the delicate balance between pathogenic factors and therapeutic interventions. Transitioning to foundational diagnostics, Kelbich et al.'s analysis of cerebrospinal fluid serves as a framework for understanding CNS impairment, laying the groundwork for unveiling molecular markers in demyelinating disorders. Lastly, Kaffe et al. scrutinize the roles of caloric restriction mimetics in central nervous system demyelination and myelin regeneration, uncovering novel therapeutic avenues to induce remyelination, a topic that has garnered significant attention in the research field [16].

In conclusion, this Editorial navigates through the complex landscape of molecular mechanisms which underlie demyelinating disorders, delineating key findings from multiple research teams. These studies offer foundational insights into oligodendrocyte dynamics and myelin origin to the elucidation of inflammation's role in MS and the contribution of glial cells, particularly microglia. The corpus of presented papers sheds light on the multifaceted nature of demyelination. Collectively, these studies advance current knowledge, provide directions for systemic and therapeutic interventions, thus, paving the way for enhanced diagnosis, management and potential treatment options for demyelinating disorders of the CNS.

Conflicts of Interest: The author declares no conflict of interest.

References

1. Stadelmann, C.; Timmler, S.; Barrantes-Freer, A.; Simons, M. Myelin in the Central Nervous System: Structure, Function, and Pathology. *Physiol. Rev.* **2019**, *99*, 1381–1431. [CrossRef] [PubMed]
2. Neely, S.A.; Lyons, D.A. Insights Into Central Nervous System Glial Cell Formation and Function From Zebrafish. *Front. Cell Dev. Biol.* **2021**, *9*, 754606. [CrossRef] [PubMed]
3. Baumann, N.; Pham-Dinh, D. Biology of Oligodendrocyte and Myelin in the Mammalian Central Nervous System. *Physiol. Rev.* **2001**, *81*, 871–927. [CrossRef] [PubMed]
4. Zeiss, C.J. Comparative Milestones in Rodent and Human Postnatal Central Nervous System Development. *Toxicol. Pathol.* **2021**, *49*, 1368–1373. [CrossRef] [PubMed]
5. Walton, C.; King, R.; Rechtman, L.; Kaye, W.; Leray, E.; Marrie, R.A.; Robertson, N.; La Rocca, N.; Uitdehaag, B.; Van Der Mei, I.; et al. Rising Prevalence of Multiple Sclerosis Worldwide: Insights from the Atlas of MS, Third Edition. *Mult. Scler. J.* **2020**, *26*, 1816–1821. [CrossRef] [PubMed]
6. Theotokis, P.; Lourbopoulos, A.; Touloumi, O.; Lagoudaki, R.; Kofidou, E.; Nousiopoulou, E.; Poulatsidou, K.-N.; Kesidou, E.; Tascos, N.; Spandou, E.; et al. Time Course and Spatial Profile of Nogo-A Expression in Experimental Autoimmune Encephalomyelitis in C57BL/6 Mice. *J. Neuropathol. Exp. Neurol.* **2012**, *71*, 907–920. [CrossRef] [PubMed]
7. Theotokis, P.; Kesidou, E.; Mitsiadou, D.; Petratos, S.; Damianidou, O.; Boziki, M.; Chatzidimitriou, A.; Grigoriadis, N. Lumbar Spine Intrathecal Transplantation of Neural Precursor Cells Promotes Oligodendrocyte Proliferation in Hot Spots of Chronic Demyelination. *Brain Pathol.* **2022**, *32*, e13040. [CrossRef] [PubMed]
8. Menassa, D.A.; Muntslag, T.A.O.; Martin-Estebané, M.; Barry-Carroll, L.; Chapman, M.A.; Adorjan, I.; Tyler, T.; Turnbull, B.; Rose-Zerilli, M.J.J.; Nicoll, J.A.R.; et al. The Spatiotemporal Dynamics of Microglia across the Human Lifespan. *Dev. Cell* **2022**, *57*, 2127–2139.e6. [CrossRef] [PubMed]
9. McNamara, N.B.; Munro, D.A.D.; Bestard-Cuche, N.; Uyeda, A.; Bogie, J.F.J.; Hoffmann, A.; Holloway, R.K.; Molina-Gonzalez, I.; Askew, K.E.; Mitchell, S.; et al. Microglia Regulate Central Nervous System Myelin Growth and Integrity. *Nature* **2023**, *613*, 120–129. [CrossRef] [PubMed]
10. Theotokis, P.; Zoupi, L.; Tremblay, M.-È.; Zhao, J.-W. Editorial: Molecular and Cellular Interactions of Myelin in Neurodevelopmental & Neurodegenerative Disorders. *Front. Cell. Neurosci.* **2024**, *17*, 1359184. [PubMed]
11. Tremblay, M.-È.; Stevens, B.; Sierra, A.; Wake, H.; Bessis, A.; Nimmerjahn, A. The Role of Microglia in the Healthy Brain: Figure 1. *J. Neurosci.* **2011**, *31*, 16064–16069. [CrossRef] [PubMed]
12. Kaur, C.; Rathnasamy, G.; Ling, E.-A. Biology of Microglia in the Developing Brain. *J. Neuropathol. Exp. Neurol.* **2017**, *76*, 736–753. [CrossRef] [PubMed]
13. Guerrero, B.L.; Sicotte, N.L. Microglia in Multiple Sclerosis: Friend or Foe? *Front. Immunol.* **2020**, *11*, 374. [CrossRef] [PubMed]
14. Li, W.; Liu, J.; Tan, W.; Zhou, Y. The Role and Mechanisms of Microglia in Neuromyelitis Optica Spectrum Disorders. *Int. J. Med. Sci.* **2021**, *18*, 3059–3065. [CrossRef] [PubMed]

15. Yoo, H.-J.; Kwon, M.-S. Aged Microglia in Neurodegenerative Diseases: Microglia Lifespan and Culture Methods. *Front. Aging Neurosci.* **2022**, *13*, 766267. [CrossRef] [PubMed]
16. Franklin, R.J.M.; Frisén, J.; Lyons, D.A. Revisiting Remyelination: Towards a Consensus on the Regeneration of CNS Myelin. *Semin. Cell Dev. Biol.* **2021**, *116*, 3–9. [CrossRef] [PubMed]

current issues in
molecular biology

MDPI

Review

Developmental Cues and Molecular Drivers in Myelinogenesis: Revisiting Early Life to Re-Evaluate the Integrity of CNS Myelin

Iasonas Dermitzakis [1], Maria Eleni Manthou [1], Soultana Meditskou [1], Dimosthenis Miliaras [1], Evangelia Kesidou [2], Marina Boziki [2], Steven Petratos [3], Nikolaos Grigoriadis [2] and Paschalis Theotokis [1,2,*]

[1] Department of Histology-Embryology, School of Medicine, Aristotle University of Thessaloniki, 54124 Thessaloniki, Greece; iasonasd@auth.gr (I.D.); mmanthou@auth.gr (M.E.M.); sefthym@auth.gr (S.M.); miliaras@auth.gr (D.M.)

[2] Laboratory of Experimental Neurology and Neuroimmunology, Second Department of Neurology, AHEPA University Hospital, 54621 Thessaloniki, Greece; bioevangelia@yahoo.gr (E.K.); bozikim@auth.gr (M.B.); ngrigoriadis@auth.gr (N.G.)

[3] Department of Neuroscience, Central Clinical School, Monash University, Prahran, VIC 3004, Australia; steven.petratos@monash.edu

* Correspondence: ptheotokis@auth.gr

Abstract: The mammalian central nervous system (CNS) coordinates its communication through saltatory conduction, facilitated by myelin-forming oligodendrocytes (OLs). Despite the fact that neurogenesis from stem cell niches has caught the majority of attention in recent years, oligodendrogenesis and, more specifically, the molecular underpinnings behind OL-dependent myelinogenesis, remain largely unknown. In this comprehensive review, we determine the developmental cues and molecular drivers which regulate normal myelination both at the prenatal and postnatal periods. We have indexed the individual stages of myelinogenesis sequentially; from the initiation of oligodendrocyte precursor cells, including migration and proliferation, to first contact with the axon that enlists positive and negative regulators for myelination, until the ultimate maintenance of the axon ensheathment and myelin growth. Here, we highlight multiple developmental pathways that are key to successful myelin formation and define the molecular pathways that can potentially be targets for pharmacological interventions in a variety of neurological disorders that exhibit demyelination.

Keywords: oligodendrogenesis; myelinogenesis; myelin formation; embryology; CNS development; neural tube development; morphogen signaling

1. Introduction

As the regulator of all cognitive, sensory, and motor activity, the nervous system is the most complex biological system in humans; the complexities of integrated neural networks are a hot area of intensive research that will require multidisciplinary investigations to address a variable array of neurological disorders that remain an unmet medical need. The main types of cells in the nervous system are neurons and glial cells with the latter performing vital supporting roles [1,2]. The glial/neuronal ratio differs uniformly across brain regions of mammalian species, underlining the pivotal role of interaction between glial cells and neurons for appropriate integration of the central nervous system (CNS) to coordinate neurophysiological and cognitive functions [3]. For propagation of action potentials to ensue in neurons, axonal myelination is crucial [4,5]. The cells responsible for myelination are the oligodendrocytes (OLs) in the CNS and Schwann cells in the peripheral nervous system (PNS). Rudolf Virchow initially designated the term "myelin" in 1854, named after the Greek word "marrow" (myelos), since it is especially plentiful in the brain's center, or marrow [6]. He posited that neurons produced myelin, but Pío del Río Hortega's better histological staining processes almost a century ago revealed that myelin is created by specific glial cells, which are OLs [7,8].

The CNS macroglia and neurons have a common embryonic origin from the neuroectoderm, most prominently from neuroepithelial cells of the telencephalic ventricular and subventricular zone (VZ and SVZ), while the spinal cord is supplied with cell derivatives exclusively from the central canal [9,10]. Newborn CNS is radically unmyelinated with a sparse developing pool of unipotent cells, namely oligodendrocyte precursor cells (OPCs), following their birth with gradual widespread functionality in the first few years of childhood [11]. Myelination persists in an asynchronous spatiotemporal pattern through adolescence towards adulthood, coinciding with the establishment and maintenance of correct circuit function and cognitive development [12,13]. Mature myelin sheaths remain stable by and large; however, they maintain the capacity to remodel and reorganize if need be [14]. As expected, aging promulgates limit resources and energy deficiency to sustain such developmental processes, thus cellular senescence is a common event [15]. Consequently, there is a variety in the patterns of myelination, with qualitative- and quantitative-ontogenic checkpoints, throughout human life.

In this review, we focus on the de novo synthesis of myelin referred to herein as myelinogenesis. This is the primordial pattern of myelination, which starts prenatally and predominates during the first two years of human life [16]. In order for myelinogenesis to happen, neural stem cells (NSCs) need to undergo specific developmental stages, with the process of oligodendrogenesis, as well as additional steps for the maintenance of these primary myelin sheaths. Interestingly, it is possible that lifelong myelinogenesis may still occur in specific CNS regions through quiescent, adult OPCs (aOPCs), based on miscellaneous factors, such as unmyelinated space, new OLs turnover, energy balance, and neural circuit activity [17]. Such processes are broadly defined as adaptive myelination or myelin remodelling/plasticity which is under fine regulation and is generally restricted. Lastly, another crucial factor that may trigger myelinogenesis is injury and disease, such as demyelination, and is discussed briefly towards the end, with a process known as remyelination.

2. Myelinogenesis and Myelin Development: A Spatiotemporal Coordination

2.1. Primordium Regions of OPCs

The mammalian CNS emerges from an ectodermal, neuroepithelial lining of the neural tube in the developing embryo [9,18]. Multiple divisions give rise to radial glia (RG), a multipotent neural stem population that colonizes the newly-formed ventricular walls (Figure 1) [18,19]. The VZ is the primary embryonic site for OPCs production through asymmetrical division of the RG cells. In mice, OPCs are firstly detected in the ventral VZ closer to the floor plate on embryonic day 12.5 (E12.5), and in humans at gestational week (GW) 6.5 (~E45) [20]. More specifically, the outer SVZ (oSVZ) is an enlarged cortical germinal zone only generated in humans [21]. In oSVZ, a distinct RG cell population termed as outer RG (oRG) is located peripherally and gives rise to a transit-amplifying population, which is an additional source of OPCs supplying the human cortex [19,21].

In the human forebrain, the first wave of OPCs originates from the medial ganglionic eminence (MGE) and the anterior entopeduncular area (AEP), while a second batch emerges postnatally from the lateral or caudal ganglionic eminences, establishing a sufficient amount of OPCs in the cerebral cortex [22]. OPCs of the human forebrain appear in the SVZ of the MGE at GW7.5, whilst at E12 in mice [19]. In the spinal cord, the majority of the nascent OPCs (about 80% of the total number) complete their formation at the motor neuron progenitor (pMN) domain of the ventral spinal cord, while the pool is enriched later at E15.5 by additional OPCs migrating from dorsal regions [23]. Lastly, the cerebellar OPCs are derived from the metencephalic ventral rhombomere 1 region, manifesting their presence at E16.5 and are reinforced additionally with a secondary population originating from the cerebellar VZ [10].

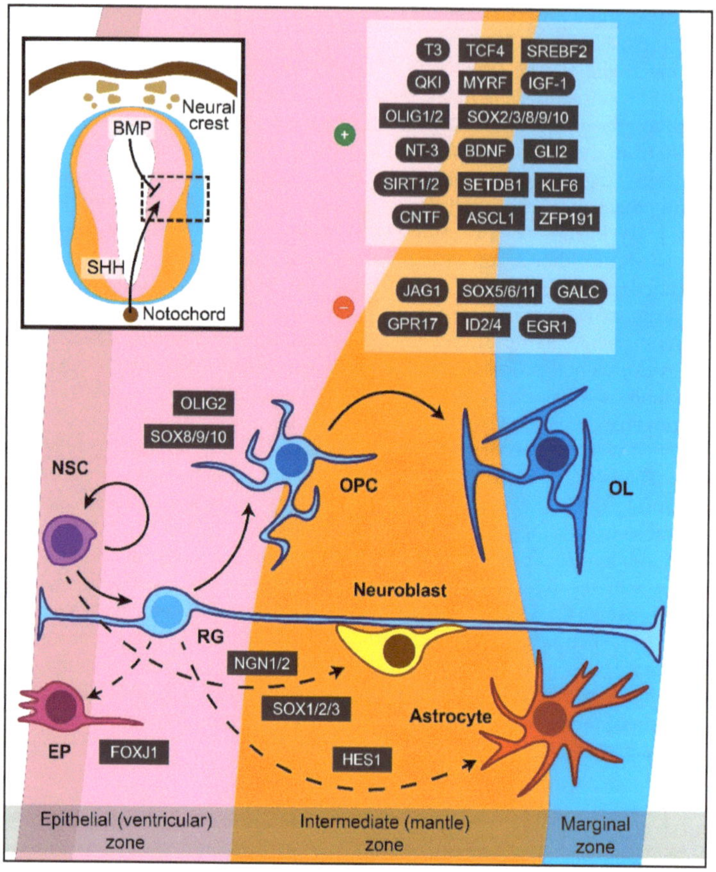

Figure 1. Major cues of OPCs generation and differentiation during myelinogenesis in the prenatal period. In the neuroepithelium lining the neural tube, NSCs are under the influence of notochord-derived SHH, which drives the cells to become OPCs through OLIG2, SOX8/9/10 or follow neuronal fate (neuroblasts) via NGN1/2 and SOX1/2/3. BMP originated from the neural crest instructing NSCs to become astrocytes, controlled by HES1 as well. FOXJ1 is a crucial transcription factor for the ependymal trajectory. The positive and negative cues controlling OPCs differentiation are displayed in the upper right boxes. The hatched box depicts a representative area around sulcus limitans (between alar and basal plates). Dashed lines showcase naturally occurring processes, albeit not addressed in detail in the current review. ASCL1: Achaete-scute family bHLH transcription factor 1, BDNF: Brain-derived neurotrophic factor, BMP: Bone morphogenetic protein, CNTF: Ciliary neurotrophic factor, EGR1: Early growth response 1, EP: Ependymal cells, FOXJ1: Transcription factor forkhead box J1, GALC: Galactosylceramidase, GLI2: Glioma-associated oncogene family zinc finger 2, GPR17: G protein-coupled receptor 17, HES1: Hes family bHLH transcription factor 1, ID2: Inhibitor of DNA binding 2, ID4: Inhibitor of DNA binding 2, IGF-1: Insulin-like growth factor 1, JAG1: Jagged canonical Notch ligand 1, KLF6: Kruppel-like factor 6, MYRF: Myelin regulatory factor, NGN1: Neurogenin-1, NGN2: Neurogenin-2, NSC: Neural stem cells, NT-3: Neurotrophin 3, OL: Oligodendrocytes, OLIG1: Oligodendrocyte transcription factor 1, OLIG2: Oligodendrocyte transcription factor 2, OPC: Oligodendrocyte precursor cell, QKI: Quaking homolog, KH domain RNA binding, RG: Radial glia, SET domain bifurcated histone lysine methyltransferase 1, SETDB1: SHH: Sonic hedgehog signaling molecule, SIRT1: Sirtuin 1, SIRT2: Sirtuin 2, SOX: Sex-determining region Y-box transcription factor, SREBF2: Sterol regulatory element-binding transcription factor 2, T3: Triiodothyronine, TCF4: Transcription factor 4, ZFP191: Zinc finger protein 191.

2.2. Molecular Signals Driving Myelinogenesis

As has been articulated from the experimental evidence, the inauguration of myelinogenesis necessitates the formation of OPCs from multipotent NSCs, which ultimately give rise to mature myelinating OLs through a multistep process (Figure 1) [18,24]. A vital step herein lies in OPCs' ability to migrate toward miscellaneous sites and proliferate, based predominately on environmental stimuli. These cells become post-mitotic, exiting the cell cycle to express a substantial amount of myelin-associated proteins and differentiate into mature pre-myelinating OLs [23]. Following the proper recognition, targeting and ensheathing specific nerve fibers is the subsequent critical milestone where each pioneer process creates lamellar extensions that stretch and elaborate circumferentially around the target axon [24]. As a new membrane is generated at the leading edge of the forming myelin sheath's inner tongue, which starts to resemble a spiral cross-sectional shape, the sheath continues to spread along the axonal length. The secured stability and maintenance of a newly-formed myelin sheath is the concluding event. Specific developmental cues and molecular drivers regulate all the aforementioned cellular activities and are enlisted in full capacity in Tables A1–A3.

2.2.1. Formation of OPCs

OPCs being generated from the ventral VZ are under the influence of the morphogen molecule Sonic hedgehog (SHH) secreted from the notochord, while the dorsal counterparts are SHH-independent [25,26]. SHH signalling drives NSCs into a neuronal or OLs lineage fate superseding the effect of bone morphogenetic proteins (BMPs) which favour astroglial generation (Figure 1) [27,28]. Early secretion of SHH promotes motor neuron lineage formation, while interaction in later time periods promotes OLs differentiation [29]. Interestingly, the concentration of SHH can be controlled by sulfatase 1 expression in the ventral neuroepithelium prior to OPCs specification [30], whereas fibroblast growth factor (FGF) signalling is of paramount importance for further OLs differentiation, especially in the spinal cord [31,32].

Oligodendrocyte transcription factor 2 (OLIG2) is the primary regulator of OPCs generation [33,34], and its gene expression can be potentially repressed throughout the pre to postnatal period by paired box 6 (PAX6), Brahma-related gene-1 (BRG1), Iroquois homeobox 3 (IRX3), histone deacetylase (HDAC) 1, HDAC2, Distal-less homeobox (DLX) 1 and DLX 2 [35–41]. On the other hand, oligodendrocyte transcription factor 1 (OLIG1) is activated in later stages of OLs development [42]. Interestingly, the Hes family bHLH transcription factor (HES1) can drive RG to an astrocytic phenotype [43], while co-occurrence of OLIG2 with neurogenin-1 or neurogenin-2 supports motor neuron production [38,44,45].

Members of the sex-determining region Y-box transcription factor (SOX) family, such as SOX1, SOX2, and SOX3, can also direct OPCs towards a neuronal fate [33], in contrast to SOX8, SOX9, and SOX10, which favour the turnover of NSCs to OPCs in an autonomous manner [34–36]. Additionally, transcription factor forkhead box J1 (FOXJ1) supports the retention of RGs as ependymal cells throughout ventricles. Lastly, glioma-associated oncogene family zinc finger 2 (GLI2), myelin transcription factor 1 (MYT1), NK2 homeobox 6 (NKX2-6), and chromodomain-helicase-DNA-binding protein 8 (CHD8), among others (Table A1), are embryonic cues for OLs specification that vary within CNS regions indicating brain region specificity [37–40].

2.2.2. Migration

SHH presence is equally catalytic to OPCs migration [41]. Platelet-derived growth factor subunit A (PDGFA) and its cognate receptor, PDGF receptor alpha (PDGFRα), are essential positive drivers for OPCs migration [42]. In line with this, SOX5, SOX6, SOX9, and SOX10 stimulate the migration, ensuring PDGF responsiveness [43,44]. Chondroitin sulfate proteoglycan neuron-glia antigen 2 (NG2) and ephrin-B2/B3 molecules control OPCs polarity and contact abilities, promoting or intercepting migration, respectively [45,46]. Nestin, neural cell adhesion molecule (NCAM), and OLIG1 can also act as chemoattractants, determining cytoskeletal plasticity as well as OPCs motility [47–51]. Other migration chemoattractants are 2′,3′-cyclic nucleotide 3′ phosphodiesterase (CNPase), OLIG2, hepatocyte growth factor (HGF), thrombospondin 1, endothelin 1 (ET-1), oligodendrocyte specific protein (OSP), OSP–associated protein (OAP-1), N-cadherin (NCAD), merosin, fibronectin, and integrin subunit beta 1 ($\alpha v\beta 1$ integrin) [52–60]. Spassky et al. suggested that netrin-1 is a candidate mediator for chemoattraction during migration [61]. However, other studies considered this molecule as a chemorepellent, antagonizing PDGF [62,63].

More growth factors and associated molecules, such as vascular endothelial growth factor A (VEGF-A) combined with VEFG receptor 2 (VEGFR2), can act as chemoattractant molecules for OPCs migration along with miscellaneous members of the transforming growth factor beta (TGF-β) family (e.g., BMP7 and BMP4), and Gαi-linked sphingosine-1-phosphate receptor (S1PR) 1 and S1PR3 [64–66]. In contrast to these specific sphingosine molecules, S1PR2 and S1PR5 negatively regulated migration [66]. Moreover, although C-X-C motif chemokine receptor (CXCR) 4, C-X-C motif chemokine ligand (CXCL) 12 and semaphorin 3F have chemoattractive effects on the OPCs migration, semaphorin 3A, CXCL1, and CXCR2 inhibit migration [61,67,68]. In addition, tenascin-c inhibited OPCs migration, whilst both claudin (CLDN) 1 and CLDN3 supported OPCs relocation, validated also in human specimens [59,69,70].

2.2.3. Proliferation

Specific driver molecules that participate in migration, such as PDGFA and PDGFRα, contribute additionally to the OPC proliferation [47,71]. Interestingly, in the spinal cord, the mitogenic effect of PDGF was enhanced by chemokine CXCL1 and CXCR2 [44,72], while CXCL12 had a proliferative effect on OPCs, mediated by its receptor CXCR4 [73]. More growth factors, such as FGF2, brain-derived neurotrophic factor (BDNF), and epidermal growth factor (EGF) are shown to play a vital role in OPCs proliferation [74–76].

Associate developmental pathways are also implicated in this step; PDGF-mediated proliferation depends largely on Wnt/β-catenin and PI3K/AKT/mTOR pathways [77,78]. Furthermore, jagged canonical Notch ligand 1 (JAG1) promotes OPCs proliferation and critically blocks the subsequent differentiation step [79]. Carrying on subcellular, CHD7 and CHD8 regulate gene expression in specific brain regions [80,81]. Another member of the SOX family, SOX9, supports the development of OLs in the cerebellum, regulating the timing of proliferation [82]. MYT1, NCAM, cyclin-dependent kinase inhibitor 1B ($p27^{KIP1}$), oligodendrocyte myelin glycoprotein (OMgp), and tubulin polymerization promoting protein (TPPP) are negative regulator cues for OPCs proliferation [83–87]. Interestingly, overexpression of inhibitor of DNA binding (ID) 2 and ID4 enhances proliferation [88,89]. Similarly, expression of SHH, HGF, neurotrophin-4 (NT-4), noggin, superoxide dismutase 1 (SOD1), neurotrophin-3 (NT-3), achaete-scute family bHLH transcription factor 1 (ASCL1), PAX6, CLDN1, and CLDN3 promotes the proliferation process [41,54,70,90–95].

Integrin-mediated signalling and, more specifically, OSP, OAP-1, $\alpha v\beta 1$ integrin, $\alpha v\beta 3$ integrin, fibronectin and laminin are pivotal mediators in cytoskeletal remodelling of proliferating OPCs [56,96,97]. Gadea et al. revealed that ET-1 is a candidate molecule for enhancing cell migration without influencing proliferation [60]. Later, Adams and colleagues underscored that loss of ET-1 reduces OPCs proliferation in the developing SVZ via directly binding to endothelin type B receptor (ETBR) [98]. A reduced OPCs proliferation is observed in *GS homeobox 1/2* (*Gsx1/2*) mutant embryos, whereas galectin-4 (GAL-4) treatment increased the proliferation [99,100]. At last, NRG1 and SOX2 induce cell division [101,102]; however, the latest data demonstrate that NRG1 acting via ErbB did not alter the proliferation state of OPCs [103].

2.2.4. Differentiation

OLIG1 and OLIG2 are heavily involved in the post-proliferating step of myelinogenesis, defining the initiation of OPCs differentiation (Figure 1) [51,53,104], while BMPs seem to inhibit this process by downregulating myelin protein expression [105]. The effect can be reversed by using a physiological antagonist of BMP4, such as noggin, which may restore differentiation [91,106,107]. OLIG2 appears to interact with a variety of factors, such as ASCL1, BRG1, transcription factor 4 (TCF4), and SET domain bifurcated histone lysine methyltransferase 1 (SETDB1) to ensure proper OPCs differentiation [108–112]. G protein-coupled receptor 17 (GPR17) can act as a downregulator of OLIG1 that negatively controls the maturation and coordinates the generation of myelinating OLs from pre-myelinating OLs through ID proteins [113]. Although overexpression of ID2 and ID4 both regulate myelin gene expression by inhibiting OLs differentiation [89,114], they are not the major in vivo repressors of differentiation [115]. Moreover, decreased levels of OLIG1 and myelin regulatory factor (MYRF) were observed under early growth response 1 (EGR1) and SOX11 overexpression, delineating the inhibitory action of the latest in OPCs differentiation [116,117]. Intriguingly, MYRF is a unique regulator participating in the late stages of OLs maturation and myelination, while the action of the other OLs' lineage transcription factors is restricted on OPCs specification or initial differentiation of OLs [118].

SOX family proteins are also participating in the OLs differentiation. In particular, SOX2 and SOX3, through negative regulation of miR145, promote OLs maturation [119], while SOX5 and SOX6 increase PDGFRα expression, maintaining OLs in their immature state [44]. For the terminal differentiation of OLs, SOX8, SOX9, and SOX10 are required [82,120–122]. The state of myelinogenesis-associated gene expression is uniformly affected by NKX2-2 and NKX2-6 [40,123,124]. Ji et al. suggested a mechanism regarding NKX2-2-mediated inhibition of OLs differentiation via regulation of sirtuin 2 (SIRT2), which generally is a positive cue for OLs maturation [125]. Similarly, sirtuin 1 (SIRT1) participates in the differentiation of OPCs during development [126] through cytoskeleton-related OLs proteins. The Kruppel-like factor 6 (KLF6) is another transcription factor promoting OPCs differentiation through glycoprotein 130 (GP130)-signal transducer and transcription activator 3 (STAT3) signalling [127]. Growth factor-wise, BDNF is a regulator of OLs differentiation operating via binding to tyrosine receptor kinase B (TrkB) and enhancing the MAPK pathway to upregulate gene expression during OLs maturation [75,77,128]. Evidently, NT-3 is important for the transition of immature OLs to myelin-forming cells by recruiting c-Fos protein-activating protein kinase C (PKC) and tyrosine kinase activities [129,130]. Insulin-like growth factor 1 (IGF-1) is another main factor in assisting the development of OPCs to mature OLs [131]. In accordance with that, GRB2 associated binding protein 1 (GAB1) absence decreased OLs differentiation, acting as a novel target of PDGF [132]. Incidentally, Canoll et al. suggested that NRG1 is a negative regulator of OPCs differentiation [101], while Brinkmann et al. later demonstrated that NRG1 is required for OPCs differentiation [103].

As far as metabolism is concerned, quaking homolog, KH domain RNA binding (QKI)-5 forms a complex with sterol regulatory element-binding transcription factor 2 (SREBF2) that regulates the transcription of genes responsible for cholesterol biosynthesis in OLs during differentiation [133]. Lack of transactive response DNA-binding protein 43 (TDP-43) results in lower SREBF2 and low-density lipoprotein receptor (LDLR) expression and cholesterol levels in vitro and in vivo, indicating the potential role of TDP-43 in cholesterol homeostasis in OLs, which is linked with the proper completion of OLs development [134]. In the same manner, ectonucleotide pyrophosphatase/phosphodiesterase 6 (ENPP6) participates in OLs maturation via a supplement of OLs with choline [135]. Most importantly, triiodothyronine (T3) is a key molecule for blocking OPCs proliferation and promoting their differentiation into mature OLs [136,137]. Thyroid hormone receptor alpha (TRα) is found both in OPCs and mature OLs, whilst thyroid hormone receptor isoform beta 1 (TRβ1) is located only in mature OLs [138]. The OPCs differentiation is mediated by the TRα, while TRβ1 is responsible for promoting myelinogenesis in later stages [77]. Overexpression of HES5 decreases the levels of TRβ1 receptors, while ASCL1 increases them, demonstrating their role in regulating OLs differentiation timing [139]. The neurogenic locus notch homolog protein 1 (NOTCH1) is another receptor that also regulates the differentiation timing [140]. Interestingly, JAG1 is a receptor's ligand responsible for inhibiting OLs differentiation, while contactin 1 (CNTN1) is another ligand with the opposite function [79,141].

Other membrane molecules which repress OPCs differentiation are NCAM and leucine-rich repeat, and Ig-like domain-containing Nogo receptor interacting protein 1 (LINGO-1) [142,143]. OLs maturation is negatively affected by GAL-4 and galactosylceramidase (GALC), while prominin-1, GLI2, p21-activated kinase 1 (PAK1), myelin-associated glycoprotein (MAG), SOD1, ciliary neurotrophic factor (CNTF), and inward rectifying potassium channel 4.1 (Kir4.1) are crucial for proper differentiation [38,95,100,144–149]. On the other hand, proper completion of OLs differentiation requires zinc finger protein 191 (ZFP191) [150]. Microtubule-associated protein 2 (MAP2), microtubule-associated protein tau (MAPT), CNPase, and TPPP may be involved in OLs differentiation by organising the microtubule system, similar to fasciculation and elongation protein zeta 1 (FEZ1), which is responsible for developing OLs processes' arbour [87,151–153]. Additionally, important molecules being involved in the completion of OLs development are OMgp, brain enriched myelin-associated protein 1 (BCAS1) and glutathione (GSH) [154–157]. Myelin proteolipid protein (PLP) and myelin basic protein (MBP) are the main myelin structural proteins, but it is suggested that they play an additional role in OLs differentiation [158,159]. CLDN1 and CLDN3 control MBP, OLIG2, PLP, and SOX10 expression: these molecules are essential for OLs differentiation, indicating that claudins are needed [70]. Finally, connexin 47 (CX47) and adenosine triphosphate binding cassette subfamily D member 1 (ABCD1) may support OLs during their differentiation, aiding in gap junction coupling and reducing oxidative stress, respectively [160–164].

2.2.5. Ensheathment

Multiple positive cues are important for the inauguration of ensheathment (Figure 2). Amongst the prime ones with a positive effect on axon-glial junction maintenance is NCAD, which regulates the interaction between OLs processes and axons [165]. The L1 cell adhesion molecule (L1-CAM) and laminin expressed in axons bind to contactin and integrin located in OLs [166]. Upon the formation of the first loops/wraps, neurofascin 155 (NF155), located in paranodal loops, forms a well-defined complex with contactin-associated protein (CASPR) and CNTN1, transmembrane proteins which are expressed in axons [167–169]. The activation of this complex has a pivotal role in myelin targeting, sheath growth, organisation of paranodal loops and, therefore, supporting the axoglial junction [170, 171]. However, CASPR does not participate in myelin targeting [170]. In juxtaparanodes, the axoglial junction is strengthened when transient axonal glycoprotein-1 (TAG-1), a crucial molecule for maintaining enrichment of Kv1.1/Kv1.2 channels [172], interacts with CASPR2. Regarding internodal axoglial adhesion, glial cell adhesion molecule (CADM) 4 binds to axonal CADM2 and CADM3, facilitating myelin targeting, axon wrapping, and myelin sheath growth [173]. Similarly, CADM1b strongly binds to axonal CADM2, positively regulating ensheathment and strengthening the junction [174]. In the same region of the myelin sheath, MAG binds to ganglioside in axons, especially ganglioside GD1a and GT1b, and enforces the junction's stability [175,176].

Based on several studies, ephrins (A, B) and cognate receptors (A, B) have dual roles that rely on location and expression. While ephrin receptor (Eph) A4 in OLs is activated by axonal ephrin-A1 ligand, which inhibits the stability of axoglial junctions needed for ensheathment, EphA4, expressed in the axon surface, interacts with ephrin-B, promoting myelin sheet formation [177,178]. In addition, EphB1 of axons is activated through ephrin-B in OLs, which in turn stimulates myelinogenesis [178]. The axonal ephrinB2 via binding with EphB OLs receptor influences integrin activation, reducing myelin sheet formation [178]. The list of negative cues includes LINGO-1, which is located in both axons and OLs, and self-interacts in trans to control the number of targeted axons inhibiting myelinogenesis [143,179]. The NCAM is a cell adhesion molecule negatively regulating myelinogenesis. The downregulation of this protein is essential for promoting myelin formation during development, as myelinogenesis occurs only on NCAM negative axons [180].

A somatodendritic protein, junctional adhesion molecule 2 (JAM2) inhibits oligodendroglial interaction, suppressing myelinogenesis [181]. Apart from the somatodendritic molecules, GAL-4 is expressed only to unmyelinated segments of neurons in hippocampal and cortical regions; this protein is demonstrated as the first identified inhibitor of myelinogenesis in axons [182]. Of particular interest is the possible role of OLIG1 in axonal recognition during myelinogenesis (Table A2) [183].

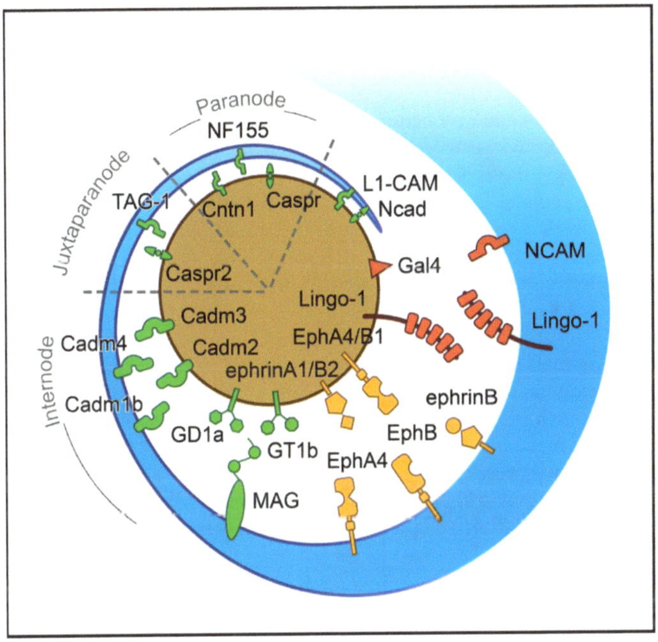

Figure 2. Axoglial driving cues for the initiation of ensheathment during myelinogenesis. A process of oligodendrocyte (blue) approaches the axon (brown) based on their surfaces' attractive and repulsive signals. The red-colored shapes represent negative surface molecules; the green ones stand for positive and the yellow for bidirectional signals. For illustrational purposes, the paranode, juxtaparanode, and internode regions are simplified. CADM1b: Cell adhesion molecule 1b, CADM2: Cell adhesion molecule 2, CADM3: Cell adhesion molecule 3, CADM4: Cell adhesion molecule 4, CASPR: Contactin-associated protein, CASPR2: Contactin-associated protein-like 2, CNTN1: Contactin 1, EphA4: Ephrin receptor A4, EphB: Ephrin receptor B, EphB1: Ephrin receptor B1, GAL-4: Galectin-4, GD1a: Ganglioside GD1a, GT1b: Ganglioside GT1b, L1-CAM: L1 cell adhesion molecule, LINGO-1: Leucine-rich repeat and Ig-like domain-containing Nogo receptor interacting protein 1, MAG: Myelin-associated glycoprotein, NCAD: N-cadherin, NCAM: Neural cell adhesion molecule, NF155: Neurofascin 155, TAG-1: Transient axonal glycoprotein-1.

2.2.6. Myelin Sheath Growth and Preservation

The long-term membrane expansion and maintenance of the newly-formed myelin sheath is the final step in completing myelinogenesis and is utterly controlled by the major myelin proteins (Table A3). The most abundant myelin proteins are PLP (>50%) and MBP (~15%), having a significant role in the stabilization of the myelin structure [24,52,184]. The disruption of PLP gene expression presents impaired membrane compaction [185]. MAG, on the other side, is the third most abundant protein in CNS myelin (~5%), and does not seem to contribute to maintenance as much as it does to the previously described initial interaction between OLs and axons [147,186]. Interestingly, myelin oligodendrocyte glycoprotein (MOG) [187,188], CNPase [52,189], myelin-associated oligodendrocyte basic protein (MOBP) [190], and OMgp [86,191,192], all minor CNS myelin proteins (<1%), need more investigation on how they influence the formation and maintenance of myelin sheaths in compact myelin.

OLs microtubule stability is mediated by MAP2 and MAPT [151], while CX32 and CX47 participate in maintenance [161]. Claudins, such as OSP, CLDN1, and CLDN3, play a pivotal role as well [70,185]. Transcription factors that participate in the lamellar extension process are SOX8, SOX10, NKX2-2, NKX6-2, and MYRF [35,122,193,194]. Transmembrane protein (TMEM) 98, which inhibits the self-cleavage of MYRF, ID4, and OLIG1, could also be involved in the process [114,195], whereas OLIG2 is expressed only until myelin membranes' production is completed [183,196]. In addition, the ERK1/2 MAP kinase pathway is indispensable in maintaining myelinated axons via FGF–FGF receptor 1 and 2 (FGFR1 and FGFR2) [197,198]. Experiments in *Hdac3*-mutant optic nerves raised the possibility that HDAC3 is also necessary for myelin integrity [199].

Proper cholesterol biosynthesis is prioritized in myelinogenesis, with QKI regulating this cholesterol production via SREBF2. Specifically, QKI-5 acts synergistically with peroxisome proliferator-activated receptor beta (PPARβ)-retinoid X receptor alpha (RXRα) activating transcription of the response in fatty acid metabolism genes. This operation of QKI-5 is significant for maintaining myelin homeostasis [133]. The ceramide galactosyl transferase (CGT) is a key enzyme for catalyzing GALC synthesis, while ceramide sulfotransferase (CST) is responsible for converting GALC to sulfatide [200,201]. Both CST and CGT mutant animals showed a regionally specific loss of myelin stability [200]. Thus, GALC and sulfatide have a pivotal role in the long-term maintenance of myelin, with the GALC being more crucial for myelin development than its assembly [200,201]. Additionally, peroxisomal metabolism also influences myelin survival [202]. For example, a peroxisomal transmembrane protein responsible for very long-chain fatty metabolism is encoded by the *ABCD1* gene and is key in maintaining myelin stability [164,203]. Lastly, the age-dependent changes of TMEM10 might be linked with its action in maintaining CNS myelin [204].

2.3. Myelin Formation after Infancy

Although myelinogenesis has been described in the nascent developmental years, myelination does naturally occur for the duration of a person's life to promote learning and memory through brain circuit plasticity [205], or as remyelination after an injury [206]. The synaptic plasticity has been studied in depth; however, a newly discovered form of brain plasticity, namely myelin plasticity or myelin remodelling, is under intensive investigation [205]. Extrinsic factors can influence, either positively or negatively, this remodelling in the toddler, adolescent, and adult brain. For example, since myelin formation is sensitive to experience, sensory stimulation may upregulate myelination, while sensory or social deprivation can potentially downregulate axon ensheathment [205,207]. Myelin remodelling initiates when pre-existing OPCs recruit or directly differentiate into newly-formed mature OLs, whereas existing OLs have the ability to engage in plasticity [205]. The principal cues for this "adaptive" myelination should not be different from the ones we scrutinize in this review.

The regenerative process following injury also presents many similarities with specific steps of myelinogenesis [208]. The neonatal OPCs are maintained in a resting, quiescent state through adulthood, and they are referred to as adult aOPCs, constituting ~6% of all cells in the CNS [206]. Interestingly, aOPCs have a transcriptome similar to mature OLs. After injury, the innate immune response activates aOPCs, transforming them into a neonatal-like transcriptome [209]. The activation of aOPCs is followed by their proliferation, migration, and final differentiation into mature OLs. Older literature describes these aOPCs as the primary remyelinating cells [210]. Nevertheless, newer research has suggested that neural progenitors in SVZ, Schwann cells, and surviving mature OLs are also implicated in the remyelinating process [211–213].

The myelination efficiency is age-dependent, as the impairment of aged OPCs to recruit and differentiate into mature OLs leads to decreased remodelling and remyelination [214]. The nutrient support of OLs is highly compromised in aging due to the presence of senescent astrocytes, leading to decreased cholesterol biosynthesis which in turn weighs in the impaired OLs membrane development [15,215,216]. This age-related energy depletion that decreases the myelination efficiency is further fed from the accumulation of DNA damage while rendering the neurons vulnerable to oxidative stress through free radicals [15,217]. Additionally, the ineffectiveness of microglia, which translates to aged phagocytes to clear out impaired myelin, is a potential aetiology for the downregulation of remyelination [218]. Taken all together, the detailed investigation of cues that drives de novo myelination could be a crucial point for revisiting them in demyelination and remyelination of the adult CNS, a concept that is discussed briefly in the following section.

3. Myelinogenesis in Disease and Beyond

Although aging is a natural process that leads to a decreased turnover of functional OLs and diminished myelin formation, the integrity of myelinogenesis can be highly compromised in pathological situations such as demyelination, characterized by extensive myelin loss [219]. This condition has to be distinguished from dysmyelination, which is a genetic-based anomaly affecting basic myelin proteins and leads to uneven/not properly compacted myelin sheaths [219]. Demyelinating diseases could be divided into many categories; according to their pathogenesis mechanism, which mostly implicate environmental factors, nutritional deficits, presence of myelinotoxic agents, or virus-mediated impairments. In quite frequent cases, immune system mediators are deregulated, leading to autoimmune inflammatory demyelination [219,220]. Among the three most prevalent inflammatory demyelinating diseases are multiple sclerosis (MS), neuromyelitis optica spectrum disorder (NMOSD), and acute disseminated encephalomyelitis (ADEM).

In this review, we summarized all the potential molecules responsible for the long-term maintenance of myelin along the axoglial junction (see Sections 2.2.5 and 2.2.6), serving simultaneously as key factors in demyelinating disease sequelae. Recent data revealed that impaired mitochondrial function and oxidative stress are also candidate pathophysiology mechanisms for demyelinating diseases [221]. Berghoff et al. demonstrated that disruption of cholesterol metabolism alters brain lipid metabolism in CNS and is associated with neurological diseases such as autoimmune inflammatory conditions, including MS [222]. Nonetheless, under such circumstances, an autoimmune attack generates myelin debris from damaged myelin [223]. These components impair the CNS remyelination by obstructing OPCs and OLs functionality while triggering additional deleterious immune responses, also known as epitope spreading [213,223,224]. The clearance of myelin debris is crucial for rearrangement since recent studies suggest that the failure of myelin clearance leads to inefficient remyelination [225,226].

Remyelination can be spontaneous or in an experimental setup, achieved by the providence of an exogenous source of neural precursor cells (NPCs) with myelinating potential [227,228]. In various transplantation paradigms, it is shown that these cells can either exert an in situ myelinating effect, as seen and applied successfully in spinal cord injury (SCI) cases [229,230], or by instructing and enhancing the capacity of endogenous cells to remyelinate, documented in experimental autoimmune encephalomyelitis (EAE) [208,231,232] (324). Proposed mechanisms of action also underline immunomodulatory effects rather than direct cell replacement [233,234]. Nevertheless, the scarce population of surviving mature OLs after demyelination is shown to be less effective in comparison to newly created ones [213,235–237]. Towards this trajectory, which is a fully functional recruitment of aOPCs to form myelinating OLs [208,238] (324, 325), it is extremely important to comprehend the developmental molecular cues and factors governing the process of myelinogenesis (see Section 2.2.1, Section 2.2.2, Section 2.2.3, Section 2.2.4), since these same molecules can be candidate targets for therapeutic intervention in demyelinating diseases.

4. Conclusions

Through this comprehensive review, we attempt to list and categorize the genes and proteins that act as developmental morphogens to the CNS development and, more specifically, those that are activated in the process of oligodendrogenesis. The fully functional OLs, originating from unspecialized stem cells, are able to identify newly-formed axons which emanate and branch in regions that need fast conduction early in life, completing their task of myelinogenesis. Some of these cells persist in adult life in an intermediate, dormant phenotype scattered or organized around the primordial niches. An argument that was intended to bring into attention is how the powerful dynamics that shape myelination, which is naturally declining as we age, can be sustained, or even re-engaged after an injury or demyelinating disease. In the current era, transcriptomic profiling or metabolomic data can potentially give an answer as to which of the enlisted molecules, drivers, and regulators should be prioritized.

Author Contributions: I.D. and P.T., writing—original draft preparation and visualization; M.E.M., S.M. and D.M., conceptualization, review and editing; E.K., M.B., S.P. and N.G., review and editing. All authors have read and agreed to the published version of the manuscript.

Funding: This research received no external funding.

Institutional Review Board Statement: Not applicable.

Informed Consent Statement: Not applicable.

Data Availability Statement: Not applicable.

Conflicts of Interest: The authors declare no conflict of interest.

Abbreviations

OPCs	Oligodendrocyte precursor cells
OLs	Oligodendrocytes
CNS	Central nervous system
NSCs	Neural stem cells
aOPCs	Adult oligodendrocyte precursor cells
E	Embryonic day
GW	Gestational week
VZ	Ventricular zone
SVZ	Subventricular zone
RG	Radial glia
oSVZ	Outer subventricular zone
MGE	Medial ganglionic eminence
MS	Multiple sclerosis
ABCD1	Adenosine triphosphate binding cassette subfamily D member 1
ASCL1	Achaete-scute family basic helix-loop-helix transcription factor 1
BDNF	Brain-derived neurotrophic factor
BMP4	Bone morphogenetic protein 4
BMP7	Bone morphogenetic protein 7
CADM1b	Cell adhesion molecule 1b
CADM2	Cell adhesion molecule 2
CADM3	Cell adhesion molecule 3
CADM4	Cell adhesion molecule 4
CASPR	Contactin-associated protein
CASPR2	Contactin-associated protein-like 2
CGT	Ceramide galactosyl transferase
CHD7	Chromodomain-helicase-DNA-binding protein 7
CHD8	Chromodomain-helicase-DNA-binding protein 8
CLDN1	Claudin 1
OSP	Oligodendrocyte specific protein
CLDN3	Claudin 3

CNPase	2′,3′-cyclic nucleotide 3′ phosphodiesterase
CNTN1	Contactin 1
CST	Ceramide sulfotransferase
CX32	Connexin 32
CX47	Connexin 47
CXCL1	C-X-C motif chemokine ligand 1
CXCL12	C-X-C motif chemokine ligand 12
CXCR2	C-X-C motif chemokine receptor 2
CXCR4	C-X-C motif chemokine receptor 4
DLX1	Distal-less homeobox 1
DLX2	Distal-less homeobox 2
EphA4	Ephrin receptor A4
EphB1	Ephrin receptor B1
EphB2	Ephrin receptor B2
ET-1	Endothelin 1
FGF2	Fibroblast growth factor 2
FGFR1	Fibroblast growth factor receptor 1
FGFR2	Fibroblast growth factor receptor 2
GAL-4	Galectin-4
GALC	Galactosylceramidase
GLI2	Glioma-associated oncogene family zinc finger 2
HDAC1	Histone deacetylase 1
HDAC2	Histone deacetylase 2
HDAC3	Histone deacetylase 3
HES5	Hairy and enhancer of split family basic helix-loop-helix transcription factor 5
HGF	Hepatocyte growth factor
ID2	Inhibitor of DNA binding 2
ID4	Inhibitor of DNA binding 4
JAG1	Jagged canonical Notch ligand 1
LINGO-1	Leucine-rich repeat and Ig-like domain-containing Nogo receptor interacting protein 1
MAG	Myelin-associated glycoprotein
MAP2	Microtubule-associated protein 2
MAPT	Microtubule-associated protein tau
MBP	Myelin basic protein
MYRF	Myelin regulatory factor
MYT1	Myelin transcription factor 1
NCAD	N-cadherin
NCAM	Neural cell adhesion molecule
NKX2-2	NK2 homeobox 2
NKX2-6	NK2 homeobox 6
NKX6-2	NK6 homeobox 2
NRG1	Neuregulin 1
NT-3	Neurotrophin 3
OAP-1	Oligodendrocyte specific protein–associated protein
OLIG1	Oligodendrocyte transcription factor 1
OLIG2	Oligodendrocyte transcription factor 2
OMgp	Oligodendrocyte myelin glycoprotein
PAX6	Paired box 6
PDGFA	Platelet-derived growth factor subunit A
PDGFRα	Platelet-derived growth factor receptor alpha
PLP	Myelin proteolipid protein
QKI	Quaking homolog, KH domain RNA binding
S1PR1	Sphingosine-1-phosphate receptor 1
S1PR2	Sphingosine-1-phosphate receptor 2
S1PR3	Sphingosine-1-phosphate receptor 3
S1PR5	Sphingosine-1-phosphate receptor 5
SHH	Sonic hedgehog signaling molecule
BRG1	Brahma-Related Gene-1
SOD1	Superoxide dismutase 1

SOX1	Sex-determining region Y-box transcription factor 1
SOX10	Sex-determining region Y-box transcription factor 10
SOX11	Sex-determining region Y-box transcription factor 11
SOX2	Sex-determining region Y-box transcription factor 2
SOX3	Sex-determining region Y-box transcription factor 3
SOX5	Sex-determining region Y-box transcription factor 5
SOX6	Sex-determining region Y-box transcription factor 6
SOX8	Sex-determining region Y-box transcription factor 8
SOX9	Sex-determining region Y-box transcription factor 9
SREBF2	Sterol regulatory element-binding transcription factor 2
TRα	Thyroid hormone receptor alpha
TRβ1	Thyroid hormone receptor isoform beta 1
TDP-43	Transactive response DNA-binding protein 43
TMEM10	Transmembrane Protein 10
TMEM98	Transmembrane protein 98
TPPP	Tubulin polymerization promoting protein
VEGF-A	Vascular endothelial growth factor A
VEGFR2	Vascular endothelial growth factor receptor 2
αvβ1 integrin	Integrin subunit beta 1
αvβ3 integrin	Integrin subunit beta 3

Appendix A

The following appendix contains all the genes and relevant chromosomal loci from proteins involved in myelinogenesis in relation to their biological role. This data is supplemental to the main text based on the current knowledge and literature on cues driving oligodendrocyte development, ensheathment and myelin maintenance.

Table A1. Molecular drivers and morphogens in specification, migration, proliferation, and differentiation of OPCs.

Gene *	Chromosomal Locus *	Protein *	Biological Role	Reference
ABCD1	Xq28	ATP binding cassette subfamily D member 1	Differentiation	[163,164]
ADGRG1	16q21	Adhesion G protein-coupled receptor G1	Proliferation	[239]
ANOS1	Xp22.31	Anosmin 1	Migration	[240]
ASCL1	12q23.2	Achaete-scute family bHLH transcription factor 1	Specification; Proliferation; Differentiation	[93,108,139,241]
BCAS1	20q13.2	Brain enriched myelin-associated protein 1	Differentiation	[156,157,242]
BDNF	11p14.1	Brain-derived neurotrophic factor	Proliferation; Differentiation	[75,128]
BMP2	20p12.3	Bone morphogenetic protein 2	Specification; Differentiation	[27,105]
BMP4	14q22.2	Bone morphogenetic protein 4	Specification; Migration; Differentiation	[28,65,105]
BMP7	20q13.31	Bone morphogenetic protein 7	Migration	[65]
CDH2	18q12.1	Cadherin 2	Migration	[57]
CDKN1B	12p13.1	Cyclin-dependent kinase inhibitor 1B	Proliferation	[85]
CHD7	8q12.2	Chromodomain-helicase-DNA-binding protein 7	Proliferation; Differentiation	[80,243]
CHD8	14q11.2	Chromodomain-helicase-DNA-binding protein 8	Specification; Proliferation; Differentiation	[80,81]

Table A1. *Cont.*

Gene *	Chromosomal Locus *	Protein *	Biological Role	Reference
CLDN1	3q28	Claudin 1	Migration; Proliferation; Differentiation	[70]
CLDN3	7q11.23	Claudin 3	Migration; Proliferation; Differentiation	[70]
CLDN11	3q26.2	Claudin 11	Migration; Proliferation	[56]
CNP	17q21.2	2′,3′-cyclic nucleotide 3′ phosphodiesterase	Migration; Differentiation	[52,153]
CNTF	11q12.1	Ciliary neurotrophic factor	Proliferation; Differentiation	[148,244]
CNTFR	9p13.3	Ciliary neurotrophic factor receptor	Proliferation	[244]
CNTN1	12q12	Contactin 1	Differentiation	[141]
CREB3L2	7q33	CAMP responsive element binding protein 3 like 2	Differentiation	[243]
CSPG4	15q24.2	Chondroitin sulfate proteoglycan 4	Proliferation	[245]
CXCL1	4q13.3	C-X-C motif chemokine ligand 1	Migration; Proliferation	[67,72]
CXCL12	10q11.21	C-X-C motif chemokine ligand 12	Migration; Proliferation	[68,73]
CXCR2	2q35	C-X-C motif chemokine receptor 2	Migration; Proliferation	[67,72]
CXCR4	2q22.1	C-X-C motif chemokine receptor 4	Migration; Proliferation	[68,73]
DLX1	2q31.1	Distal-less homeobox 1	Specification	[246]
DLX2	2q31.1	Distal-less homeobox 2	Specification	[246]
DUSP15	20q11.21	Dual specificity phosphatase 15	Differentiation	[247]
EDN1	6p24.1	Endothelin 1	Migration; Proliferation	[60,98]
EDNRB	13q22.3	Endothelin receptor type B	Proliferation	[98]
EFNB2	13q33.3	Ephrin B2	Migration; Proliferation	[46,248]
EFNB3	17p13.1	Ephrin B3	Migration	[46]
EGF	4q25	Epidermal growth factor	Proliferation	[76]
EGR1	5q31.2	Early growth response 1	Differentiation	[116]
ENPP6	4q35.1	Ectonucleotide pyrophosphatase/phosphodiesterase 6	Differentiation	[135]
EPHB2	1p36.12	Ephrin receptor B2	Migration; Proliferation	[46,248]
FEZ1	11q24.2	Fasciculation and elongation protein zeta 1	Differentiation	[152]
FGF2	4q28.1	Fibroblast growth factor 2	Specification; Migration; Proliferation	[240,249]
FGFR1	8p11.23	Fibroblast growth factor receptor 1	Migration; Proliferation	[240,249]
FGFR2	10q26.13	Fibroblast growth factor receptor 2	Specification	[31,249]
FGFR3	4p16.3	Fibroblast growth factor receptor 3	Proliferation	[249]
FLT1	13q12.3	Fms related receptor tyrosine kinase 1	Proliferation	[250]
FN1	2q35	Fibronectin 1	Migration; Proliferation	[59,96]
GAB1	4q31.21	GRB2-associated binding protein 1	Differentiation	[132]
GALC	14q31.3	Galactosylceramidase	Differentiation	[144]
GDPD2	Xq13.1	Glycerophosphodiester phosphodiesterase domain containing 2	Proliferation	[244]
GJC2	1q42.13	Gap junction protein gamma 2	Differentiation	[160–162,251]
GLI2	2q14.2	GLI family zinc finger 2	Specification; Differentiation	[38]
GPR17	2q14.3	G protein-coupled receptor 17	Differentiation	[113]
GPR37	7q31.33	G protein-coupled receptor 37	Differentiation	[252]
GSX1	13q12.2	GS homeobox 1	Proliferation	[99]
GSX2	4q12	GS homeobox 2	Specification; Proliferation	[99,253]
HDAC1	1p35.2-p35.1	Histone deacetylase 1	Specification	[254,255]
HDAC2	6q21	Histone deacetylase 2	Specification	[254]
HES1	3q29	Hes family bHLH transcription factor 1	Specification	[256]
HES5	1p36.32	Hes family bHLH transcription factor 5	Differentiation	[139]

Table A1. *Cont.*

Gene *	Chromosomal Locus *	Protein *	Biological Role	Reference
HEY1	8q21.13	Hes related family bHLH transcription factor with YRPW motif 1	Differentiation	[257]
HGF	7q21.11	Hepatocyte growth factor	Migration; Proliferation	[54]
ID2	2p25.1	Inhibitor of DNA binding 2	Proliferation; Differentiation	[89,113,115]
ID4	6p22.3	Inhibitor of DNA binding 4, HLH protein	Proliferation; Differentiation	[88,113–115]
IGF1	12q23.2	Insulin-like growth factor 1	Proliferation; Differentiation	[74,131]
IRX3	16q12.2	Iroquois homeobox 3	Specification	[37]
ITGB1	10p11.22	Integrin subunit beta 1	Migration; Proliferation; Differentiation	[56,58,258]
ITGB3	17q21.32	Integrin subunit beta 3	Proliferation	[69,97]
JAG1	20p12.2	Jagged canonical Notch ligand 1	Proliferation; Differentiation	[79]
JUN	1p32.1	Jun proto-oncogene, AP-1 transcription factor subunit	Proliferation	[259,260]
KCNJ10	1q23.2	Potassium inwardly rectifying channel subfamily J member 10	Differentiation	[149]
KDR	4q12	Kinase insert domain receptor	Migration; Proliferation	[64,250]
KLF6	10p15.2	Kruppel-like factor 6	Differentiation	[127]
LAMA2	6q22.33	Laminin subunit alpha 2	Migration; Proliferation	[96,261]
LAMA4	6q21	Laminin subunit alpha 4	Migration; Proliferation	[96,261]
LAMA5	20q13.33	Laminin subunit alpha 5	Migration; Proliferation	[96,261]
LGALS4	19q13.2	Galectin-4	Proliferation; Differentiation	[100]
LINGO1	15q24.3	Leucine rich repeat and Ig domain containing 1	Differentiation	[143]
MAG	19q13.12	Myelin-associated glycoprotein	Differentiation	[147]
MAP2	2q34	Microtubule-associated protein 2	Differentiation	[151]
MAPT	17q21.31	Microtubule-associated protein tau	Differentiation	[151]
MBP	18q23	Myelin basic protein	Differentiation	[159]
MOBP	3p22.1	Myelin associated oligodendrocyte basic protein	Differentiation	[190]
MYOC	1q24.3	Myocilin	Differentiation	[262]
MYRF	11q12.2	Myelin regulatory factor	Differentiation	[117]
MYT1	20q13.33	Myelin transcription factor 1	Specification; Proliferation	[39,83]
NCAM1	11q23.2	Neural cell adhesion molecule 1	Migration; Proliferation	[47,48,84,142]
NES	1q23.1	Nestin	Migration; Proliferation	[49,263]
NEUROG1	5q31.1	Neurogenin 1	Specification	[37,264,265]
NEUROG2	4q25	Neurogenin 2	Specification	[37,264,265]
NFIA	1p31.3	Nuclear factor I A	Specification	[37,266]
NGF	1p13.2	Nerve growth factor	Proliferation	[92,267]
NKX2-2	20p11.22	NK2 homeobox 2	Specification; Proliferation; Differentiation	[37,108,123,124, 268]
NKX2-6	8p21.2	NK2 homeobox 6	Specification; Differentiation	[40]
NKX6-1	4q21.23	NK6 homeobox 1	Specification	[26]
NKX6-2	10q26.3	NK6 homeobox 2	Specification	[26]
NOG	17q22	Noggin	Proliferation; Differentiation	[91,106,107]
NOTCH1	9q34.3	Notch receptor 1	Proliferation; Differentiation	[79,140]

Table A1. *Cont.*

Gene *	Chromosomal Locus *	Protein *	Biological Role	Reference
NRG1	8p12	Neuregulin 1	Migration; Proliferation; Differentiation	[101,103,269]
NTF3	12p13.31	Neurotrophin 3	Proliferation; Differentiation	[92,129,130]
NTF4	19q13.33	Neurotrophin 4	Proliferation	[90]
NTN1	17p13.1	Netrin 1	Migration	[61–63]
NTRK2	9q21.33	Neurotrophic receptor tyrosine kinase 2	Proliferation; Differentiation	[75,270]
OLIG1	21q22.11	Oligodendrocyte transcription factor 1	Migration; Differentiation	[50,51,104,271]
OLIG2	21q22.11	Oligodendrocyte transcription factor 2	Specification; Migration; Differentiation	[51,53,271]
OMG	17q11.2	Oligodendrocyte myelin glycoprotein	Proliferation; Differentiation	[155]
OPALIN	10q24.1	Oligodendrocytic myelin paranodal and inner loop protein	Differentiation	[272,273]
PAK1	11q13.5-q14.1	P21 (RAC1) activated kinase 1	Differentiation	[146]
PAX6	11p13	Paired box 6	Specification; Proliferation	[94,274,275]
PDE5	4q26	Phosphodiesterase 5A	Differentiation	[276]
PDGFA	7p22.3	Platelet-derived growth factor subunit A	Migration; Proliferation; Differentiation	[42,277]
PDGFRA	4q12	Platelet-derived growth factor receptor alpha	Migration; Proliferation; Differentiation	[42,47,71,277]
PLP1	Xq22.2	Proteolipid protein 1	Differentiation	[158]
PRMT5	14q11.2	Protein arginine methyltransferase 5	Differentiation	[278]
PROM1	4p15.32	Prominin 1	Differentiation	[145]
QKI	6q26	QKI, KH domain containing RNA binding	Differentiation	[133,279]
RTN4	2p16.1	Reticulon 4	Migration	[280]
S1PR1	1p21.2	Sphingosine-1-phosphate receptor 1	Migration	[66]
S1PR2	19p13.2	Sphingosine-1-phosphate receptor 2	Migration	[66]
S1PR3	9q22.1	Sphingosine-1-phosphate receptor 3	Migration	[66]
S1PR5	19p13.2	Sphingosine-1-phosphate receptor 5	Migration	[66]
SEMA3A	7q21.11	Semaphorin 3A	Migration	[61]
SEMA3F	3p21.31	Semaphorin 3F	Migration; Proliferation	[61]
SETDB1	1q21.3	SET domain bifurcated histone lysine methyltransferase 1	Differentiation	[112]
SHH	7q36.3	Sonic hedgehog signaling molecule	Specification; Migration; Proliferation	[27–30,32,41]
SIRT1	10q21.3	Sirtuin 1	Differentiation	[126]
SIRT2	19q13.2	Sirtuin 2	Differentiation	[125]
SMARCA4	19p13.2	SWI/SNF related, matrix associated, actin-dependent regulator of chromatin, subfamily a, member 4	Specification; Differentiation	[109,243]
SOD1	21q22.11	Superoxide dismutase 1	Proliferation; Differentiation	[95]
SOX1	13q34	SRY-box transcription factor 1	Specification	[33]
SOX2	3q26.33	SRY-box transcription factor 2	Specification; Proliferation; Differentiation	[33,102,119]
SOX3	Xq27.1	SRY-box transcription factor 3	Specification; Differentiation	[33,119]

Table A1. *Cont.*

Gene *	Chromosomal Locus *	Protein *	Biological Role	Reference
SOX5	12p12.1	SRY-box transcription factor 5	Migration; Proliferation; Differentiation	[44]
SOX6	11p15.2	SRY-box transcription factor 6	Migration; Proliferation; Differentiation	[44]
SOX8	16p13.3	SRY-box transcription factor 8	Specification; Differentiation	[34–36,120]
SOX9	17q24.3	SRY-box transcription factor 9	Specification; Migration; Proliferation; Differentiation	[36,44,82]
SOX10	22q13.1	SRY-box transcription factor 10	Specification; Migration; Differentiation	[43,44,122,281]
SOX11	2p25.2	SRY-box transcription factor 11	Differentiation	[116]
SP7	12q13.13	Sp7 transcription factor	Differentiation	[243]
SREBF2	22q13.2	Sterol regulatory element-binding transcription factor 2	Differentiation	[133]
STAT3	17q21.2	Signal transducer and activator of transcription 3	Differentiation	[282]
SULF1	8q13.2-q13.3	Sulfatase 1	Specification	[30]
TARDBP	1p36.22	TAR DNA binding protein	Differentiation	[134]
TCF4	18q21.2	Transcription factor 4	Differentiation	[110]
TCF7L2	10q25.2-q25.3	Transcription factor 7 like 2	Differentiation	[111]
THBS1	15q14	Thrombospondin 1	Migration	[55]
THRA	17q21.1	Thyroid hormone receptor alpha	Differentiation	[136–138]
TMEM98	17q11.2	Transmembrane protein 98	Differentiation	[195]
TNC	9q33.1	Tenascin C	Migration; Proliferation	[59,69]
TPPP	5p15.33	Tubulin polymerization promoting protein	Proliferation; Differentiation	[87]
TSPAN3	15q24.3	Tetraspanin 3	Migration; Proliferation	[56]
VEGFA	6p21.1	Vascular endothelial growth factor A	Migration; Proliferation	[64,250]
WDR1	4p16.1	WD repeat domain 1	Differentiation	[279]
YY1	14q32.2	YY1 transcription factor	Differentiation	[283]
ZBTB33	Xq24	Zinc finger and BTB domain containing 33	Differentiation	[111]
ZDHHC5	11q12.1	Zinc finger DHHC-type palmitoyltransferase 5	Differentiation	[282]
ZEB2	2q22.3	Zinc finger E-box binding homeobox 2	Differentiation	[284]
ZNF24	18q12.2	Zinc finger protein 24	Differentiation	[150]

* Data are retrieved from "The Human Protein Atlas" [285]. OPCs: Oligodendrocyte precursor cells.

Table A2. Regulators of axoglial interactions in myelin ensheathment.

Gene *	Chromosomal Locus *	Protein *	Reference
CADM1	11q23.3	Cell adhesion molecule 1	[174]
CADM2	3p12.1	Cell adhesion molecule 2	[173,174]
CADM3	1q23.2	Cell adhesion molecule 3	[173]
CADM4	19q13.31	Cell adhesion molecule 4	[173]
CDH2	18q12.1	Cadherin 2	[165]
CNTN1	12q12	Contactin 1	[167–169,171]
CNTN2	1q32.1	Contactin 2	[172]
CNTNAP1	17q21.2	Contactin-associated protein 1	[167–170]
CNTNAP2	7q35–q36.1	Contactin-associated protein 2	[172]

Table A2. *Cont.*

Gene *	Chromosomal Locus *	Protein *	Reference
EFNA1	1q22	Ephrin A1	[177]
EFNB2	13q33.3	Ephrin B2	[178]
EPHA4	2q36.1	Ephrin receptor A4	[177,178]
EPHB1	3q22.2	Ephrin receptor B1	[178]
JAM2	21q21.3	Junctional adhesion molecule 2	[181]
L1CAM	Xq28	L1 cell adhesion molecule	[166]
LGALS4	19q13.2	Galectin-4	[182]
LINGO1	15q24.3	Leucine rich repeat and Ig domain containing 1	[143,179]
MAG	19q13.12	Myelin-associated glycoprotein	[176]
NCAM1	11q23.2	Neural cell adhesion molecule 1	[180]
NFASC	1q32.1	Neurofascin	[167–170]
NRG1	8p12	Neuregulin 1	[286,287]
OLIG1	21q22.11	Oligodendrocyte transcription factor 1	[183]
ST3GAL2	16q22.1	ST3 beta-galactoside alpha-2,3-sialyltransferase 2	[175,176]
ST3GAL3	1p34.1	ST3 beta-galactoside alpha-2,3-sialyltransferase 3	[175,176]
WASL	7q31.32	WASP-like actin nucleation promoting factor	[288,289]

* Data are retrieved from "The Human Protein Atlas" [285].

Table A3. Molecules implicated in myelin growth and preservation.

Gene *	Chromosomal Locus *	Protein *	Reference
ABCD1	Xq28	ATP binding cassette subfamily D member 1	[164,203]
AGPS	2q31.2	Alkylglycerone phosphate synthase	[24,290]
CA2	8q21.2	Carbonic anhydrase 2	[291]
CLDN1	3q28	Claudin 1	[70]
CLDN3	7q11.23	Claudin 3	[70]
CLDN11	3q26.2	Claudin 11	[185]
CNP	17q21.2	2′,3′-cyclic nucleotide 3′ phosphodiesterase	[52,189]
DUSP15	20q11.21	Dual specificity phosphatase 15	[247]
FGF1	5q31.3	Fibroblast growth factor 1	[198]
FGF2	4q28.1	Fibroblast growth factor 2	[198]
FGFR1	8p11.23	Fibroblast growth factor receptor 1	[197,198]
FGFR2	10q26.13	Fibroblast growth factor receptor 2	[197,198]
GAL3ST1	22q12.2	Galactose-3-O-sulfotransferase 1	[200]
GALC	14q31.3	Galactosylceramidase	[200,201]
GFAP	17q21.31	Glial fibrillary acidic protein	[292]
GJB1	Xq13.1	Gap junction protein beta 1	[161]
GJC2	1q42.13	Gap junction protein gamma 2	[161]
GNPAT	1q42.2	Glyceronephosphate O-acyltransferase	[290]
HDAC3	5q31.3	Histone deacetylase 3	[199]
ID4	6p22.3	Inhibitor of DNA binding 4, HLH protein	[114]
MAG	19q13.12	Myelin-associated glycoprotein	[147,186]
MAL	2q11.1	Mal, T cell differentiation protein	[293]
MAP2	2q34	Microtubule-associated protein 2	[151]
MAPT	17q21.31	Microtubule-associated protein tau	[151]
MBP	18q23	Myelin basic protein	[52]
MOBP	3p22.1	Myelin-associated oligodendrocyte basic protein	[190]
MOG	6p22.1	Myelin oligodendrocyte glycoprotein	[187,188]
MYRF	11q12.2	Myelin regulatory factor	[193]
NCAM1	11q23.2	Neural cell adhesion molecule 1	[294]
NKX2-2	20p11.22	NK2 homeobox 2	[194]
NKX2-6	8p21.2	NK2 homeobox 6	[194]
NPC1	18q11.2	NPC intracellular cholesterol transporter 1	[295]

Table A3. *Cont.*

Gene *	Chromosomal Locus *	Protein *	Reference
OLIG1	21q22.11	Oligodendrocyte transcription factor 1	[183,196]
OLIG2	21q22.11	Oligodendrocyte transcription factor 2	[112,196]
OMG	17q11.2	Oligodendrocyte myelin glycoprotein	[86,191,192]
OPALIN	10q24.1	Oligodendrocytic myelin paranodal and inner loop protein	[204]
PEX5	12p13.31	Peroxisomal biogenesis factor 5	[202]
PLP1	Xq22.2	Proteolipid protein 1	[184,185]
PROM1	4p15.32	Prominin 1	[296]
QKI	6q26	QKI, KH domain containing RNA binding	[133]
SETDB1	1q21.3	SET domain bifurcated histone lysine methyltransferase 1	[112]
SOX8	16p13.3	SRY-box transcription factor 8	[35]
SOX10	22q13.1	SRY-box transcription factor 10	[35,122]
SREBF2	22q13.2	Sterol regulatory element-binding transcription factor 2	[133]
TMEM98	17q11.2	Transmembrane protein 98	[195]
TPPP	5p15.33	Tubulin polymerization promoting protein	[297]
UGT8	4q26	UDP glycosyltransferase 8	[200,201]

* Data are retrieved from "The Human Protein Atlas" [285].

References

1. Allen, N.J.; Barres, B.A. Glia—More than Just Brain Glue. *Nature* **2009**, *457*, 675–677. [CrossRef] [PubMed]
2. Simons, M.; Nave, K.-A. Oligodendrocytes: Myelination and Axonal Support. *Cold Spring Harb. Perspect. Biol.* **2016**, *8*, a020479. [CrossRef]
3. Herculano-Houzel, S. The Glia/Neuron Ratio: How It Varies Uniformly across Brain Structures and Species and What That Means for Brain Physiology and Evolution: The Glia/Neuron Ratio. *Glia* **2014**, *62*, 1377–1391. [CrossRef] [PubMed]
4. Bercury, K.K.; Macklin, W.B. Dynamics and Mechanisms of CNS Myelination. *Dev. Cell* **2015**, *32*, 447–458. [CrossRef]
5. Nave, K.-A.; Werner, H.B. Myelination of the Nervous System: Mechanisms and Functions. *Annu. Rev. Cell Dev. Biol.* **2014**, *30*, 503–533. [CrossRef] [PubMed]
6. Boullerne, A.I. The History of Myelin. *Exp. Neurol.* **2016**, *283*, 431–445. [CrossRef]
7. Edgar, J.M.; McGowan, E.; Chapple, K.J.; Möbius, W.; Lemgruber, L.; Insall, R.H.; Nave, K.; Boullerne, A. Río-Hortega's Drawings Revisited with Fluorescent Protein Defines a Cytoplasm-filled Channel System of CNS Myelin. *J. Anat.* **2021**, *239*, 1241–1255. [CrossRef]
8. Pérez-Cerdá, F.; Sánchez-Gómez, M.V.; Matute, C. Pío Del Río Hortega and the Discovery of the Oligodendrocytes. *Front. Neuroanat.* **2015**, *9*, 92. [CrossRef]
9. Martínez-Cerdeño, V.; Noctor, S.C. Neural Progenitor Cell Terminology. *Front. Neuroanat.* **2018**, *12*, 104. [CrossRef]
10. Van Tilborg, E.; de Theije, C.G.M.; van Hal, M.; Wagenaar, N.; de Vries, L.S.; Benders, M.J.; Rowitch, D.H.; Nijboer, C.H. Origin and Dynamics of Oligodendrocytes in the Developing Brain: Implications for Perinatal White Matter Injury. *Glia* **2018**, *66*, 221–238. [CrossRef]
11. Nishiyama, A.; Shimizu, T.; Sherafat, A.; Richardson, W.D. Life-Long Oligodendrocyte Development and Plasticity. *Semin. Cell Dev. Biol.* **2021**, *116*, 25–37. [CrossRef] [PubMed]
12. Scantlebury, N.; Cunningham, T.; Dockstader, C.; Laughlin, S.; Gaetz, W.; Rockel, C.; Dickson, J.; Mabbott, D. Relations between White Matter Maturation and Reaction Time in Childhood. *J. Int. Neuropsychol. Soc.* **2014**, *20*, 99–112. [CrossRef]
13. Mabbott, D.J.; Noseworthy, M.; Bouffet, E.; Laughlin, S.; Rockel, C. White Matter Growth as a Mechanism of Cognitive Development in Children. *NeuroImage* **2006**, *33*, 936–946. [CrossRef] [PubMed]
14. Young, K.M.; Psachoulia, K.; Tripathi, R.B.; Dunn, S.-J.; Cossell, L.; Attwell, D.; Tohyama, K.; Richardson, W.D. Oligodendrocyte Dynamics in the Healthy Adult CNS: Evidence for Myelin Remodeling. *Neuron* **2013**, *77*, 873–885. [CrossRef] [PubMed]
15. Sams, E.C. Oligodendrocytes in the Aging Brain. *Neuronal Signal.* **2021**, *5*, NS20210008. [CrossRef] [PubMed]
16. Kinney, H.C.; Volpe, J.J. Chapter 8—Myelination Events. In *Volpe's Neurology of the Newborn*, 6th ed.; Volpe, J.J., Inder, T.E., Darras, B.T., de Vries, L.S., du Plessis, A.J., Neil, J.J., Perlman, J.M., Eds.; Elsevier: Amsterdam, The Netherlands, 2018; pp. 176–188, ISBN 978-0-323-42876-7.
17. Hughes, E.G.; Orthmann-Murphy, J.L.; Langseth, A.J.; Bergles, D.E. Myelin Remodeling through Experience-Dependent Oligodendrogenesis in the Adult Somatosensory Cortex. *Nat. Neurosci.* **2018**, *21*, 696–706. [CrossRef]
18. Grabel, L. Developmental Origin of Neural Stem Cells: The Glial Cell That Could. *Stem Cell Rev. Rep.* **2012**, *8*, 577–585. [CrossRef]
19. Fletcher, J.L.; Makowiecki, K.; Cullen, C.L.; Young, K.M. Oligodendrogenesis and Myelination Regulate Cortical Development, Plasticity and Circuit Function. *Semin. Cell Dev. Biol.* **2021**, *118*, 14–23. [CrossRef]

20. Bergles, D.E.; Richardson, W.D. Oligodendrocyte Development and Plasticity. *Cold Spring Harb. Perspect. Biol.* **2015**, *8*, a020453. [CrossRef]
21. Huang, W.; Bhaduri, A.; Velmeshev, D.; Wang, S.; Wang, L.; Rottkamp, C.A.; Alvarez-Buylla, A.; Rowitch, D.H.; Kriegstein, A.R. Origins and Proliferative States of Human Oligodendrocyte Precursor Cells. *Cell* **2020**, *182*, 594–608.e11. [CrossRef]
22. Kessaris, N.; Fogarty, M.; Iannarelli, P.; Grist, M.; Wegner, M.; Richardson, W.D. Competing Waves of Oligodendrocytes in the Forebrain and Postnatal Elimination of an Embryonic Lineage. *Nat. Neurosci.* **2006**, *9*, 173–179. [CrossRef] [PubMed]
23. Bradl, M.; Lassmann, H. Oligodendrocytes: Biology and Pathology. *Acta Neuropathol.* **2010**, *119*, 37–53. [CrossRef] [PubMed]
24. Baumann, N.; Pham-Dinh, D. Biology of Oligodendrocyte and Myelin in the Mammalian Central Nervous System. *Physiol. Rev.* **2001**, *81*, 871–927. [CrossRef] [PubMed]
25. Tripathi, R.B.; Clarke, L.E.; Burzomato, V.; Kessaris, N.; Anderson, P.N.; Attwell, D.; Richardson, W.D. Dorsally and Ventrally Derived Oligodendrocytes Have Similar Electrical Properties but Myelinate Preferred Tracts. *J. Neurosci.* **2011**, *31*, 6809–6819. [CrossRef]
26. Cai, J.; Qi, Y.; Hu, X.; Tan, M.; Liu, Z.; Zhang, J.; Li, Q.; Sander, M.; Qiu, M. Generation of Oligodendrocyte Precursor Cells from Mouse Dorsal Spinal Cord Independent of Nkx6 Regulation and Shh Signaling. *Neuron* **2005**, *45*, 41–53. [CrossRef] [PubMed]
27. Zhu, G.; Mehler, M.F.; Zhao, J.; Yu Yung, S.; Kessler, J.A. Sonic Hedgehog and BMP2 Exert Opposing Actions on Proliferation and Differentiation of Embryonic Neural Progenitor Cells. *Dev. Biol.* **1999**, *215*, 118–129. [CrossRef] [PubMed]
28. Gomes, W.A.; Mehler, M.F.; Kessler, J.A. Transgenic Overexpression of BMP4 Increases Astroglial and Decreases Oligodendroglial Lineage Commitment. *Dev. Biol.* **2003**, *255*, 164–177. [CrossRef]
29. Orentas, D.M.; Hayes, J.E.; Dyer, K.L.; Miller, R.H. Sonic Hedgehog Signaling Is Required during the Appearance of Spinal Cord Oligodendrocyte Precursors. *Dev. Camb. Engl.* **1999**, *126*, 2419–2429. [CrossRef]
30. Danesin, C.; Agius, E.; Escalas, N.; Ai, X.; Emerson, C.; Cochard, P.; Soula, C. Ventral Neural Progenitors Switch toward an Oligodendroglial Fate in Response to Increased Sonic Hedgehog (Shh) Activity: Involvement of Sulfatase 1 in Modulating Shh Signaling in the Ventral Spinal Cord. *J. Neurosci. Off. J. Soc. Neurosci.* **2006**, *26*, 5037–5048. [CrossRef]
31. Farreny, M.-A.; Agius, E.; Bel-Vialar, S.; Escalas, N.; Khouri-Farah, N.; Soukkarieh, C.; Danesin, C.; Pituello, F.; Cochard, P.; Soula, C. FGF Signaling Controls Shh-Dependent Oligodendroglial Fate Specification in the Ventral Spinal Cord. *Neural Develop.* **2018**, *13*, 3. [CrossRef]
32. Kearns, C.A.; Walker, M.; Ravanelli, A.M.; Scott, K.; Arzbecker, M.R.; Appel, B. Zebrafish Spinal Cord Oligodendrocyte Formation Requires Boc Function. *Genetics* **2021**, *218*, iyab082. [CrossRef] [PubMed]
33. Bylund, M.; Andersson, E.; Novitch, B.G.; Muhr, J. Vertebrate Neurogenesis Is Counteracted by Sox1–3 Activity. *Nat. Neurosci.* **2003**, *6*, 1162–1168. [CrossRef] [PubMed]
34. Stolt, C.C.; Schmitt, S.; Lommes, P.; Sock, E.; Wegner, M. Impact of Transcription Factor Sox8 on Oligodendrocyte Specification in the Mouse Embryonic Spinal Cord. *Dev. Biol.* **2005**, *281*, 309–317. [CrossRef] [PubMed]
35. Turnescu, T.; Arter, J.; Reiprich, S.; Tamm, E.R.; Waisman, A.; Wegner, M. Sox8 and Sox10 Jointly Maintain Myelin Gene Expression in Oligodendrocytes. *Glia* **2018**, *66*, 279–294. [CrossRef]
36. Pozniak, C.D.; Langseth, A.J.; Dijkgraaf, G.J.P.; Choe, Y.; Werb, Z.; Pleasure, S.J. Sox10 Directs Neural Stem Cells toward the Oligodendrocyte Lineage by Decreasing Suppressor of Fused Expression. *Proc. Natl. Acad. Sci. USA* **2010**, *107*, 21795–21800. [CrossRef]
37. Wegner, M. Specification of Oligodendrocytes. In *Patterning and Cell Type Specification in the Developing CNS and PNS*; Elsevier: Amsterdam, The Netherlands, 2020; pp. 847–866, ISBN 978-0-12-814405-3.
38. Qi, Y.; Tan, M.; Hui, C.-C.; Qiu, M. Gli2 Is Required for Normal Shh Signaling and Oligodendrocyte Development in the Spinal Cord. *Mol. Cell. Neurosci.* **2003**, *23*, 440–450. [CrossRef]
39. Hudson, L.D.; Romm, E.; Berndt, J.A.; Nielsen, J.A. A Tool for Examining the Role of the Zinc Finger Myelin Transcription Factor 1 (Myt1) in Neural Development: Myt1 Knock-in Mice. *Transgenic Res.* **2011**, *20*, 951–961. [CrossRef]
40. Miron, V.E.; Kuhlmann, T.; Antel, J.P. Cells of the Oligodendroglial Lineage, Myelination, and Remyelination. *Biochim. Biophys. Acta BBA—Mol. Basis Dis.* **2011**, *1812*, 184–193. [CrossRef]
41. Merchán, P.; Bribián, A.; Sánchez-Camacho, C.; Lezameta, M.; Bovolenta, P.; de Castro, F. Sonic Hedgehog Promotes the Migration and Proliferation of Optic Nerve Oligodendrocyte Precursors. *Mol. Cell. Neurosci.* **2007**, *36*, 355–368. [CrossRef] [PubMed]
42. Frost, E.E.; Zhou, Z.; Krasnesky, K.; Armstrong, R.C. Initiation of Oligodendrocyte Progenitor Cell Migration by a PDGF-A Activated Extracellular Regulated Kinase (ERK) Signaling Pathway. *Neurochem. Res.* **2009**, *34*, 169–181. [CrossRef]
43. Finzsch, M.; Stolt, C.C.; Lommes, P.; Wegner, M. Sox9 and Sox10 Influence Survival and Migration of Oligodendrocyte Precursors in the Spinal Cord by Regulating PDGF Receptor Aexpression. *Development* **2008**, *135*, 637–646. [CrossRef] [PubMed]
44. Baroti, T.; Zimmermann, Y.; Schillinger, A.; Liu, L.; Lommes, P.; Wegner, M.; Stolt, C.C. Transcription Factors Sox5 and Sox6 Exert Direct and Indirect Influences on Oligodendroglial Migration in Spinal Cord and Forebrain: SoxD Proteins in Oligodendrocyte Progenitors. *Glia* **2016**, *64*, 122–138. [CrossRef] [PubMed]
45. Biname, F.; Sakry, D.; Dimou, L.; Jolivel, V.; Trotter, J. NG2 Regulates Directional Migration of Oligodendrocyte Precursor Cells via Rho GTPases and Polarity Complex Proteins. *J. Neurosci.* **2013**, *33*, 10858–10874. [CrossRef] [PubMed]
46. Prestoz, L.; Chatzopoulou, E.; Lemkine, G.; Spassky, N.; Lebras, B.; Kagawa, T.; Ikenaka, K.; Zalc, B.; Thomas, J.-L. Control of Axonophilic Migration of Oligodendrocyte Precursor Cells by Eph–Ephrin Interaction. *Neuron Glia Biol.* **2004**, *1*, 73–83. [CrossRef]

47. Grinspan, J.B.; Franceschini, B. Platelet-Derived Growth Factor Is a Survival Factor for PSA-NCAM+ Oligodendrocyte Pre-Progenitor Cells. *J. Neurosci. Res.* **1995**, *41*, 540–551. [CrossRef]
48. Decker, L.; Avellana-Adalid, V.; Nait-Oumesmar, B.; Durbec, P.; Baron-Van Evercooren, A. Oligodendrocyte Precursor Migration and Differentiation: Combined Effects of PSA Residues, Growth Factors, and Substrates. *Mol. Cell. Neurosci.* **2000**, *16*, 422–439. [CrossRef]
49. Gallo, V.; Armstrong, R. Developmental and Growth Factor-Induced Regulation of Nestin in Oligodendrocyte Lineage Cells. *J. Neurosci.* **1995**, *15*, 394–406. [CrossRef]
50. Motizuki, M.; Isogaya, K.; Miyake, K.; Ikushima, H.; Kubota, T.; Miyazono, K.; Saitoh, M.; Miyazawa, K. Oligodendrocyte Transcription Factor 1 (Olig1) Is a Smad Cofactor Involved in Cell Motility Induced by Transforming Growth Factor-β. *J. Biol. Chem.* **2013**, *288*, 18911–18922. [CrossRef]
51. Zhou, Q.; Anderson, D.J. The BHLH Transcription Factors OLIG2 and OLIG1 Couple Neuronal and Glial Subtype Specification. *Cell* **2002**, *109*, 61–73. [CrossRef]
52. Yin, X.; Peterson, J.; Gravel, M.; Braun, P.E.; Trapp, B.D. CNP Overexpression Induces Aberrant Oligodendrocyte Membranes and Inhibits MBP Accumulation and Myelin Compaction. *J. Neurosci. Res.* **1997**, *50*, 238–247. [CrossRef]
53. Wegener, A.; Deboux, C.; Bachelin, C.; Frah, M.; Kerninon, C.; Seilhean, D.; Weider, M.; Wegner, M.; Nait-Oumesmar, B. Gain of Olig2 Function in Oligodendrocyte Progenitors Promotes Remyelination. *Brain* **2015**, *138*, 120–135. [CrossRef] [PubMed]
54. Yan, H.; Rivkees, S.A. Hepatocyte Growth Factor Stimulates the Proliferation and Migration of Oligodendrocyte Precursor Cells. *J. Neurosci. Res.* **2002**, *69*, 597–606. [CrossRef] [PubMed]
55. Scott-Drew, S.; ffrench-Constant, C. Expression and Function of Thrombospondin-1 in Myelinating Glial Cells of the Central Nervous System. *J. Neurosci. Res.* **1997**, *50*, 202–214. [CrossRef]
56. Tiwari-Woodruff, S.K.; Buznikov, A.G.; Vu, T.Q.; Micevych, P.E.; Chen, K.; Kornblum, H.I.; Bronstein, J.M. OSP/Claudin-11 Forms a Complex with a Novel Member of the Tetraspanin Super Family and Beta1 Integrin and Regulates Proliferation and Migration of Oligodendrocytes. *J. Cell Biol.* **2001**, *153*, 295–305. [CrossRef]
57. Payne, H.R.; Hemperly, J.J.; Lemmon, V. N-Cadherin Expression and Function in Cultured Oligodendrocytes. *Dev. Brain Res.* **1996**, *97*, 9–15. [CrossRef]
58. Milner, R.; Edwards, G.; Streuli, C.; Ffrench-Constant, C. A Role in Migration for the Alpha V Beta 1 Integrin Expressed on Oligodendrocyte Precursors. *J. Neurosci. Off. J. Soc. Neurosci.* **1996**, *16*, 7240–7252. [CrossRef]
59. Frost, E.; Kiernan, B.W.; Faissner, A.; ffrench-Constant, C. Regulation of Oligodendrocyte Precursor Migration by Extracellular Matrix: Evidence for Substrate-Specific Inhibition of Migration by Tenascin-C. *Dev. Neurosci.* **1996**, *18*, 266–273. [CrossRef]
60. Gadea, A.; Aguirre, A.; Haydar, T.F.; Gallo, V. Endothelin-1 Regulates Oligodendrocyte Development. *J. Neurosci.* **2009**, *29*, 10047–10062. [CrossRef]
61. Spassky, N.; de Castro, F.; Le Bras, B.; Heydon, K.; Quéraud-LeSaux, F.; Bloch-Gallego, E.; Chédotal, A.; Zalc, B.; Thomas, J.-L. Directional Guidance of Oligodendroglial Migration by Class 3 Semaphorins and Netrin-1. *J. Neurosci.* **2002**, *22*, 5992–6004. [CrossRef]
62. Jarjour, A.A.; Manitt, C.; Moore, S.W.; Thompson, K.M.; Yuh, S.-J.; Kennedy, T.E. Netrin-1 Is a Chemorepellent for Oligodendrocyte Precursor Cells in the Embryonic Spinal Cord. *J. Neurosci.* **2003**, *23*, 3735–3744. [CrossRef]
63. Tsai, H.-H.; Tessier-Lavigne, M.; Miller, R.H. Netrin 1 Mediates Spinal Cord Oligodendrocyte Precursor Dispersal. *Development* **2003**, *130*, 2095–2105. [CrossRef] [PubMed]
64. Zhang, H.; Vutskits, L.; Pepper, M.S.; Kiss, J.Z. VEGF Is a Chemoattractant for FGF-2–Stimulated Neural Progenitors. *J. Cell Biol.* **2003**, *163*, 1375–1384. [CrossRef] [PubMed]
65. Choe, Y.; Huynh, T.; Pleasure, S.J. Migration of Oligodendrocyte Progenitor Cells Is Controlled by Transforming Growth Factor Family Proteins during Corticogenesis. *J. Neurosci.* **2014**, *34*, 14973–14983. [CrossRef] [PubMed]
66. Novgorodov, A.S.; El-Awani, M.; Bielawski, J.; Obeid, L.M.; Gudz, T.I. Activation of Sphingosine-1-phosphate Receptor S1P5 Inhibits Oligodendrocyte Progenitor Migration. *FASEB J.* **2007**, *21*, 1503–1514. [CrossRef]
67. Tsai, H.-H.; Frost, E.; To, V.; Robinson, S.; Ffrench-Constant, C.; Geertman, R.; Ransohoff, R.M.; Miller, R.H. The Chemokine Receptor CXCR2 Controls Positioning of Oligodendrocyte Precursors in Developing Spinal Cord by Arresting Their Migration. *Cell* **2002**, *110*, 373–383. [CrossRef]
68. Dziembowska, M.; Tham, T.N.; Lau, P.; Vitry, S.; Lazarini, F.; Dubois-Dalcq, M. A Role for CXCR4 Signaling in Survival and Migration of Neural and Oligodendrocyte Precursors. *Glia* **2005**, *50*, 258–269. [CrossRef] [PubMed]
69. Garcion, E.; Faissner, A.; ffrench-Constant, C. Knockout Mice Reveal a Contribution of the Extracellular Matrix Molecule Tenascin-C to Neural Precursor Proliferation and Migration. *Dev. Camb. Engl.* **2001**, *128*, 2485–2496. [CrossRef]
70. Chen, Y.; Zheng, Z.; Mei, A.; Huang, H.; Lin, F. Claudin-1 and Claudin-3 as Molecular Regulators of Myelination in Leukoaraiosis Patients. *Clinics* **2021**, *76*, e2167. [CrossRef]
71. Calver, A.R.; Hall, A.C.; Yu, W.-P.; Walsh, F.S.; Heath, J.K.; Betsholtz, C.; Richardson, W.D. Oligodendrocyte Population Dynamics and the Role of PDGF In Vivo. *Neuron* **1998**, *20*, 869–882. [CrossRef]
72. Robinson, S.; Tani, M.; Strieter, R.M.; Ransohoff, R.M.; Miller, R.H. The Chemokine Growth-Regulated Oncogene-Alpha Promotes Spinal Cord Oligodendrocyte Precursor Proliferation. *J. Neurosci. Off. J. Soc. Neurosci.* **1998**, *18*, 10457–10463. [CrossRef]
73. Kadi, L.; Selvaraju, R.; de Lys, P.; Proudfoot, A.E.I.; Wells, T.N.C.; Boschert, U. Differential Effects of Chemokines on Oligodendrocyte Precursor Proliferation and Myelin Formation in Vitro. *J. Neuroimmunol.* **2006**, *174*, 133–146. [CrossRef] [PubMed]

74. Frederick, T.J.; Min, J.; Altieri, S.C.; Mitchell, N.E.; Wood, T.L. Synergistic Induction of Cyclin D1 in Oligodendrocyte Progenitor Cells by IGF-I and FGF-2 Requires Differential Stimulation of Multiple Signaling Pathways. *Glia* **2007**, *55*, 1011–1022. [CrossRef] [PubMed]
75. Van't Veer, A.; Du, Y.; Fischer, T.Z.; Boetig, D.R.; Wood, M.R.; Dreyfus, C.F. Brain-Derived Neurotrophic Factor Effects on Oligodendrocyte Progenitors of the Basal Forebrain Are Mediated through TrkB and the MAP Kinase Pathway. *J. Neurosci. Res.* **2009**, *87*, 69–78. [CrossRef]
76. Yang, J.; Cheng, X.; Qi, J.; Xie, B.; Zhao, X.; Zheng, K.; Zhang, Z.; Qiu, M. EGF Enhances Oligodendrogenesis from Glial Progenitor Cells. *Front. Mol. Neurosci.* **2017**, *10*, 106. [CrossRef] [PubMed]
77. Pukos, N.; Yoseph, R.; McTigue, D.M. To Be or Not to Be: Environmental Factors That Drive Myelin Formation during Development and after CNS Trauma. *Neuroglia* **2018**, *1*, 63–90. [CrossRef]
78. Hill, R.A.; Patel, K.D.; Medved, J.; Reiss, A.M.; Nishiyama, A. NG2 Cells in White Matter but Not Gray Matter Proliferate in Response to PDGF. *J. Neurosci.* **2013**, *33*, 14558–14566. [CrossRef]
79. Wang, S.; Sdrulla, A.D.; diSibio, G.; Bush, G.; Nofziger, D.; Hicks, C.; Weinmaster, G.; Barres, B.A. Notch Receptor Activation Inhibits Oligodendrocyte Differentiation. *Neuron* **1998**, *21*, 63–75. [CrossRef]
80. Marie, C.; Clavairoly, A.; Frah, M.; Hmidan, H.; Yan, J.; Zhao, C.; Van Steenwinckel, J.; Daveau, R.; Zalc, B.; Hassan, B.; et al. Oligodendrocyte Precursor Survival and Differentiation Requires Chromatin Remodeling by Chd7 and Chd8. *Proc. Natl. Acad. Sci. USA* **2018**, *115*, E8246–E8255. [CrossRef]
81. Zhao, C.; Dong, C.; Frah, M.; Deng, Y.; Marie, C.; Zhang, F.; Xu, L.; Ma, Z.; Dong, X.; Lin, Y.; et al. Dual Requirement of CHD8 for Chromatin Landscape Establishment and Histone Methyltransferase Recruitment to Promote CNS Myelination and Repair. *Dev. Cell* **2018**, *45*, 753–768.e8. [CrossRef]
82. Hashimoto, R.; Hori, K.; Owa, T.; Miyashita, S.; Dewa, K.; Masuyama, N.; Sakai, K.; Hayase, Y.; Seto, Y.; Inoue, Y.U.; et al. Origins of Oligodendrocytes in the Cerebellum, Whose Development Is Controlled by the Transcription Factor, Sox9. *Mech. Dev.* **2016**, *140*, 25–40. [CrossRef]
83. Nielsen, J.A.; Berndt, J.A.; Hudson, L.D.; Armstrong, R.C. Myelin Transcription Factor 1 (Myt1) Modulates the Proliferation and Differentiation of Oligodendrocyte Lineage Cells. *Mol. Cell. Neurosci.* **2004**, *25*, 111–123. [CrossRef] [PubMed]
84. Amoureux, M.-C.; Cunningham, B.A.; Edelman, G.M.; Crossin, K.L. N-CAM Binding Inhibits the Proliferation of Hippocampal Progenitor Cells and Promotes Their Differentiation to a Neuronal Phenotype. *J. Neurosci.* **2000**, *20*, 3631–3640. [CrossRef] [PubMed]
85. Casaccia-Bonnefil, P.; Hardy, R.J.; Teng, K.K.; Levine, J.M.; Koff, A.; Chao, M.V. Loss of P27Kip1 Function Results in Increased Proliferative Capacity of Oligodendrocyte Progenitors but Unaltered Timing of Differentiation. *Development* **1999**, *126*, 4027–4037. [CrossRef] [PubMed]
86. Vourc'h, P.; Dessay, S.; Mbarek, O.; Marouillat Védrine, S.; Müh, J.-P.; Andres, C. The Oligodendrocyte-Myelin Glycoprotein Gene Is Highly Expressed during the Late Stages of Myelination in the Rat Central Nervous System. *Brain Res. Dev. Brain Res.* **2003**, *144*, 159–168. [CrossRef]
87. Lehotzky, A.; Lau, P.; Tokési, N.; Muja, N.; Hudson, L.D.; Ovádi, J. Tubulin Polymerization-Promoting Protein (TPPP/P25) Is Critical for Oligodendrocyte Differentiation. *Glia* **2010**, *58*, 157–168. [CrossRef]
88. Kondo, T. The Id4 HLH Protein and the Timing of Oligodendrocyte Differentiation. *EMBO J.* **2000**, *19*, 1998–2007. [CrossRef]
89. Wang, S.; Sdrulla, A.; Johnson, J.E.; Yokota, Y.; Barres, B.A. A Role for the Helix-Loop-Helix Protein Id2 in the Control of Oligodendrocyte Development. *Neuron* **2001**, *29*, 603–614. [CrossRef]
90. Scarisbrick, I.A.; Asakura, K.; Rodriguez, M. Neurotrophin-4/5 Promotes Proliferation of Oligodendrocyte-Type-2 Astrocytes (O-2A). *Dev. Brain Res.* **2000**, *123*, 87–90. [CrossRef]
91. Kondo, T.; Raff, M.C. A Role for Noggin in the Development of Oligodendrocyte Precursor Cells. *Dev. Biol.* **2004**, *267*, 242–251. [CrossRef]
92. Cohen, R.I.; Marmur, R.; Norton, W.T.; Mehler, M.F.; Kessler, J.A. Nerve Growth Factor and Neurotrophin-3 Differentially Regulate the Proliferation and Survival of Developing Rat Brain Oligodendrocytes. *J. Neurosci.* **1996**, *16*, 6433–6442. [CrossRef]
93. Castro, D.S.; Martynoga, B.; Parras, C.; Ramesh, V.; Pacary, E.; Johnston, C.; Drechsel, D.; Lebel-Potter, M.; Garcia, L.G.; Hunt, C.; et al. A Novel Function of the Proneural Factor Ascl1 in Progenitor Proliferation Identified by Genome-Wide Characterization of Its Targets. *Genes Dev.* **2011**, *25*, 930–945. [CrossRef]
94. Warren, N.; Price, D.J. Roles of Pax-6 in Murine Diencephalic Development. *Dev. Camb. Engl.* **1997**, *124*, 1573–1582. [CrossRef] [PubMed]
95. Veiga, S.; Ly, J.; Chan, P.H.; Bresnahan, J.C.; Beattie, M.S. SOD1 Overexpression Improves Features of the Oligodendrocyte Precursor Response in Vitro. *Neurosci. Lett.* **2011**, *503*, 10–14. [CrossRef] [PubMed]
96. Hu, J.; Deng, L.; Wang, X.; Xu, X.-M. Effects of Extracellular Matrix Molecules on the Growth Properties of Oligodendrocyte Progenitor Cells in Vitro. *J. Neurosci. Res.* **2009**, *87*, 2854–2862. [CrossRef] [PubMed]
97. Blaschuk, K.L.; Frost, E.E.; ffrench-Constant, C. The Regulation of Proliferation and Differentiation in Oligodendrocyte Progenitor Cells by AlphaV Integrins. *Dev. Camb. Engl.* **2000**, *127*, 1961–1969. [CrossRef]
98. Adams, K.L.; Riparini, G.; Banerjee, P.; Breur, M.; Bugiani, M.; Gallo, V. Endothelin-1 Signaling Maintains Glial Progenitor Proliferation in the Postnatal Subventricular Zone. *Nat. Commun.* **2020**, *11*, 2138. [CrossRef]

99. Chapman, H.; Riesenberg, A.; Ehrman, L.A.; Kohli, V.; Nardini, D.; Nakafuku, M.; Campbell, K.; Waclaw, R.R. Gsx Transcription Factors Control Neuronal versus Glial Specification in Ventricular Zone Progenitors of the Mouse Lateral Ganglionic Eminence. *Dev. Biol.* **2018**, *442*, 115–126. [CrossRef]
100. Stancic, M.; Slijepcevic, D.; Nomden, A.; Vos, M.J.; de Jonge, J.C.; Sikkema, A.H.; Gabius, H.-J.; Hoekstra, D.; Baron, W. Galectin-4, a Novel Neuronal Regulator of Myelination. *Glia* **2012**, *60*, 919–935. [CrossRef]
101. Canoll, P.D.; Musacchio, J.M.; Hardy, R.; Reynolds, R.; Marchionni, M.A.; Salzer, J.L. GGF/Neuregulin Is a Neuronal Signal That Promotes the Proliferation and Survival and Inhibits the Differentiation of Oligodendrocyte Progenitors. *Neuron* **1996**, *17*, 229–243. [CrossRef]
102. Zhang, S.; Zhu, X.; Gui, X.; Croteau, C.; Song, L.; Xu, J.; Wang, A.; Bannerman, P.; Guo, F. Sox2 Is Essential for Oligodendroglial Proliferation and Differentiation during Postnatal Brain Myelination and CNS Remyelination. *J. Neurosci.* **2018**, *38*, 1802–1820. [CrossRef]
103. Brinkmann, B.G.; Agarwal, A.; Sereda, M.W.; Garratt, A.N.; Müller, T.; Wende, H.; Stassart, R.M.; Nawaz, S.; Humml, C.; Velanac, V.; et al. Neuregulin-1/ErbB Signaling Serves Distinct Functions in Myelination of the Peripheral and Central Nervous System. *Neuron* **2008**, *59*, 581–595. [CrossRef] [PubMed]
104. Dai, J.; Bercury, K.K.; Ahrendsen, J.T.; Macklin, W.B. Olig1 Function Is Required for Oligodendrocyte Differentiation in the Mouse Brain. *J. Neurosci. Off. J. Soc. Neurosci.* **2015**, *35*, 4386–4402. [CrossRef] [PubMed]
105. See, J.; Zhang, X.; Eraydin, N.; Mun, S.-B.; Mamontov, P.; Golden, J.A.; Grinspan, J.B. Oligodendrocyte Maturation Is Inhibited by Bone Morphogenetic Protein. *Mol. Cell. Neurosci.* **2004**, *26*, 481–492. [CrossRef] [PubMed]
106. Harnisch, K.; Teuber-Hanselmann, S.; Macha, N.; Mairinger, F.; Fritsche, L.; Soub, D.; Meinl, E.; Junker, A. Myelination in Multiple Sclerosis Lesions Is Associated with Regulation of Bone Morphogenetic Protein 4 and Its Antagonist Noggin. *Int. J. Mol. Sci.* **2019**, *20*, 154. [CrossRef]
107. Izrael, M.; Zhang, P.; Kaufman, R.; Shinder, V.; Ella, R.; Amit, M.; Itskovitz-Eldor, J.; Chebath, J.; Revel, M. Human Oligodendrocytes Derived from Embryonic Stem Cells: Effect of Noggin on Phenotypic Differentiation in vitro and on Myelination in vivo. *Mol. Cell. Neurosci.* **2007**, *34*, 310–323. [CrossRef]
108. Sugimori, M.; Nagao, M.; Parras, C.M.; Nakatani, H.; Lebel, M.; Guillemot, F.; Nakafuku, M. Ascl1 Is Required for Oligodendrocyte Development in the Spinal Cord. *Dev. Camb. Engl.* **2008**, *135*, 1271–1281. [CrossRef]
109. Matsumoto, S.; Banine, F.; Feistel, K.; Foster, S.; Xing, R.; Struve, J.; Sherman, L.S. Brg1 Directly Regulates Olig2 Transcription and Is Required for Oligodendrocyte Progenitor Cell Specification. *Dev. Biol.* **2016**, *413*, 173–187. [CrossRef] [PubMed]
110. Wedel, M.; Fröb, F.; Elsesser, O.; Wittmann, M.-T.; Lie, D.C.; Reis, A.; Wegner, M. Transcription Factor Tcf4 Is the Preferred Heterodimerization Partner for Olig2 in Oligodendrocytes and Required for Differentiation. *Nucleic Acids Res.* **2020**, *48*, 4839–4857. [CrossRef]
111. Zhao, C.; Deng, Y.; Liu, L.; Yu, K.; Zhang, L.; Wang, H.; He, X.; Wang, J.; Lu, C.; Wu, L.N.; et al. Dual Regulatory Switch through Interactions of Tcf7l2/Tcf4 with Stage-Specific Partners Propels Oligodendroglial Maturation. *Nat. Commun.* **2016**, *7*, 10883. [CrossRef]
112. Zhang, K.; Chen, S.; Yang, Q.; Guo, S.; Chen, Q.; Liu, Z.; Li, L.; Jiang, M.; Li, H.; Hu, J.; et al. The Oligodendrocyte Transcription Factor 2 OLIG2 Regulates Transcriptional Repression during Myelinogenesis in Rodents. *Nat. Commun.* **2022**, *13*, 1423. [CrossRef]
113. Chen, Y.; Wu, H.; Wang, S.; Koito, H.; Li, J.; Ye, F.; Hoang, J.; Escobar, S.S.; Gow, A.; Arnett, H.A.; et al. The Oligodendrocyte-Specific G Protein–Coupled Receptor GPR17 Is a Cell-Intrinsic Timer of Myelination. *Nat. Neurosci.* **2009**, *12*, 1398–1406. [CrossRef] [PubMed]
114. Marin-Husstege, M.; He, Y.; Li, J.; Kondo, T.; Sablitzky, F.; Casaccia-Bonnefil, P. Multiple Roles of Id4 in Developmental Myelination: Predicted Outcomes and Unexpected Findings. *Glia* **2006**, *54*, 285–296. [CrossRef] [PubMed]
115. Huang, H.; Wu, H.; He, W.; Zhou, F.; Yu, X.; Yi, M.; Du, J.; Xie, B.; Qiu, M. Id2 and Id4 Are Not the Major Negative Regulators of Oligodendrocyte Differentiation during Early Central Nervous System Development. *Glia* **2022**, *70*, 590–601. [CrossRef] [PubMed]
116. Swiss, V.A.; Nguyen, T.; Dugas, J.; Ibrahim, A.; Barres, B.; Androulakis, I.P.; Casaccia, P. Identification of a Gene Regulatory Network Necessary for the Initiation of Oligodendrocyte Differentiation. *PLoS ONE* **2011**, *6*, e18088. [CrossRef] [PubMed]
117. Bujalka, H.; Koenning, M.; Jackson, S.; Perreau, V.M.; Pope, B.; Hay, C.M.; Mitew, S.; Hill, A.F.; Lu, Q.R.; Wegner, M.; et al. MYRF Is a Membrane-Associated Transcription Factor That Autoproteolytically Cleaves to Directly Activate Myelin Genes. *PLoS Biol.* **2013**, *11*, e1001625. [CrossRef]
118. Emery, B.; Agalliu, D.; Cahoy, J.D.; Watkins, T.A.; Dugas, J.C.; Mulinyawe, S.B.; Ibrahim, A.; Ligon, K.L.; Rowitch, D.H.; Barres, B.A. Myelin Gene Regulatory Factor Is a Critical Transcriptional Regulator Required for CNS Myelination. *Cell* **2009**, *138*, 172–185. [CrossRef]
119. Hoffmann, S.A.; Hos, D.; Küspert, M.; Lang, R.A.; Lovell-Badge, R.; Wegner, M.; Reiprich, S. Stem Cell Factor Sox2 and Its Close Relative Sox3 Have Differentiation Functions in Oligodendrocytes. *Development* **2014**, *141*, 39–50. [CrossRef]
120. Stolt, C.C.; Lommes, P.; Friedrich, R.P.; Wegner, M. Transcription Factors Sox8 and Sox10 Perform Non-Equivalent Roles during Oligodendrocyte Development despite Functional Redundancy. *Development* **2004**, *131*, 2349–2358. [CrossRef]
121. Stolt, C.C.; Rehberg, S.; Ader, M.; Lommes, P.; Riethmacher, D.; Schachner, M.; Bartsch, U.; Wegner, M. Terminal Differentiation of Myelin-Forming Oligodendrocytes Depends on the Transcription Factor Sox10. *Genes Dev.* **2002**, *16*, 165–170. [CrossRef]

122. Takada, N.; Kucenas, S.; Appel, B. Sox10 Is Necessary for Oligodendrocyte Survival Following Axon Wrapping. *Glia* **2010**, *58*, 996–1006. [CrossRef]
123. Zhang, C.; Huang, H.; Chen, Z.; Zhang, Z.; Lu, W.; Qiu, M. The Transcription Factor NKX2-2 Regulates Oligodendrocyte Differentiation through Domain-Specific Interactions with Transcriptional Corepressors. *J. Biol. Chem.* **2020**, *295*, 1879–1888. [CrossRef] [PubMed]
124. Qi, Y.; Cai, J.; Wu, Y.; Wu, R.; Lee, J.; Fu, H.; Rao, M.; Sussel, L.; Rubenstein, J.; Qiu, M. Control of Oligodendrocyte Differentiation by the Nkx2.2 Homeodomain Transcription Factor. *Dev. Camb. Engl.* **2001**, *128*, 2723–2733. [CrossRef] [PubMed]
125. Ji, S.; Doucette, J.R.; Nazarali, A.J. Sirt2 Is a Novel in Vivo Downstream Target of Nkx2.2 and Enhances Oligodendroglial Cell Differentiation. *J. Mol. Cell Biol.* **2011**, *3*, 351–359. [CrossRef] [PubMed]
126. Hisahara, S.; Iwahara, N.; Matsushita, T.; Suzuki, S.; Matsumura, A.; Fujikura, M.; Yokokawa, K.; Saito, T.; Manabe, T.; Kawamata, J.; et al. SIRT1 Decelerates Morphological Processing of Oligodendrocyte Cell Lines and Regulates the Expression of Cytoskeleton-Related Oligodendrocyte Proteins. *Biochem. Biophys. Res. Commun.* **2021**, *546*, 7–14. [CrossRef]
127. Laitman, B.M.; Asp, L.; Mariani, J.N.; Zhang, J.; Liu, J.; Sawai, S.; Chapouly, C.; Horng, S.; Kramer, E.G.; Mitiku, N.; et al. The Transcriptional Activator Krüppel-like Factor-6 Is Required for CNS Myelination. *PLOS Biol.* **2016**, *14*, e1002467. [CrossRef]
128. Vondran, M.W.; Clinton-Luke, P.; Honeywell, J.Z.; Dreyfus, C.F. BDNF+/- Mice Exhibit Deficits in Oligodendrocyte Lineage Cells of the Basal Forebrain. *Glia* **2010**, *58*, 848–856. [CrossRef] [PubMed]
129. Heinrich, M.; Gorath, M.; Richter-Landsberg, C. Neurotrophin-3 (NT-3) Modulates Early Differentiation of Oligodendrocytes in Rat Brain Cortical Cultures. *Glia* **1999**, *28*, 244–255. [CrossRef]
130. Yan, H.; Wood, P.M. NT-3 Weakly Stimulates Proliferation of Adult Rat O1(−)O4(+) Oligodendrocyte-Lineage Cells and Increases Oligodendrocyte Myelination in vitro. *J. Neurosci. Res.* **2000**, *62*, 329–335. [CrossRef]
131. McMorris, F.A.; Dubois-Dalcq, M. Insulin-like Growth Factor I Promotes Cell Proliferation and Oligodendroglial Commitment in Rat Glial Progenitor Cells Developing in vitro. *J. Neurosci. Res.* **1988**, *21*, 199–209. [CrossRef]
132. Zhou, L.; Shao, C.-Y.; Xie, Y.-J.; Wang, N.; Xu, S.-M.; Luo, B.-Y.; Wu, Z.-Y.; Ke, Y.H.; Qiu, M.; Shen, Y. Gab1 Mediates PDGF Signaling and Is Essential to Oligodendrocyte Differentiation and CNS Myelination. *eLife* **2020**, *9*, e52056. [CrossRef]
133. Zhou, X.; Shin, S.; He, C.; Zhang, Q.; Rasband, M.N.; Ren, J.; Dai, C.; Zorrilla-Veloz, R.I.; Shingu, T.; Yuan, L.; et al. Qki Regulates Myelinogenesis through Srebp2-Dependent Cholesterol Biosynthesis. *eLife* **2021**, *10*, e60467. [CrossRef] [PubMed]
134. Ho, W.Y.; Chang, J.-C.; Lim, K.; Cazenave-Gassiot, A.; Nguyen, A.T.; Foo, J.C.; Muralidharan, S.; Viera-Ortiz, A.; Ong, S.J.M.; Hor, J.H.; et al. TDP-43 Mediates SREBF2-Regulated Gene Expression Required for Oligodendrocyte Myelination. *J. Cell Biol.* **2021**, *220*, e201910213. [CrossRef] [PubMed]
135. Morita, J.; Kano, K.; Kato, K.; Takita, H.; Sakagami, H.; Yamamoto, Y.; Mihara, E.; Ueda, H.; Sato, T.; Tokuyama, H.; et al. Structure and Biological Function of ENPP6, a Choline-Specific Glycerophosphodiester-Phosphodiesterase. *Sci. Rep.* **2016**, *6*, 20995. [CrossRef] [PubMed]
136. Baas, D.; Bourbeau, D.; Sarliève, L.L.; Ittel, M.E.; Dussault, J.H.; Puymirat, J. Oligodendrocyte Maturation and Progenitor Cell Proliferation Are Independently Regulated by Thyroid Hormone. *Glia* **1997**, *19*, 324–332. [CrossRef]
137. Barres, B.A.; Lazar, M.A.; Raff, M.C. A Novel Role for Thyroid Hormone, Glucocorticoids and Retinoic Acid in Timing Oligodendrocyte Development. *Dev. Camb. Engl.* **1994**, *120*, 1097–1108. [CrossRef] [PubMed]
138. Baas, D.; Fressinaud, C.; Ittel, M.E.; Reeber, A.; Dalençon, D.; Puymirat, J.; Sarliève, L.L. Expression of Thyroid Hormone Receptor Isoforms in Rat Oligodendrocyte Cultures. Effect of 3,5,3′-Triiodo-l-Thyronine. *Neurosci. Lett.* **1994**, *176*, 47–51. [CrossRef]
139. Kondo, T.; Raff, M. Basic Helix-Loop-Helix Proteins and the Timing of Oligodendrocyte Differentiation. *Dev. Camb. Engl.* **2000**, *127*, 2989–2998. [CrossRef]
140. Genoud, S.; Lappe-Siefke, C.; Goebbels, S.; Radtke, F.; Aguet, M.; Scherer, S.S.; Suter, U.; Nave, K.-A.; Mantei, N. Notch1 Control of Oligodendrocyte Differentiation in the Spinal Cord. *J. Cell Biol.* **2002**, *158*, 709–718. [CrossRef]
141. Hu, Q.-D.; Ang, B.-T.; Karsak, M.; Hu, W.-P.; Cui, X.-Y.; Duka, T.; Takeda, Y.; Chia, W.; Sankar, N.; Ng, Y.-K.; et al. F3/Contactin Acts as a Functional Ligand for Notch during Oligodendrocyte Maturation. *Cell* **2003**, *115*, 163–175. [CrossRef]
142. Emery, B. Regulation of Oligodendrocyte Differentiation and Myelination. *Science* **2010**, *330*, 779–782. [CrossRef]
143. Jepson, S.; Vought, B.; Gross, C.H.; Gan, L.; Austen, D.; Frantz, J.D.; Zwahlen, J.; Lowe, D.; Markland, W.; Krauss, R. LINGO-1, a Transmembrane Signaling Protein, Inhibits Oligodendrocyte Differentiation and Myelination through Intercellular Self-Interactions. *J. Biol. Chem.* **2012**, *287*, 22184–22195. [CrossRef] [PubMed]
144. Hirahara, Y.; Bansal, R.; Honke, K.; Ikenaka, K.; Wada, Y. Sulfatide Is a Negative Regulator of Oligodendrocyte Differentiation: Development in Sulfatide-Null Mice. *Glia* **2004**, *45*, 269–277. [CrossRef] [PubMed]
145. Choi, M.-H.; Na, J.E.; Yoon, Y.R.; Rhyu, I.J.; Ko, Y.-G.; Baik, J.-H. Hypomyelination and Cognitive Impairment in Mice Lacking CD133 (Prominin-1). *Biochem. Biophys. Res. Commun.* **2018**, *502*, 291–298. [CrossRef]
146. Brown, T.L.; Hashimoto, H.; Finseth, L.T.; Wood, T.L.; Macklin, W.B. PAK1 Positively Regulates Oligodendrocyte Morphology and Myelination. *J. Neurosci.* **2021**, *41*, 1864–1877. [CrossRef] [PubMed]
147. Quarles, R.H. Myelin-Associated Glycoprotein (MAG): Past, Present and Beyond. *J. Neurochem.* **2007**, *100*, 1431–1448. [CrossRef] [PubMed]
148. Stankoff, B.; Aigrot, M.-S.; Noël, F.; Wattilliaux, A.; Zalc, B.; Lubetzki, C. Ciliary Neurotrophic Factor (CNTF) Enhances Myelin Formation: A Novel Role for CNTF and CNTF-Related Molecules. *J. Neurosci.* **2002**, *22*, 9221–9227. [CrossRef] [PubMed]

149. Kalsi, A.S.; Greenwood, K.; Wilkin, G.; Butt, A.M. Kir4.1 Expression by Astrocytes and Oligodendrocytes in CNS White Matter: A Developmental Study in the Rat Optic Nerve. *J. Anat.* **2004**, *204*, 475–485. [CrossRef]
150. Howng, S.Y.B.; Avila, R.L.; Emery, B.; Traka, M.; Lin, W.; Watkins, T.; Cook, S.; Bronson, R.; Davisson, M.; Barres, B.A.; et al. ZFP191 Is Required by Oligodendrocytes for CNS Myelination. *Genes Dev.* **2010**, *24*, 301–311. [CrossRef]
151. Müller, R.; Heinrich, M.; Heck, S.; Blohm, D.; Richter-Landsberg, C. Expression of Microtubule-Associated Proteins MAP2 and Tau in Cultured Rat Brain Oligodendrocytes. *Cell Tissue Res.* **1997**, *288*, 239–249. [CrossRef]
152. Chen, X.; Ku, L.; Mei, R.; Liu, G.; Xu, C.; Wen, Z.; Zhao, X.; Wang, F.; Xiao, L.; Feng, Y. Novel Schizophrenia Risk Factor Pathways Regulate FEZ1 to Advance Oligodendroglia Development. *Transl. Psychiatry* **2017**, *7*, 1293. [CrossRef]
153. Lee, J.; Gravel, M.; Zhang, R.; Thibault, P.; Braun, P.E. Process Outgrowth in Oligodendrocytes Is Mediated by CNP, a Novel Microtubule Assembly Myelin Protein. *J. Cell Biol.* **2005**, *170*, 661–673. [CrossRef] [PubMed]
154. Monin, A.; Baumann, P.S.; Griffa, A.; Xin, L.; Mekle, R.; Fournier, M.; Butticaz, C.; Klaey, M.; Cabungcal, J.H.; Steullet, P.; et al. Glutathione Deficit Impairs Myelin Maturation: Relevance for White Matter Integrity in Schizophrenia Patients. *Mol. Psychiatry* **2015**, *20*, 827–838. [CrossRef] [PubMed]
155. Lee, X.; Hu, Y.; Zhang, Y.; Yang, Z.; Shao, Z.; Qiu, M.; Pepinsky, B.; Miller, R.H.; Mi, S. Oligodendrocyte Differentiation and Myelination Defects in OMgp Null Mice. *Mol. Cell. Neurosci.* **2011**, *46*, 752–761. [CrossRef] [PubMed]
156. Kaji, S.; Maki, T.; Ueda, J.; Ishimoto, T.; Inoue, Y.; Yasuda, K.; Sawamura, M.; Hikawa, R.; Ayaki, T.; Yamakado, H.; et al. BCAS1-Positive Immature Oligodendrocytes Are Affected by the α-Synuclein-Induced Pathology of Multiple System Atrophy. *Acta Neuropathol. Commun.* **2020**, *8*, 120. [CrossRef] [PubMed]
157. Fard, M.K.; van der Meer, F.; Sánchez, P.; Cantuti-Castelvetri, L.; Mandad, S.; Jäkel, S.; Fornasiero, E.F.; Schmitt, S.; Ehrlich, M.; Starost, L.; et al. BCAS1 Expression Defines a Population of Early Myelinating Oligodendrocytes in Multiple Sclerosis Lesions. *Sci. Transl. Med.* **2017**, *9*, eaam7816. [CrossRef] [PubMed]
158. Ikenaka, K.; Kagawa, T.; Mikoshiba, K. Selective Expression of DM-20, an Alternatively Spliced Myelin Proteolipid Protein Gene Product, in Developing Nervous System and in Nonglial Cells. *J. Neurochem.* **1992**, *58*, 2248–2253. [CrossRef] [PubMed]
159. Galiano, M.R.; Andrieux, A.; Deloulme, J.C.; Bosc, C.; Schweitzer, A.; Job, D.; Hallak, M.E. Myelin Basic Protein Functions as a Microtubule Stabilizing Protein in Differentiated Oligodendrocytes. *J. Neurosci. Res.* **2006**, *84*, 534–541. [CrossRef]
160. Uhlenberg, B.; Schuelke, M.; Rüschendorf, F.; Ruf, N.; Kaindl, A.M.; Henneke, M.; Thiele, H.; Stoltenburg-Didinger, G.; Aksu, F.; Topaloğlu, H.; et al. Mutations in the Gene Encoding Gap Junction Protein Alpha 12 (Connexin 46.6) Cause Pelizaeus-Merzbacher-like Disease. *Am. J. Hum. Genet.* **2004**, *75*, 251–260. [CrossRef]
161. Menichella, D.M.; Goodenough, D.A.; Sirkowski, E.; Scherer, S.S.; Paul, D.L. Connexins Are Critical for Normal Myelination in the CNS. *J. Neurosci.* **2003**, *23*, 5963–5973. [CrossRef]
162. Wasseff, S.K.; Scherer, S.S. Cx32 and Cx47 Mediate Oligodendrocyte:Astrocyte and Oligodendrocyte:Oligodendrocyte Gap Junction Coupling. *Neurobiol. Dis.* **2011**, *42*, 506–513. [CrossRef]
163. Mosser, J.; Douar, A.M.; Sarde, C.O.; Kioschis, P.; Feil, R.; Moser, H.; Poustka, A.M.; Mandel, J.L.; Aubourg, P. Putative X-Linked Adrenoleukodystrophy Gene Shares Unexpected Homology with ABC Transporters. *Nature* **1993**, *361*, 726–730. [CrossRef] [PubMed]
164. Strachan, L.R.; Stevenson, T.J.; Freshner, B.; Keefe, M.D.; Miranda Bowles, D.; Bonkowsky, J.L. A Zebrafish Model of X-Linked Adrenoleukodystrophy Recapitulates Key Disease Features and Demonstrates a Developmental Requirement for Abcd1 in Oligodendrocyte Patterning and Myelination. *Hum. Mol. Genet.* **2017**, *26*, 3600–3614. [CrossRef] [PubMed]
165. Schnädelbach, O.; Ozen, I.; Blaschuk, O.W.; Meyer, R.L.; Fawcett, J.W. N-Cadherin Is Involved in Axon-Oligodendrocyte Contact and Myelination. *Mol. Cell. Neurosci.* **2001**, *17*, 1084–1093. [CrossRef] [PubMed]
166. Laursen, L.S.; Chan, C.W.; ffrench-Constant, C. An Integrin–Contactin Complex Regulates CNS Myelination by Differential Fyn Phosphorylation. *J. Neurosci.* **2009**, *29*, 9174–9185. [CrossRef]
167. Charles, P.; Tait, S.; Faivre-Sarrailh, C.; Barbin, G.; Gunn-Moore, F.; Denisenko-Nehrbass, N.; Guennoc, A.-M.; Girault, J.-A.; Brophy, P.J.; Lubetzki, C. Neurofascin Is a Glial Receptor for the Paranodin/Caspr-Contactin Axonal Complex at the Axoglial Junction. *Curr. Biol.* **2002**, *12*, 217–220. [CrossRef]
168. Thaxton, C.; Pillai, A.M.; Pribisko, A.L.; Labasque, M.; Dupree, J.L.; Faivre-Sarrailh, C.; Bhat, M.A. In Vivo Deletion of Immunoglobulin Domains 5 and 6 in Neurofascin (Nfasc) Reveals Domain-Specific Requirements in Myelinated Axons. *J. Neurosci. Off. J. Soc. Neurosci.* **2010**, *30*, 4868–4876. [CrossRef] [PubMed]
169. Labasque, M.; Hivert, B.; Nogales-Gadea, G.; Querol, L.; Illa, I.; Faivre-Sarrailh, C. Specific Contactin N-Glycans Are Implicated in Neurofascin Binding and Autoimmune Targeting in Peripheral Neuropathies. *J. Biol. Chem.* **2014**, *289*, 7907–7918. [CrossRef]
170. Klingseisen, A.; Ristoiu, A.-M.; Kegel, L.; Sherman, D.L.; Rubio-Brotons, M.; Almeida, R.G.; Koudelka, S.; Benito-Kwiecinski, S.K.; Poole, R.J.; Brophy, P.J.; et al. Oligodendrocyte Neurofascin Independently Regulates Both Myelin Targeting and Sheath Growth in the CNS. *Dev. Cell* **2019**, *51*, 730–744.e6. [CrossRef]
171. Çolakoğlu, G.; Bergstrom-Tyrberg, U.; Berglund, E.O.; Ranscht, B. Contactin-1 Regulates Myelination and Nodal/Paranodal Domain Organization in the Central Nervous System. *Proc. Natl. Acad. Sci. USA* **2014**, *111*, E394–E403. [CrossRef]
172. Traka, M.; Goutebroze, L.; Denisenko, N.; Bessa, M.; Nifli, A.; Havaki, S.; Iwakura, Y.; Fukamauchi, F.; Watanabe, K.; Soliven, B.; et al. Association of TAG-1 with Caspr2 Is Essential for the Molecular Organization of Juxtaparanodal Regions of Myelinated Fibers. *J. Cell Biol.* **2003**, *162*, 1161–1172. [CrossRef]

173. Elazar, N.; Vainshtein, A.; Golan, N.; Vijayaragavan, B.; Schaeren-Wiemers, N.; Eshed-Eisenbach, Y.; Peles, E. Axoglial Adhesion by Cadm4 Regulates CNS Myelination. *Neuron* **2019**, *101*, 224–231.e5. [CrossRef] [PubMed]
174. Hughes, A.N.; Appel, B. Oligodendrocytes Express Synaptic Proteins That Modulate Myelin Sheath Formation. *Nat. Commun.* **2019**, *10*, 4125. [CrossRef] [PubMed]
175. Sturgill, E.R.; Aoki, K.; Lopez, P.H.; Colacurcio, D.; Vajn, K.; Lorenzini, I.; Majić, S.; Yang, W.H.; Heffer, M.; Tiemeyer, M.; et al. Biosynthesis of the Major Brain Gangliosides GD1a and GT1b. *Glycobiology* **2012**, *22*, 1289–1301. [CrossRef] [PubMed]
176. Schnaar, R.L. Brain Gangliosides in Axon-Myelin Stability and Axon Regeneration. *FEBS Lett.* **2010**, *584*, 1741–1747. [CrossRef]
177. Harboe, M.; Torvund-Jensen, J.; Kjaer-Sorensen, K.; Laursen, L.S. Ephrin-A1-EphA4 Signaling Negatively Regulates Myelination in the Central Nervous System. *Glia* **2018**, *66*, 934–950. [CrossRef]
178. Linneberg, C.; Harboe, M.; Laursen, L.S. Axo-Glia Interaction Preceding CNS Myelination Is Regulated by Bidirectional Eph-Ephrin Signaling. *ASN Neuro* **2015**, *7*, 1759091415602859. [CrossRef]
179. Almeida, R.G. The Rules of Attraction in Central Nervous System Myelination. *Front. Cell. Neurosci.* **2018**, *12*, 367. [CrossRef]
180. Charles, P.; Hernandez, M.P.; Stankoff, B.; Aigrot, M.S.; Colin, C.; Rougon, G.; Zalc, B.; Lubetzki, C. Negative Regulation of Central Nervous System Myelination by Polysialylated-Neural Cell Adhesion Molecule. *Proc. Natl. Acad. Sci. USA* **2000**, *97*, 7585–7590. [CrossRef]
181. Redmond, S.A.; Mei, F.; Eshed-Eisenbach, Y.; Osso, L.A.; Leshkowitz, D.; Shen, Y.-A.A.; Kay, J.N.; Aurrand-Lions, M.; Lyons, D.A.; Peles, E.; et al. Somatodendritic Expression of JAM2 Inhibits Oligodendrocyte Myelination. *Neuron* **2016**, *91*, 824–836. [CrossRef]
182. Díez-Revuelta, N.; Higuero, A.M.; Velasco, S.; Peñas-de-la-Iglesia, M.; Gabius, H.-J.; Abad-Rodríguez, J. Neurons Define Non-Myelinated Axon Segments by the Regulation of Galectin-4-Containing Axon Membrane Domains. *Sci. Rep.* **2017**, *7*, 12246. [CrossRef]
183. Xin, M.; Yue, T.; Ma, Z.; Wu, F.; Gow, A.; Lu, Q.R. Myelinogenesis and Axonal Recognition by Oligodendrocytes in Brain Are Uncoupled in Olig1-Null Mice. *J. Neurosci. Off. J. Soc. Neurosci.* **2005**, *25*, 1354–1365. [CrossRef] [PubMed]
184. Lüders, K.A.; Nessler, S.; Kusch, K.; Patzig, J.; Jung, R.B.; Möbius, W.; Nave, K.-A.; Werner, H.B. Maintenance of High Proteolipid Protein Level in Adult Central Nervous System Myelin Is Required to Preserve the Integrity of Myelin and Axons. *Glia* **2019**, *67*, 634–649. [CrossRef] [PubMed]
185. Chow, E.; Mottahedeh, J.; Prins, M.; Ridder, W.; Nusinowitz, S.; Bronstein, J.M. Disrupted Compaction of CNS Myelin in an OSP/Claudin-11 and PLP/DM20 Double Knockout Mouse. *Mol. Cell. Neurosci.* **2005**, *29*, 405–413. [CrossRef]
186. Schachner, M.; Bartsch, U. Multiple Functions of the Myelin-Associated Glycoprotein MAG (Siglec-4a) in Formation and Maintenance of Myelin. *Glia* **2000**, *29*, 154–165. [CrossRef]
187. Clements, C.S.; Reid, H.H.; Beddoe, T.; Tynan, F.E.; Perugini, M.A.; Johns, T.G.; Bernard, C.C.A.; Rossjohn, J. The Crystal Structure of Myelin Oligodendrocyte Glycoprotein, a Key Autoantigen in Multiple Sclerosis. *Proc. Natl. Acad. Sci. USA* **2003**, *100*, 11059–11064. [CrossRef]
188. Johns, T.G.; Bernard, C.C.A. The Structure and Function of Myelin Oligodendrocyte Glycoprotein. *J. Neurochem.* **1999**, *72*, 1–9. [CrossRef] [PubMed]
189. Rasband, M.N.; Tayler, J.; Kaga, Y.; Yang, Y.; Lappe-Siefke, C.; Nave, K.-A., Bansal, R. CNP Is Required for Maintenance of Axon-Glia Interactions at Nodes of Ranvier in the CNS. *Glia* **2005**, *50*, 86–90. [CrossRef]
190. Schäfer, I.; Müller, C.; Luhmann, H.J.; White, R. MOBP Levels Are Regulated by Fyn Kinase and Affect the Morphological Differentiation of Oligodendrocytes. *J. Cell Sci.* **2016**, *129*, 930–942. [CrossRef]
191. Vourc'h, P.; Andres, C. Oligodendrocyte Myelin Glycoprotein (OMgp): Evolution, Structure and Function. *Brain Res. Rev.* **2004**, *45*, 115–124. [CrossRef]
192. Chang, K.-J.; Susuki, K.; Dours-Zimmermann, M.T.; Zimmermann, D.R.; Rasband, M.N. Oligodendrocyte Myelin Glycoprotein Does Not Influence Node of Ranvier Structure or Assembly. *J. Neurosci.* **2010**, *30*, 14476–14481. [CrossRef]
193. Koenning, M.; Jackson, S.; Hay, C.M.; Faux, C.; Kilpatrick, T.J.; Willingham, M.; Emery, B. Myelin Gene Regulatory Factor Is Required for Maintenance of Myelin and Mature Oligodendrocyte Identity in the Adult CNS. *J. Neurosci.* **2012**, *32*, 12528–12542. [CrossRef] [PubMed]
194. Cai, J.; Zhu, Q.; Zheng, K.; Li, H.; Qi, Y.; Cao, Q.; Qiu, M. Co-Localization of Nkx6.2 and Nkx2.2 Homeodomain Proteins in Differentiated Myelinating Oligodendrocytes. *Glia* **2010**, *58*, 458–468. [CrossRef]
195. Huang, H.; Teng, P.; Du, J.; Meng, J.; Hu, X.; Tang, T.; Zhang, Z.; Qi, Y.B.; Qiu, M. Interactive Repression of MYRF Self-Cleavage and Activity in Oligodendrocyte Differentiation by TMEM98 Protein. *J. Neurosci.* **2018**, *38*, 9829–9839. [CrossRef] [PubMed]
196. Othman, A.; Frim, D.M.; Polak, P.; Vujicic, S.; Arnason, B.G.W.; Boullerne, A.I. Olig1 Is Expressed in Human Oligodendrocytes during Maturation and Regeneration. *Glia* **2011**, *59*, 914–926. [CrossRef] [PubMed]
197. Ishii, A.; Furusho, M.; Dupree, J.L.; Bansal, R. Role of ERK1/2 MAPK Signaling in the Maintenance of Myelin and Axonal Integrity in the Adult CNS. *J. Neurosci.* **2014**, *34*, 16031–16045. [CrossRef]
198. Furusho, M.; Ishii, A.; Bansal, R. Signaling by FGF Receptor 2, Not FGF Receptor 1, Regulates Myelin Thickness through Activation of ERK1/2–MAPK, Which Promotes MTORC1 Activity in an Akt-Independent Manner. *J. Neurosci.* **2017**, *37*, 2931–2946. [CrossRef] [PubMed]
199. Zhang, L.; He, X.; Liu, L.; Jiang, M.; Zhao, C.; Wang, H.; He, D.; Zheng, T.; Zhou, X.; Hassan, A.; et al. Hdac3 Interaction with P300 Histone Acetyltransferase Regulates the Oligodendrocyte and Astrocyte Lineage Fate Switch. *Dev. Cell* **2016**, *36*, 316–330. [CrossRef] [PubMed]

200. Marcus, J.; Honigbaum, S.; Shroff, S.; Honke, K.; Rosenbluth, J.; Dupree, J.L. Sulfatide Is Essential for the Maintenance of CNS Myelin and Axon Structure. *Glia* **2006**, *53*, 372–381. [CrossRef]
201. Coetzee, T.; Dupree, J.L.; Popko, B. Demyelination and Altered Expression of Myelin-Associated Glycoprotein Isoforms in the Central Nervous System of Galactolipid-Deficient Mice. *J. Neurosci. Res.* **1998**, *54*, 613–622. [CrossRef]
202. Hulshagen, L.; Krysko, O.; Bottelbergs, A.; Huyghe, S.; Klein, R.; Van Veldhoven, P.P.; De Deyn, P.P.; D'Hooge, R.; Hartmann, D.; Baes, M. Absence of Functional Peroxisomes from Mouse CNS Causes Dysmyelination and Axon Degeneration. *J. Neurosci.* **2008**, *28*, 4015–4027. [CrossRef]
203. Morita, M.; Shinbo, S.; Asahi, A.; Imanaka, T. Very Long Chain Fatty Acid β-Oxidation in Astrocytes: Contribution of the ABCD1-Dependent and -Independent Pathways. *Biol. Pharm. Bull.* **2012**, *35*, 1972–1979. [CrossRef] [PubMed]
204. Sato, Y.; Yoshikawa, F.; Sadakata, T.; Shinoda, Y.; Koebis, M.; Furuichi, T. Age-Dependent Redistribution and Hypersialylation of the Central Myelin Paranodal Loop Membrane Protein Opalin in the Mouse Brain. *Neurosci. Lett.* **2014**, *581*, 14–19. [CrossRef] [PubMed]
205. Xin, W.; Chan, J.R. Myelin Plasticity: Sculpting Circuits in Learning and Memory. *Nat. Rev. Neurosci.* **2020**, *21*, 682–694. [CrossRef] [PubMed]
206. Franklin, R.J.M.; ffrench-Constant, C. Regenerating CNS Myelin—From Mechanisms to Experimental Medicines. *Nat. Rev. Neurosci.* **2017**, *18*, 753–769. [CrossRef] [PubMed]
207. Craig, G.A.; Yoo, S.; Du, T.Y.; Xiao, J. Plasticity in Oligodendrocyte Lineage Progression: An OPC Puzzle on Our Nerves. *Eur. J. Neurosci.* **2021**, *54*, 5747–5761. [CrossRef]
208. Franklin, R.J.M.; ffrench-Constant, C. Remyelination in the CNS: From Biology to Therapy. *Nat. Rev. Neurosci.* **2008**, *9*, 839–855. [CrossRef]
209. Moyon, S.; Dubessy, A.L.; Aigrot, M.S.; Trotter, M.; Huang, J.K.; Dauphinot, L.; Potier, M.C.; Kerninon, C.; Melik Parsadaniantz, S.; Franklin, R.J.M.; et al. Demyelination Causes Adult CNS Progenitors to Revert to an Immature State and Express Immune Cues That Support Their Migration. *J. Neurosci.* **2015**, *35*, 4–20. [CrossRef]
210. Ffrench-Constant, C.; Raff, M.C. Proliferating Bipotential Glial Progenitor Cells in Adult Rat Optic Nerve. *Nature* **1986**, *319*, 499–502. [CrossRef]
211. Butt, A.M.; Rivera, A.D.; Fulton, D.; Azim, K. Targeting the Subventricular Zone to Promote Myelin Repair in the Aging Brain. *Cells* **2022**, *11*, 1809. [CrossRef]
212. Zawadzka, M.; Rivers, L.E.; Fancy, S.P.J.; Zhao, C.; Tripathi, R.; Jamen, F.; Young, K.; Goncharevich, A.; Pohl, H.; Rizzi, M.; et al. CNS-Resident Glial Progenitor/Stem Cells Produce Schwann Cells as Well as Oligodendrocytes during Repair of CNS Demyelination. *Cell Stem Cell* **2010**, *6*, 578–590. [CrossRef]
213. Duncan, I.D.; Radcliff, A.B.; Heidari, M.; Kidd, G.; August, B.K.; Wierenga, L.A. The Adult Oligodendrocyte Can Participate in Remyelination. *Proc. Natl. Acad. Sci. USA* **2018**, *115*, E11807–E11816. [CrossRef] [PubMed]
214. Sim, F.J.; Zhao, C.; Penderis, J.; Franklin, R.J.M. The Age-Related Decrease in CNS Remyelination Efficiency Is Attributable to an Impairment of Both Oligodendrocyte Progenitor Recruitment and Differentiation. *J. Neurosci.* **2002**, *22*, 2451–2459. [CrossRef] [PubMed]
215. Palmer, A.L.; Ousman, S.S. Astrocytes and Aging. *Front. Aging Neurosci.* **2018**, *10*, 337. [CrossRef]
216. Thelen, K.M.; Falkai, P.; Bayer, T.A.; Lütjohann, D. Cholesterol Synthesis Rate in Human Hippocampus Declines with Aging. *Neurosci. Lett.* **2006**, *403*, 15–19. [CrossRef] [PubMed]
217. Tse, K.-H.; Herrup, K. DNA Damage in the Oligodendrocyte Lineage and Its Role in Brain Aging. *Mech. Ageing Dev.* **2017**, *161*, 37–50. [CrossRef] [PubMed]
218. Cantuti-Castelvetri, L.; Fitzner, D.; Bosch-Queralt, M.; Weil, M.-T.; Su, M.; Sen, P.; Ruhwedel, T.; Mitkovski, M.; Trendelenburg, G.; Lütjohann, D.; et al. Defective Cholesterol Clearance Limits Remyelination in the Aged Central Nervous System. *Science* **2018**, *359*, 684–688. [CrossRef] [PubMed]
219. Love, S. Demyelinating Diseases. *J. Clin. Pathol.* **2006**, *59*, 1151–1159. [CrossRef]
220. Seil, F.J. Demyelination. In *Advances in Cellular Neurobiology*; Elsevier: Amsterdam, The Netherlands, 1982; Volume 3, pp. 235–274, ISBN 978-0-12-008303-9.
221. Zhao, J.-W.; Wang, D.-X.; Ma, X.-R.; Dong, Z.-J.; Wu, J.-B.; Wang, F.; Wu, Y. Impaired Metabolism of Oligodendrocyte Progenitor Cells and Axons in Demyelinated Lesion and in the Aged CNS. *Curr. Opin. Pharmacol.* **2022**, *64*, 102205. [CrossRef]
222. Berghoff, S.A.; Spieth, L.; Saher, G. Local Cholesterol Metabolism Orchestrates Remyelination. *Trends Neurosci.* **2022**, *45*, 272–283. [CrossRef] [PubMed]
223. Liu, Y.; Hammel, G.; Shi, M.; Cheng, Z.; Zivkovic, S.; Wang, X.; Xu, P.; He, X.; Guo, B.; Ren, Y.; et al. Myelin Debris Stimulates NG2/CSPG4 Expression in Bone Marrow-Derived Macrophages in the Injured Spinal Cord. *Front. Cell. Neurosci.* **2021**, *15*, 651827. [CrossRef] [PubMed]
224. Kotter, M.R. Myelin Impairs CNS Remyelination by Inhibiting Oligodendrocyte Precursor Cell Differentiation. *J. Neurosci.* **2006**, *26*, 328–332. [CrossRef] [PubMed]
225. Napoli, I.; Neumann, H. Protective Effects of Microglia in Multiple Sclerosis. *Exp. Neurol.* **2010**, *225*, 24–28. [CrossRef] [PubMed]
226. Lampron, A.; Larochelle, A.; Laflamme, N.; Préfontaine, P.; Plante, M.-M.; Sánchez, M.G.; Yong, V.W.; Stys, P.K.; Tremblay, M.-È.; Rivest, S. Inefficient Clearance of Myelin Debris by Microglia Impairs Remyelinating Processes. *J. Exp. Med.* **2015**, *212*, 481–495. [CrossRef] [PubMed]

227. Ben-Hur, T.; Einstein, O.; Bulte, J.W.M. Stem Cell Therapy for Myelin Diseases. *Curr. Drug Targets* **2005**, *6*, 3–19. [CrossRef]
228. Ottoboni, L.; Merlini, A.; Martino, G. Neural Stem Cell Plasticity: Advantages in Therapy for the Injured Central Nervous System. *Front. Cell Dev. Biol.* **2017**, *5*, 52. [CrossRef]
229. Nagoshi, N.; Khazaei, M.; Ahlfors, J.-E.; Ahuja, C.S.; Nori, S.; Wang, J.; Shibata, S.; Fehlings, M.G. Human Spinal Oligodendrogenic Neural Progenitor Cells Promote Functional Recovery After Spinal Cord Injury by Axonal Remyelination and Tissue Sparing. *Stem Cells Transl. Med.* **2018**, *7*, 806–818. [CrossRef]
230. Sankavaram, S.R.; Hakim, R.; Covacu, R.; Frostell, A.; Neumann, S.; Svensson, M.; Brundin, L. Adult Neural Progenitor Cells Transplanted into Spinal Cord Injury Differentiate into Oligodendrocytes, Enhance Myelination, and Contribute to Recovery. *Stem Cell Rep.* **2019**, *12*, 950–966. [CrossRef]
231. Theotokis, P.; Kesidou, E.; Mitsiadou, D.; Petratos, S.; Damianidou, O.; Boziki, M.; Chatzidimitriou, A.; Grigoriadis, N. Lumbar Spine Intrathecal Transplantation of Neural Precursor Cells Promotes Oligodendrocyte Proliferation in Hot Spots of Chronic Demyelination. *Brain Pathol. Zurich Switz.* **2021**, *32*, e13040. [CrossRef]
232. Theotokis, P.; Kleopa, K.A.; Touloumi, O.; Lagoudaki, R.; Lourbopoulos, A.; Nousiopoulou, E.; Kesidou, E.; Poulatsidou, K.-N.; Dardiotis, E.; Hadjigeorgiou, G.; et al. Connexin43 and Connexin47 Alterations after Neural Precursor Cells Transplantation in Experimental Autoimmune Encephalomyelitis. *Glia* **2015**, *63*, 1772–1783. [CrossRef]
233. Einstein, O.; Grigoriadis, N.; Mizrachi-Kol, R.; Reinhartz, E.; Polyzoidou, E.; Lavon, I.; Milonas, I.; Karussis, D.; Abramsky, O.; Ben-Hur, T. Transplanted Neural Precursor Cells Reduce Brain Inflammation to Attenuate Chronic Experimental Autoimmune Encephalomyelitis. *Exp. Neurol.* **2006**, *198*, 275–284. [CrossRef]
234. Pluchino, S.; Gritti, A.; Blezer, E.; Amadio, S.; Brambilla, E.; Borsellino, G.; Cossetti, C.; Del Carro, U.; Comi, G.; 't Hart, B.; et al. Human Neural Stem Cells Ameliorate Autoimmune Encephalomyelitis in Non-Human Primates. *Ann. Neurol.* **2009**, *66*, 343–354. [CrossRef] [PubMed]
235. Yeung, M.S.Y.; Djelloul, M.; Steiner, E.; Bernard, S.; Salehpour, M.; Possnert, G.; Brundin, L.; Frisén, J. Dynamics of Oligodendrocyte Generation in Multiple Sclerosis. *Nature* **2019**, *566*, 538–542. [CrossRef] [PubMed]
236. Bacmeister, C.M.; Barr, H.J.; McClain, C.R.; Thornton, M.A.; Nettles, D.; Welle, C.G.; Hughes, E.G. Motor Learning Promotes Remyelination via New and Surviving Oligodendrocytes. *Nat. Neurosci.* **2020**, *23*, 819–831. [CrossRef] [PubMed]
237. Neely, S.A.; Williamson, J.M.; Klingseisen, A.; Zoupi, L.; Early, J.J.; Williams, A.; Lyons, D.A. New Oligodendrocytes Exhibit More Abundant and Accurate Myelin Regeneration than Those That Survive Demyelination. *Nat. Neurosci.* **2022**, *25*, 415–420. [CrossRef]
238. Baaklini, C.S.; Rawji, K.S.; Duncan, G.J.; Ho, M.F.S.; Plemel, J.R. Central Nervous System Remyelination: Roles of Glia and Innate Immune Cells. *Front. Mol. Neurosci.* **2019**, *12*, 225. [CrossRef]
239. Chiou, B.; Gao, C.; Giera, S.; Folts, C.J.; Kishore, P.; Yu, D.; Oak, H.C.; Jiang, R.; Piao, X. Cell Type-Specific Evaluation of ADGRG1/GPR56 Function in Developmental Central Nervous System Myelination. *Glia* **2021**, *69*, 413–423. [CrossRef]
240. Murcia-Belmonte, V.; Medina-Rodríguez, E.M.; Bribián, A.; de Castro, F.; Esteban, P.F. ERK1/2 Signaling Is Essential for the Chemoattraction Exerted by Human FGF2 and Human Anosmin-1 on Newborn Rat and Mouse OPCs via FGFR1: Chemotactic Effect of Anosmin-1 on OPCs. *Glia* **2014**, *62*, 374–386. [CrossRef]
241. Nakatani, H.; Martin, E.; Hassani, H.; Clavairoly, A.; Maire, C.L.; Viadieu, A.; Kerninon, C.; Delmasure, A.; Frah, M.; Weber, M.; et al. Ascl1/Mash1 Promotes Brain Oligodendrogenesis during Myelination and Remyelination. *J. Neurosci.* **2013**, *33*, 9752–9768. [CrossRef]
242. Ulloa-Navas, M.J.; Pérez-Borredá, P.; Morales-Gallel, R.; Saurí-Tamarit, A.; García-Tárraga, P.; Gutiérrez-Martín, A.J.; Herranz-Pérez, V.; García-Verdugo, J.M. Ultrastructural Characterization of Human Oligodendrocytes and Their Progenitor Cells by Pre-Embedding Immunogold. *Front. Neuroanat.* **2021**, *15*, 696376. [CrossRef]
243. He, D.; Marie, C.; Zhao, C.; Kim, B.; Wang, J.; Deng, Y.; Clavairoly, A.; Frah, M.; Wang, H.; He, X.; et al. Chd7 Cooperates with Sox10 and Regulates the Onset of CNS Myelination and Remyelination. *Nat. Neurosci.* **2016**, *19*, 678–689. [CrossRef]
244. Dobrowolski, M.; Cave, C.; Levy-Myers, R.; Lee, C.; Park, S.; Choi, B.-R.; Xiao, B.; Yang, W.; Sockanathan, S. GDE3 Regulates Oligodendrocyte Precursor Proliferation via Release of Soluble CNTFRα. *Dev. Camb. Engl.* **2020**, *147*, dev180695. [CrossRef]
245. Kucharova, K.; Stallcup, W.B. The NG2 Proteoglycan Promotes Oligodendrocyte Progenitor Proliferation and Developmental Myelination. *Neuroscience* **2010**, *166*, 185–194. [CrossRef] [PubMed]
246. Petryniak, M.A.; Potter, G.B.; Rowitch, D.H.; Rubenstein, J.L.R. Dlx1 and Dlx2 Control Neuronal versus Oligodendroglial Cell Fate Acquisition in the Developing Forebrain. *Neuron* **2007**, *55*, 417–433. [CrossRef] [PubMed]
247. Muth, K.N.; Piefke, S.; Weider, M.; Sock, E.; Hermans-Borgmeyer, I.; Wegner, M.; Küspert, M. The Dual-Specificity Phosphatase Dusp15 Is Regulated by Sox10 and Myrf in Myelinating Oligodendrocytes: Dusp15 as a Common Target of Sox10 and Myrf. *Glia* **2016**, *64*, 2120–2132. [CrossRef]
248. Conover, J.C.; Doetsch, F.; Garcia-Verdugo, J.-M.; Gale, N.W.; Yancopoulos, G.D.; Alvarez-Buylla, A. Disruption of Eph/Ephrin Signaling Affects Migration and Proliferation in the Adult Subventricular Zone. *Nat. Neurosci.* **2000**, *3*, 1091–1097. [CrossRef]
249. Azim, K.; Raineteau, O.; Butt, A.M. Intraventricular Injection of FGF-2 Promotes Generation of Oligodendrocyte-Lineage Cells in the Postnatal and Adult Forebrain. *Glia* **2012**, *60*, 1977–1990. [CrossRef]
250. Hayakawa, K.; Pham, L.-D.D.; Som, A.T.; Lee, B.J.; Guo, S.; Lo, E.H.; Arai, K. Vascular Endothelial Growth Factor Regulates the Migration of Oligodendrocyte Precursor Cells. *J. Neurosci.* **2011**, *31*, 10666–10670. [CrossRef]

251. Fasciani, I.; Pluta, P.; González-Nieto, D.; Martínez-Montero, P.; Molano, J.; Paíno, C.L.; Millet, O.; Barrio, L.C. Directional Coupling of Oligodendrocyte Connexin-47 and Astrocyte Connexin-43 Gap Junctions. *Glia* **2018**, *66*, 2340–2352. [CrossRef]
252. Yang, H.-J.; Vainshtein, A.; Maik-Rachline, G.; Peles, E. G Protein-Coupled Receptor 37 Is a Negative Regulator of Oligodendrocyte Differentiation and Myelination. *Nat. Commun.* **2016**, *7*, 10884. [CrossRef]
253. Chapman, H.; Waclaw, R.R.; Pei, Z.; Nakafuku, M.; Campbell, K. The Homeobox Gene Gsx2 Controls the Timing of Oligodendroglial Fate Specification in Mouse Lateral Ganglionic Eminence Progenitors. *Dev. Camb. Engl.* **2013**, *140*, 2289–2298. [CrossRef]
254. Ye, F.; Chen, Y.; Hoang, T.; Montgomery, R.L.; Zhao, X.; Bu, H.; Hu, T.; Taketo, M.M.; van Es, J.H.; Clevers, H.; et al. HDAC1 and HDAC2 Regulate Oligodendrocyte Differentiation by Disrupting the β-Catenin–TCF Interaction. *Nat. Neurosci.* **2009**, *12*, 829–838. [CrossRef]
255. Cunliffe, V.T.; Casaccia-Bonnefil, P. Histone Deacetylase 1 Is Essential for Oligodendrocyte Specification in the Zebrafish CNS. *Mech. Dev.* **2006**, *123*, 24–30. [CrossRef]
256. Wu, Y.; Liu, Y.; Levine, E.M.; Rao, M.S. Hes1 but Not Hes5 Regulates an Astrocyte versus Oligodendrocyte Fate Choice in Glial Restricted Precursors. *Dev. Dyn. Off. Publ. Am. Assoc. Anat.* **2003**, *226*, 675–689. [CrossRef]
257. Havrda, M.C.; Paolella, B.R.; Ran, C.; Jering, K.S.; Wray, C.M.; Sullivan, J.M.; Nailor, A.; Hitoshi, Y.; Israel, M.A. Id2 Mediates Oligodendrocyte Precursor Cell Maturation Arrest and Is Tumorigenic in a PDGF-Rich Microenvironment. *Cancer Res.* **2014**, *74*, 1822–1832. [CrossRef]
258. Malek-Hedayat, S.; Rome, L.H. Expression of a Beta 1-Related Integrin by Oligodendroglia in Primary Culture: Evidence for a Functional Role in Myelination. *J. Cell Biol.* **1994**, *124*, 1039–1046. [CrossRef]
259. Barres, B.A.; Raff, M.C. Control of Oligodendrocyte Number in the Developing Rat Optic Nerve. *Neuron* **1994**, *12*, 935–942. [CrossRef]
260. Miller, R.H. Regulation of Oligodendrocyte Development in the Vertebrate CNS. *Prog. Neurobiol.* **2002**, *67*, 451–467. [CrossRef]
261. Suzuki, N.; Hyodo, M.; Hayashi, C.; Mabuchi, Y.; Sekimoto, K.; Onchi, C.; Sekiguchi, K.; Akazawa, C. Laminin A2, A4, and A5 Chains Positively Regulate Migration and Survival of Oligodendrocyte Precursor Cells. *Sci. Rep.* **2019**, *9*, 19882. [CrossRef]
262. Kwon, H.S.; Nakaya, N.; Abu-Asab, M.; Kim, H.S.; Tomarev, S.I. Myocilin Is Involved in NgR1/Lingo-1-Mediated Oligodendrocyte Differentiation and Myelination of the Optic Nerve. *J. Neurosci.* **2014**, *34*, 5539–5551. [CrossRef]
263. Almazán, G.; Vela, J.M.; Molina-Holgado, E.; Guaza, C. Re-Evaluation of Nestin as a Marker of Oligodendrocyte Lineage Cells: Nestin in Oligodendroglial Lineage. *Microsc. Res. Tech.* **2001**, *52*, 753–765. [CrossRef]
264. Nieto, M.; Schuurmans, C.; Britz, O.; Guillemot, F. Neural BHLH Genes Control the Neuronal versus Glial Fate Decision in Cortical Progenitors. *Neuron* **2001**, *29*, 401–413. [CrossRef]
265. Mizuguchi, R.; Sugimori, M.; Takebayashi, H.; Kosako, H.; Nagao, M.; Yoshida, S.; Nabeshima, Y.; Shimamura, K.; Nakafuku, M. Combinatorial Roles of Olig2 and Neurogenin2 in the Coordinated Induction of Pan-Neuronal and Subtype-Specific Properties of Motoneurons. *Neuron* **2001**, *31*, 757–771. [CrossRef]
266. Deneen, B.; Ho, R.; Lukaszewicz, A.; Hochstim, C.J.; Gronostajski, R.M.; Anderson, D.J. The Transcription Factor NFIA Controls the Onset of Gliogenesis in the Developing Spinal Cord. *Neuron* **2006**, *52*, 953–968. [CrossRef] [PubMed]
267. Althaus, H.H.; Klöppner, S.; Schmidt-Schultz, T.; Schwartz, P. Nerve Growth Factor Induces Proliferation and Enhances Fiber Regeneration in Oligodendrocytes Isolated from Adult Pig Brain. *Neurosci. Lett.* **1992**, *135*, 219–223. [CrossRef]
268. Kucenas, S.; Snell, H.; Appel, B. Nkx2.2a Promotes Specification and Differentiation of a Myelinating Subset of Oligodendrocyte Lineage Cells in Zebrafish. *Neuron Glia Biol.* **2008**, *4*, 71–81. [CrossRef]
269. Ortega, M.C.; Bribián, A.; Peregrín, S.; Gil, M.T.; Marín, O.; de Castro, F. Neuregulin-1/ErbB4 Signaling Controls the Migration of Oligodendrocyte Precursor Cells during Development. *Exp. Neurol.* **2012**, *235*, 610–620. [CrossRef] [PubMed]
270. Wong, A.W.; Xiao, J.; Kemper, D.; Kilpatrick, T.J.; Murray, S.S. Oligodendroglial Expression of TrkB Independently Regulates Myelination and Progenitor Cell Proliferation. *J. Neurosci. Off. J. Soc. Neurosci.* **2013**, *33*, 4947–4957. [CrossRef]
271. Liu, Y.; Long, Z.; Yang, C. The Effects of the Olig Family on the Regulation of Spinal Cord Development and Regeneration. *Neurochem. Res.* **2021**, *46*, 2776–2782. [CrossRef]
272. Golan, N.; Adamsky, K.; Kartvelishvily, E.; Brockschnieder, D.; Möbius, W.; Spiegel, I.; Roth, A.D.; Thomson, C.E.; Rechavi, G.; Peles, E. Identification of Tmem10/Opalin as an Oligodendrocyte Enriched Gene Using Expression Profiling Combined with Genetic Cell Ablation. *Glia* **2008**, *56*, 1176–1186. [CrossRef]
273. De Faria, O.; Dhaunchak, A.S.; Kamen, Y.; Roth, A.D.; Kuhlmann, T.; Colman, D.R.; Kennedy, T.E. TMEM10 Promotes Oligodendrocyte Differentiation and Is Expressed by Oligodendrocytes in Human Remyelinating Multiple Sclerosis Plaques. *Sci. Rep.* **2019**, *9*, 3606. [CrossRef]
274. Sun, T.; Pringle, N.P.; Hardy, A.P.; Richardson, W.D.; Smith, H.K. Pax6 Influences the Time and Site of Origin of Glial Precursors in the Ventral Neural Tube. *Mol. Cell. Neurosci.* **1998**, *12*, 228–239. [CrossRef] [PubMed]
275. Jang, E.S.; Goldman, J.E. Pax6 Expression Is Sufficient to Induce a Neurogenic Fate in Glial Progenitors of the Neonatal Subventricular Zone. *PLoS ONE* **2011**, *6*, e20894. [CrossRef] [PubMed]
276. Muñoz-Esquivel, J.; Göttle, P.; Aguirre-Cruz, L.; Flores-Rivera, J.; Corona, T.; Reyes-Terán, G.; Küry, P.; Torres, K.J. Sildenafil Inhibits Myelin Expression and Myelination of Oligodendroglial Precursor Cells. *ASN Neuro* **2019**, *11*, 175909141983244. [CrossRef] [PubMed]

277. Butt, A.M.; Hornby, M.F.; Kirvell, S.; Berry, M. Platelet-Derived Growth Factor Delays Oligodendrocyte Differentiation and Axonal Myelination in Vivo in the Anterior Medullary Velum of the Developing Rat. *J. Neurosci. Res.* **1997**, *48*, 588–596. [CrossRef]
278. Scaglione, A.; Patzig, J.; Liang, J.; Frawley, R.; Bok, J.; Mela, A.; Yattah, C.; Zhang, J.; Teo, S.X.; Zhou, T.; et al. PRMT5-Mediated Regulation of Developmental Myelination. *Nat. Commun.* **2018**, *9*, 2840. [CrossRef]
279. Doukhanine, E.; Gavino, C.; Haines, J.D.; Almazan, G.; Richard, S. The QKI-6 RNA Binding Protein Regulates Actin-Interacting Protein-1 MRNA Stability during Oligodendrocyte Differentiation. *Mol. Biol. Cell* **2010**, *21*, 3029–3040. [CrossRef]
280. Chong, S.Y.C.; Rosenberg, S.S.; Fancy, S.P.J.; Zhao, C.; Shen, Y.-A.A.; Hahn, A.T.; McGee, A.W.; Xu, X.; Zheng, B.; Zhang, L.I.; et al. Neurite Outgrowth Inhibitor Nogo-A Establishes Spatial Segregation and Extent of Oligodendrocyte Myelination. *Proc. Natl. Acad. Sci. USA* **2012**, *109*, 1299–1304. [CrossRef]
281. Hornig, J.; Fröb, F.; Vogl, M.R.; Hermans-Borgmeyer, I.; Tamm, E.R.; Wegner, M. The Transcription Factors Sox10 and Myrf Define an Essential Regulatory Network Module in Differentiating Oligodendrocytes. *PLoS Genet.* **2013**, *9*, e1003907. [CrossRef]
282. Ma, Y.; Liu, H.; Ou, Z.; Qi, C.; Xing, R.; Wang, S.; Han, Y.; Zhao, T.-J.; Chen, Y. DHHC5 Facilitates Oligodendrocyte Development by Palmitoylating and Activating STAT3. *Glia* **2022**, *70*, 379–392. [CrossRef]
283. He, Y.; Dupree, J.; Wang, J.; Sandoval, J.; Li, J.; Liu, H.; Shi, Y.; Nave, K.A.; Casaccia-Bonnefil, P. The Transcription Factor Yin Yang1 Is Essential for Oligodendrocyte Progenitor Differentiation. *Neuron* **2007**, *55*, 217–230. [CrossRef]
284. Weng, Q.; Chen, Y.; Wang, H.; Xu, X.; Yang, B.; He, Q.; Shou, W.; Chen, Y.; Higashi, Y.; van den Berghe, V.; et al. Dual-Mode Modulation of Smad Signaling by Smad-Interacting Protein Sip1 Is Required for Myelination in the Central Nervous System. *Neuron* **2012**, *73*, 713–728. [CrossRef] [PubMed]
285. The Human Protein Atlas. Available online: https://www.proteinatlas.org/ (accessed on 22 June 2022).
286. Taveggia, C.; Thaker, P.; Petrylak, A.; Caporaso, G.L.; Toews, A.; Falls, D.L.; Einheber, S.; Salzer, J.L. Type III Neuregulin-1 Promotes Oligodendrocyte Myelination. *Glia* **2008**, *56*, 284–293. [CrossRef] [PubMed]
287. Bare, D.J.; Becker-Catania, S.G.; DeVries, G.H. Differential Localization of Neuregulin-1 Type III in the Central and Peripheral Nervous System. *Brain Res.* **2011**, *1369*, 10–20. [CrossRef] [PubMed]
288. Katanov, C.; Novak, N.; Vainshtein, A.; Golani, O.; Dupree, J.L.; Peles, E. N-Wasp Regulates Oligodendrocyte Myelination. *J. Neurosci.* **2020**, *40*, 6103–6111. [CrossRef] [PubMed]
289. Bacon, C.; Lakics, V.; Machesky, L.; Rumsby, M. N-WASP Regulates Extension of Filopodia and Processes by Oligodendrocyte Progenitors, Oligodendrocytes, and Schwann Cells—Implications for Axon Ensheathment at Myelination. *Glia* **2007**, *55*, 844–858. [CrossRef] [PubMed]
290. Malheiro, A.R.; Correia, B.; Ferreira da Silva, T.; Bessa-Neto, D.; Van Veldhoven, P.P.; Brites, P. Leukodystrophy Caused by Plasmalogen Deficiency Rescued by Glyceryl 1-myristyl Ether Treatment. *Brain Pathol.* **2019**, *29*, 622–639. [CrossRef]
291. Kida, E.; Palminiello, S.; Golabek, A.A.; Walus, M.; Wierzba-Bobrowicz, T.; Rabe, A.; Albertini, G.; Wisniewski, K.E. Carbonic Anhydrase II in the Developing and Adult Human Brain. *J. Neuropathol. Exp. Neurol.* **2006**, *65*, 664–674. [CrossRef]
292. Liedtke, W.; Edelmann, W.; Bieri, P.L.; Chiu, F.-C.; Cowan, N.J.; Kucherlapati, R.; Raine, C.S. GFAP Is Necessary for the Integrity of CNS White Matter Architecture and Long-Term Maintenance of Myelination. *Neuron* **1996**, *17*, 607–615. [CrossRef]
293. Schaeren-Wiemers, N.; Bonnet, A.; Erb, M.; Erne, B.; Bartsch, U.; Kern, F.; Mantei, N.; Sherman, D.; Suter, U. The Raft-Associated Protein MAL Is Required for Maintenance of Proper Axon–Glia Interactions in the Central Nervous System. *J. Cell Biol.* **2004**, *166*, 731–742. [CrossRef]
294. Fewou, S.N.; Ramakrishnan, H.; Büssow, H.; Gieselmann, V.; Eckhardt, M. Down-Regulation of Polysialic Acid Is Required for Efficient Myelin Formation. *J. Biol. Chem.* **2007**, *282*, 16700–16711. [CrossRef]
295. Yu, T.; Lieberman, A.P. Npc1 Acting in Neurons and Glia Is Essential for the Formation and Maintenance of CNS Myelin. *PLoS Genet.* **2013**, *9*, e1003462. [CrossRef] [PubMed]
296. Corbeil, D.; Joester, A.; Fargeas, C.A.; Jászai, J.; Garwood, J.; Hellwig, A.; Werner, H.B.; Huttner, W.B. Expression of Distinct Splice Variants of the Stem Cell Marker Prominin-1 (CD133) in Glial Cells. *Glia* **2009**, *57*, 860–874. [CrossRef] [PubMed]
297. Fu, M.-M.; McAlear, T.S.; Nguyen, H.; Oses-Prieto, J.A.; Valenzuela, A.; Shi, R.D.; Perrino, J.J.; Huang, T.-T.; Burlingame, A.L.; Bechstedt, S.; et al. The Golgi Outpost Protein TPPP Nucleates Microtubules and Is Critical for Myelination. *Cell* **2019**, *179*, 132–146.e14. [CrossRef] [PubMed]

current issues in molecular biology

MDPI

Article

Basic Analysis of the Cerebrospinal Fluid: An Important Framework for Laboratory Diagnostics of the Impairment of the Central Nervous System

Petr Kelbich [1,2,3,*], Karel Hrach [1,4], Jan Spicka [1], Petr Vachata [5,6], Tomas Radovnicky [5], Eva Hanuljakova [1,3] and Jan Krejsek [2]

1 Department of Biomedicine and Laboratory Diagnostics, University J.E. Purkinje and Masaryk Hospital, 401 13 Usti nad Labem, Czech Republic
2 Department of Clinical Immunology and Allergology, Faculty of Medicine and University Hospital, Charles University, 500 03 Hradec Kralove, Czech Republic
3 Laboratory for Cerebrospinal Fluid, Neuroimmunology, Pathology and Special Diagnostics Topelex, 190 00 Prague, Czech Republic
4 Faculty of Health Studies, University J.E. Purkinje, 400 96 Usti nad Labem, Czech Republic
5 Department of Neurosurgery, University J.E. Purkinje and Masaryk Hospital, 401 13 Usti nad Labem, Czech Republic
6 Department of Neurosurgery, Faculty of Medicine and University Hospital, Charles University, 301 00 Pilsen, Czech Republic
* Correspondence: petr.kelbich@kzcr.eu

Abstract: Laboratory analysis of basic cerebrospinal fluid (CSF) parameters is considered as essential for any CSF evaluation. It can provide rapidly very valuable information about the status of the central nervous system (CNS). Our retrospective study evaluated parameters of basic CSF analysis in cases of either infectious or non-infectious CNS involvement. Neutrophils are effector cells of innate immunity. Predominance of neutrophils was found in 98.2% of patients with purulent inflammation in CNS. Lymphocytes are cellular substrate of adaptive immunity. We found their predominance in 94.8% of patients with multiple sclerosis (MS), 66.7% of patients with tick-borne encephalitis (TBE), 92.2% of patients with neuroborreliosis, 83.3% of patients with inflammatory response with oxidative burst of macrophages in CNS and 75.0% of patients with malignant infiltration of meninges (MIM). The simultaneous assessment of aerobic and anaerobic metabolism in CSF using the coefficient of energy balance (KEB) allows us to specify the type of inflammation in CNS. We found predominantly aerobic metabolism (KEB > 28.0) in 100.0% CSF of patients with normal CSF findings and in 92.8% CSF of patients with MS. Predominant faintly anaerobic metabolism (28.0 > KEB > 20.0) in CSF was found in 71.8% patients with TBE and in 64.7% patients with neuroborreliosis. Strong anaerobic metabolism (KEB < 10.0) was found in the CSF of 99.1% patients with purulent inflammation, 100.0% patients with inflammatory response with oxidative burst of macrophages and in 80.6% patients with MIM. Joint evaluation of basic CSF parameters provides sufficient information about the immune response in the CSF compartment for rapid and reliable diagnosis of CNS involvement.

Keywords: cerebrospinal fluid; cytological-energy analysis; coefficient of energy balance; blood-cerebrospinal fluid barrier; blood-brain barrier; aspartate aminotransferase

1. Introduction

Basic cerebrospinal fluid (CSF) analysis is a very important approach to quickly assess the current state of the central nervous system (CNS). Despite this fact, basic CSF examination is often underestimated. The aim of this study is to present our scheme of basic CSF examination, to show the interpretation of results in several subgroups of patients with different CNS involvement and to stimulate interest in this important part of CSF analysis.

Our basic CSF examination consists of a simultaneous assessment of the blood-cerebrospinal fluid barrier (BCB) permeability (see 1.1.), cytological composition (see 1.2.), energy ratios (see 1.2.) and detection of CNS tissue damage (see 1.3.). Measurement of total CSF protein concentration or albumin quotient is used to assess BCB permeability. Cytological analysis provides the essential information, especially addressing the presence of immunocompetent cells in CSF, possibly also the presence of tumor cells, signs of tissue damage, bleeding, presence of microbial pathogens, etc. Energy parameters, i.e., the simultaneous assessment of immunocompetent cells and KEB values in CSF is called cytological-energy analysis and allows us to determine intensity and the type of local inflammatory response in the CNS. CNS tissue damage at the level of baseline CSF examination is evidenced by aspartate aminotransferase (AST) catalytic activity determination.

1.1. Cerebrospinal Fluid Production and Blood-Cerebrospinal Fluid Barrier Permeability (Figure 1)

Approximately 80% of cerebrospinal fluid (CSF) is produced by ultrafiltration of blood plasma through the endothelium of the choroid plexus vessels. This structure is called the blood-cerebrospinal fluid barrier (BCB) and regulates the flow of immune system components into the CSF. The absence of pathological processes in the CSF is accompanied by the influx of a limited number of immunocompetent cells and a low concentration of proteins. In contrast, pathological processes in the CSF are associated with an increased number of cells and changes in the concentration of humoral components in the CSF. This condition is usually referred to as "increased BCB permeability". It is evidenced as elevated concentration of total protein in CSF or albumin quotient (Qalb. = albumin in CSF/albumin in blood) (Figure 1) [1–5].

The brain parenchyma is highly vascularized. The endothelial cells of the brain capillaries are one from the key components of blood-brain barrier (BBB), which significantly influences the composition of the extracellular fluid in the brain. After crossing the ventricular wall, the fluid replenishes the remaining approximately 20% volume of the CSF. Therefore, CSF is thus an important source of information about the physiology or pathophysiology of the brain parenchyma (Figure 1) [2,5–7].

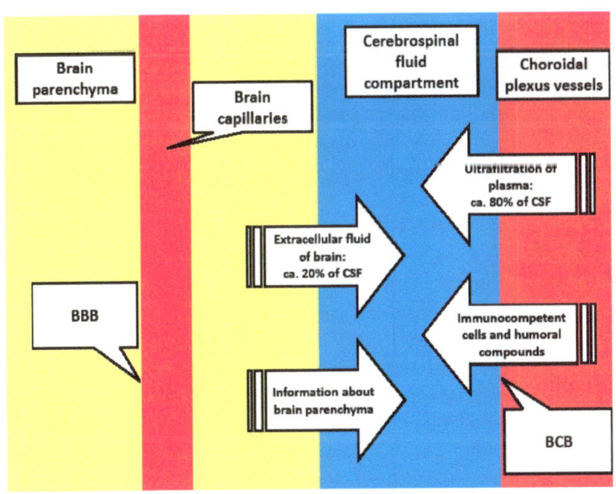

Figure 1. Schematic representation of CSF production. BCB: Blood-Cerebrospinal Fluid Barrier; BBB: Blood-Brain Barrier.

1.2. Cytological-Energy Analysis of the CSF

The evaluation of cytological and energy parameters in the CSF compartment is performed in two steps. The first is to determine the number and composition of immunocompetent cells in the CSF. The second is to determine the level of their activation by examining energy parameters in the CSF. To determine energy parameters, we have recently proposed so-called coefficient of energy balance (KEB; in Czech "Koeficient energetické bilance"). KEB is calculated using the molar concentrations of glucose and lactate in CSF and calculate as followed:

$$\text{KEB} = 38 - 18\frac{[\text{lactate}]}{[\text{glucose}]}$$

KEB is defined as the theoretical average number of adenosine triphosphate (ATP) molecules that are produced from one glucose molecule under the appropriate energy conditions in the CSF compartment. Activation of immunocompetent cells correlates with an increase in glucose and oxygen consumption and the development of anaerobic metabolism in CSF. The decrease in ATP production is reflected by a decrease in KEB values [8–17].

Based on the KEB values, we stratified our cases as follows:

- 28.0 to 38.0: aerobic metabolism in the CSF.
- 20.0 to 28.0: slight anaerobic metabolism in the CSF.
- 10.0 to 20.0: moderate anaerobic metabolism in the CSF.
- <10.0: strong anaerobic metabolism in the CSF.

1.3. *Detection of CNS Tissue Injury*

We consider aspartate aminotransferase (AST) catalytic activity in the CSF to be a readily available, easily measurable and inexpensive parameter for reliable assessment of CNS injury. This enzyme is present in all nucleated cells. Cellular damage is characterized by release of AST with subsequent elevation of AST activity in body fluids including CSF [8,18].

1.4. *Absence of Pathology in the CSF*

The absence of a pathological process in the CNS is characterized by no significant immune response in the CSF. There is the only basal immune surveillance there. The cellular and humoral components of the immune system in the CSF are at a basic level. The maximum leukocyte count in CSF is 4 cells/1 μL with predominance of resting lymphocytes (about 70%) and a minority of resting monocytes (about 30%). The low concentration of total protein in the CSF (<430.0 mg/L) indicates normal permeability of the BCB or the absence of any disturbance in the CSF circulation. Energy metabolism in CSF is aerobic with KEB values above 28.0. AST catalytic activity below 18.0 IU/L is not indicating tissue destruction in the CNS. No signs of hemorrhage are detected by CSF cytology [8,10,12,14,18–20].

1.5. *Inflammatory Response in the CSF Compartment*

The inflammatory response in the CSF compartment is followed by mobilization of cellular and humoral components into the CSF. The consequence of increased BCB permeability is increase in total protein concentration in CSF. The number of cells in the CSF is increased and their composition is reflecting the type of inflammatory response. Immunocompetent cells are activated, and more energy is required. Glucose and oxygen consumption is increased in this way. The concentration of glucose in the CSF is decreased. There is the switch from aerobic glucose metabolism to anaerobic one. Energy production in the form of adenosine triphosphate (ATP) molecules is decreased. This process is revealed as decrease in KEB values. In addition, local inflammation in the CNS may be associated with tissue destruction resulting in increased AST catalytic activity in the CSF [8,10,12,14,15,18–20].

1.6. *Infectious Impairment of the CNS*

Precise determination of the nature of the inflammatory reaction in the CSF can define the spectrum of causes of CNS pathologies.

Neutrophils represent the major population of phagocytic cells and are the final effector cells of innate immunity, with a primary role to clear extracellular pathogens [16]. The progression of purulent inflammation is based on the neutrophils oxidative burst with the production of reactive oxygen species (ROS). This is responsible for enhanced oxygen consumption. In sum, extensive accumulation of neutrophils and strong anaerobic metabolism in the CSF (KEB < 10.0) together with increased BCB permeability reveal purulent inflammation induced by the presence of extracellular bacteria in the CNS [8–10,12,14,15,17,21–28].

Increased BCB permeability, pleiocytosis with lymphocytes predominance, and aerobic or faintly anaerobic metabolism in the CSF compartment (28.0 > KEB > 20.0) usually represent the presence of serous inflammatory response in the CSF induced by either virus or spirochetes present in the CNS [10,12,14,19,29–41].

Very similar findings in CSF corresponding to mononuclear or lymphocytic pleiocytosis, hyperproteinorhachia, hypoglycorhachia and hyperlactatorhachia have been described in patients with neurotuberculosis, neurolisteriosis and cryptococcal meningitis [10,19,32,42–49]. In contrary, Bicanic and Harrison (2004) reported normal CSF white cell counts in HIV-associated cryptococcal meningitis, probably reflecting inability to mount protective immune response in these patients [49].

1.7. *Inflammatory Response in the CNS to Non Infectious Stimuli*

There are also numerous non-infectious causes of inflammatory response in CSF, such as autoimmunity, injury, hemorrhage, ischemia, tumors and neurodegenerative disorders [4,6,9,10,50–55].

1.8. *Multiple Sclerosis*

Multiple sclerosis (MS) is an autoimmune immunopathological disease affecting primarily white matter of the brain and spinal cord. Immunopathological inflammation targets myeline sheets of neurons thus impairing nerve signal transduction with ultimate axonal loss. Other CNS structures, including oligodendrocytes, are also targeted. Blood-brain barrier (BBB) contributes significantly to the pathogenesis of multiple sclerosis. It is a gateway for autoreactive lymphocytes entry into brain parenchyma. Basic analysis of CSF of patients with multiple sclerosis usually shows only subtle nonspecific changes. Total protein concentrations are often within normal limits, leukocyte counts are low or only slightly elevated, CSF energy ratios are usually insignificant, and CNS tissue destruction is not apparent. Lymphocytic oligocytosis or slight lymphocytic pleiocytosis with predominance of activated lymphocytes and the presence of plasmocytes in the CSF are frequently found. The gold standard of laboratory analyses in multiple sclerosis is still detection of intrathecal oligoclonal immunoglobulin synthesis by isoelectric focusing of CSF and blood [4,10,11,54–58]. However, this approach is not used in our present study.

1.9. *Malignant Infiltration of Meninges*

Cytological analysis of CSF plays a key role in the detection of malignant infiltration of the brain meninges (MIM). Deep analysis of inflammatory parameters can identify the presence of malignancy in CNS even if tumor cells in the CSF cytology are absent. Elevated proteins, pleiocytosis with predominance of lymphocytes and hypoglycorrhachia are characteristic in CSF patients with malignant infiltration of meninges [51,53,59–61].

2. Material and Methods

This retrospective study was approved by the local Ethics Committee of the Masaryk Hospital Usti nad Labem, Czech Republic (reference number: 305/19). No informed consent was required for this study as this work did not involve any human experiment. All patient records and information were anonymized and deidentified.

We performed a basic analysis of 524 cerebrospinal fluid samples evaluated as normal serving as controls for this study (Normal). In total, 304 CSF samples from patients with multiple sclerosis (MS), 39 CSF samples from patients with tick-borne encephalitis (TBE),

51 CSF samples from patients with central neuroborreliosis (NB), 113 CSF samples from patients with purulent inflammation (P) in the CNS induced by extracellular bacteria, and 31 CSF samples from patients with malignant infiltration of meninges (MIM) were enrolled to this study. We separately evaluated 6 CSF samples taken from 1 patient with cryptococcal meningitis, 1 patient with neurotuberculosis, 1 patient with neurolisteriosis and 3 patients with neuroborreliosis. These CSF samples were evaluated as "serous" inflammation in terms of cytological analysis and "purulent" in terms of energy analysis (Table 1).

Table 1. A review of CSF analysis in several patients with neuroinfection caused by intracellular bacteria and yeasts.

	Patient 1 Cryptococcal Meningitis	**Patient 2 Neurotuberculosis**	**Patient 3 Neurolisteriosis**	**Patient 4 Neuroborreliosis**	**Patient 5 Neuroborreliosis**	**Patient 6 Neuroborreliosis**
Total protein [mg/L]	6926.0	3240.0	3925.0	3970.0	2060.0	3310.0
Leukocytes/1 μL	15.3	78.7	180.0	159.0	209.0	156.7
Lymphocytes [%]	15.0	94.5	95.8	89.0	90.0	92.0
Monocytes [%]	81.0	3.1	1.4	8.0	10.0	4.0
Neutrophils [%]	4.0	2.4	2.8	3.0	0.0	4.0
Glucose [mmol/L]	1.51	3.20	2.93	1.46	1.36	2.53
Lactate [mmol/L]	10.85	8.42	6.37	3.86	3.60	4.12
KEB	−91.34	−9.36	−1.13	−9.59	−9.65	8.69
AST [IU/L]	256.8	16.8	37.2	10.8	not tested	21.6

2.1. Determination of the Blood-Cerebrospinal Fluid Barrier Permeability

BCB permeability was assessed using only cerebrospinal fluid total protein concentrations. We did not evaluate the albumin quotient because in some emergency cases cerebrospinal fluid samples only without blood samples were analyzed.

Cerebrospinal fluid samples were centrifuged, and the mass concentration of total protein was determined by the turbidimetry method with bensetonium chloride on a Cobas 6000 analyzer (Roche Diagnostics, Basel, Switzerland).

2.2. Cytological-Energy Analysis of CSF

The samples of CSF were collected into tubes without anticoagulants and immediately transported to our clinical laboratory. The total number of elements in these samples was enumerated using a Fuchs-Rosenthal chamber under the optical microscope. Cytological smear using cytocentrifuge method was prepared immediately after receiving the sample in all cases. Permanent cytological smears were stained using Hemacolor (Merck Co., Gernsheim, Germany). Microscopic analyses to determine cellular composition of CSF were performed by trained laboratory personal using Olympus BX40 microscope (Olympus, Tokyo, Japan).

Another aliquot of the samples was centrifuged and the molar concentrations of glucose using the hexokinase method and lactate using the lactate-oxidase and peroxidase method on a Cobas 6000 analyzer (Roche Diagnostics, Basel, Switzerland) were determined.

KEB values were calculated for all samples, including rare cases with very low glucose concentrations below the measurement limit (=0.11 mmol/L). Glucose concentration of 0.11 mmol/L was used to calculate KEB values in all these anaerobic cases.

2.3. Assessment of CNS Tissue Injury

The cerebrospinal fluid samples were centrifuged, and the catalytic activities of aspartate aminotransferase (AST) were determined by the IFCC method on a Cobas 6000 analyzer (Roche Diagnostics, Basel, Switzerland). Catalytic activities of AST in CSF exceeding 18.0 IU/L were identified as evidence of CNS tissue damage [13].

2.4. Statistical Methods

Concentrations of total protein, numbers of leukocytes, the percentages of lymphocytes, neutrophils and monocytes and AST catalytic activities in the CSF are in box plots expressed as a median, the 1st and 3rd interquartile range and non-outlier range of values. KEB values are divided into subgroups with aerobic metabolism (>28.0), slight anaerobic metabolism (20.0 to 28.0), moderate anaerobic metabolism (10.0 to 20.0), and strong anaerobic metabolism (<10.0) in CSF in the bar graph. The nonparametric Mann-Whitney two sample tests were performed to compare each patients group with our control group. The variables were age-adjusted before testing. The 5% level was the criterion of significance.

All statistical tests were carried out using Statistica 14.0 software (StatSoft Inc., Tulsa, OK, USA).

3. Results

Using the Mann-Whitney two-sample test, we compared the CSF findings of our patients with CNS involvement to normal CSF findings.

3.1. BCB Permeability

Compared to normal CSF findings (Normal), we found significantly higher total protein concentrations and leukocyte counts in the CSF of patients with multiple sclerosis (MS; $p < 0.001$), tick-borne encephalitis (TBE; $p < 0.001$), central neuroborreliosis (NB; $p < 0.001$), purulent inflammation (P; $p < 0.001$), intensive inflammation with oxidative burst of macrophages (MF; $p < 0.001$), and malignant infiltration of meninges (MIM; $p < 0.001$) (Figures 2 and 3).

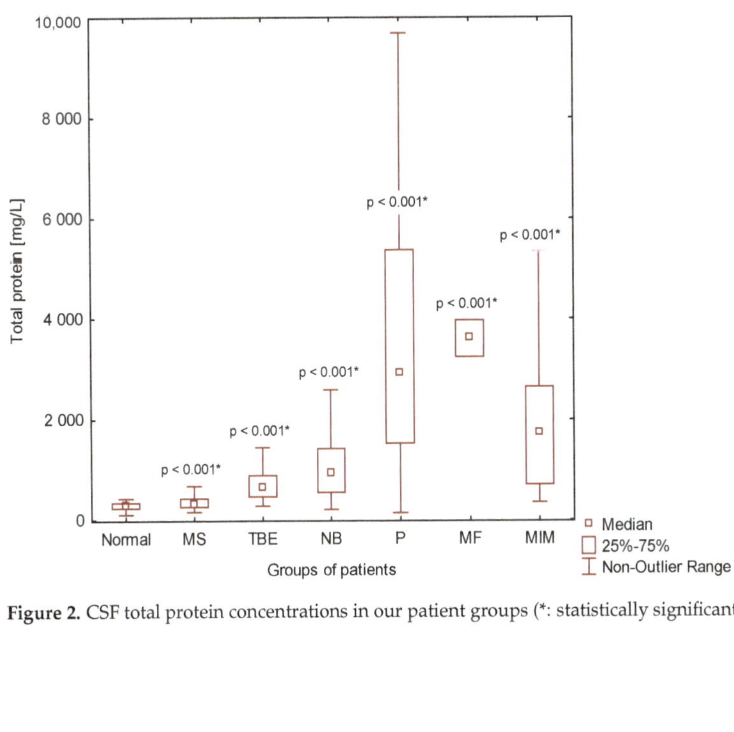

Figure 2. CSF total protein concentrations in our patient groups (*: statistically significant).

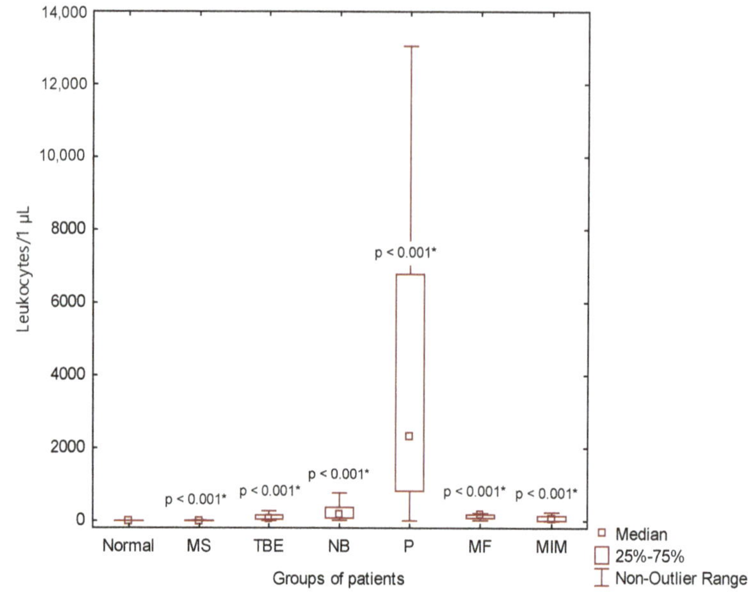

Figure 3. CSF leukocyte counts in our patient groups (*: statistically significant).

3.2. Cytological Parameters

A significantly higher percentage of lymphocytes in CSF compared to normal CSF findings was found in patients with MS ($p < 0.001$) and NB ($p < 0.001$), and a significantly lower percentage of lymphocytes was found in patients with purulent inflammation (P) in the CNS ($p < 0.001$ *) (Figure 4).

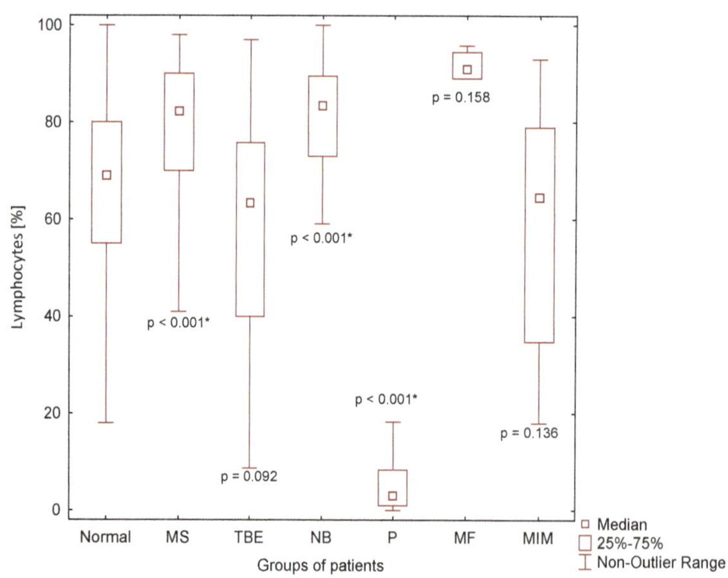

Figure 4. Percentage of lymphocytes in CSF in our patient groups (*: statistically significant).

A significantly higher percentage of neutrophils in CSF compared to normal CSF findings was found in patients with TBE ($p < 0.001$), NB ($p = 0.003$), P ($p < 0.001$) and MIM ($p > 0.001$). The absolute highest neutrophil count is typical for patients with purulent inflammation in the CNS (P) (Figure 5).

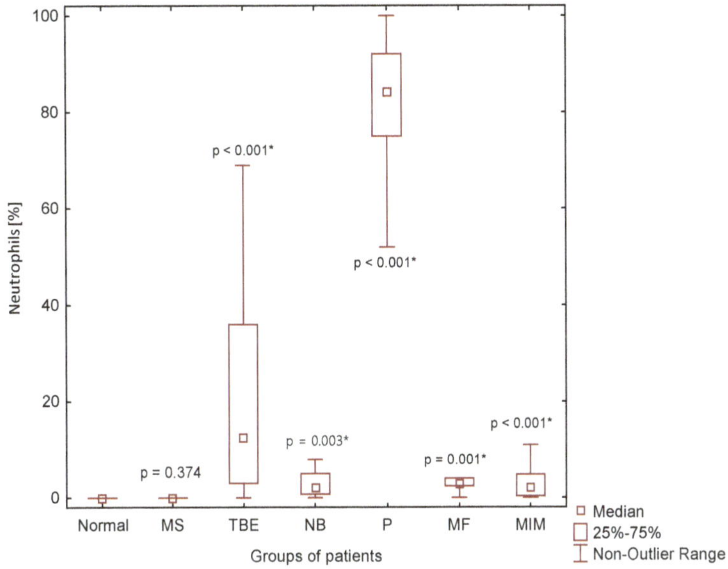

Figure 5. Percentage of neutrophils in CSF in our patient groups (*: statistically significant).

A significantly lower percentage of monocytes in CSF compared to normal CSF findings was found in CSF of patients with MS ($p < 0.001$), TBE ($p < 0.001$), NB ($p < 0.001$) and P ($p < 0.001$) (Figure 6).

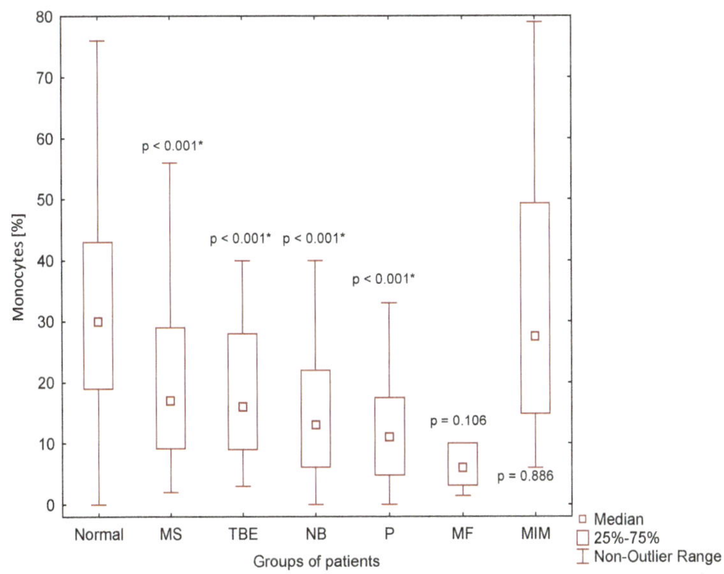

Figure 6. Percentage of monocytes in CSF in our patient groups (*: statistically significant).

3.3. Energy Parameters

Figure 7 shows the overwhelming preponderance of cases with strongly anaerobic metabolism in the CSF (KEB < 10.0) in patients with purulent inflammation (P) and intensive inflammation with oxidative burst of macrophages (MF), and its predominance in patients with malignant infiltration of the meninges (MIM). Predominantly slight anaerobic metabolism (28.0 > KEB > 20.0) was found in CSF of patients with tick-borne encephalitis (TBE) and central neuroborreliosis (NB). We found only a few cases of mild anaerobic metabolism in CSF in patients with multiple sclerosis (MS) and 100% of cases of aerobic metabolism in CSF (KEB > 28.0) in patients with normal findings (Normal) (Figure 7).

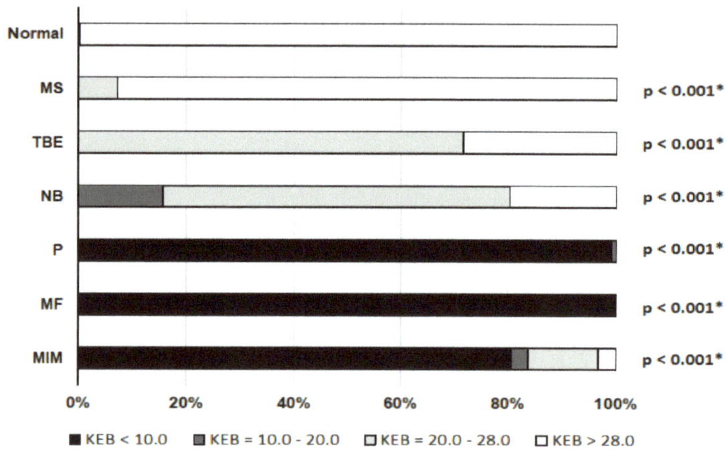

Figure 7. Distribution of KEB values in subgroups of our patients (*: statistically significant).

3.4. Tissue Damage

We found significantly higher AST catalytic activities in the CSF of patients with NB ($p = 0.005$), P ($p < 0.001$), MF ($p = 0.012$) and MIM ($p < 0.001$) compared to normal findings (Normal) (Figure 8).

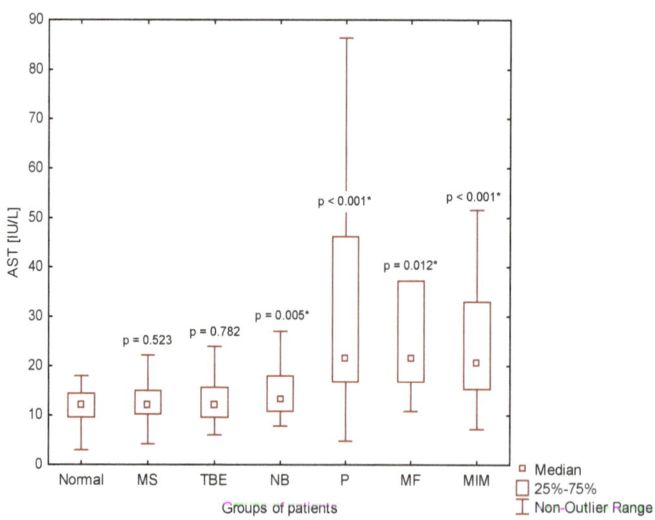

Figure 8. Catalytic activities of AST in CSF in our patient groups (*: statistically significant).

4. Discussion

We consider basic CSF examination to be a very important part of complex CSF analysis. Its results provide key information about the current status of the CSF compartment and CNS. Many CNS impairments can be reliably detected by basic CSF analysis.

4.1. Inflammations in the CNS with Predominance of Lymphocytes in CSF

Lymphocytes are immunocompetent cells of adaptive immunity. Consistent with observations of many authors, we found predominance of these cells in the CSF of patients with multiple sclerosis, thick-borne encephalitis, central neuroborreliosis, malignant infiltration of meninges and a very small group of several patients with cytologically proven "serous inflammation" and energy proven "purulent inflammation" in the CSF (Table 1, Figure 4) [10,19,29–32,35,37,40,41].

4.2. CNS Inflammation in Multiple Sclerosis

Energy parameters, especially KEB values, allows us to distinguish multiple sclerosis patients with predominantly aerobic metabolism in the CSF (KEB > 28.0) of patients with tick-borne encephalitis and central neuroborreliosis with predominantly slightly anaerobic metabolism in the CSF (28.0 > KEB > 20.0), and in patients with malignant infiltration of meninges or in a very small group of several patients with cytologically proven "serous inflammation" and energy proven "purulent inflammation" in the CSF with strongly anaerobic metabolism in the CSF (KEB < 10.0) (Figure 7). The same delineation can almost identically be observed when assessing BCB permeability by total protein concentration in CSF and CNS tissue destruction by catalytic activities of AST in CSF (Figures 2 and 8) [8,9,12,14]. Predominantly aerobic metabolism in the CSF (92.8%) of patients with multiple sclerosis is associated with predominantly normal BCB permeability (73.9%) and absence of tissue destruction in the CNS (93.0%).

We are convinced that important cause for moderate expression of inflammatory response in the CSF of patients with multiple sclerosis is the lower contribution of BCB in the pathogenesis of this disease. Autoreactive lymphocytes are migrating from the blood into the brain parenchyma across the blood-brain barrier (BBB) (Figure 1). Autoimmune immunopathological inflammation in patients with multiple sclerosis is targeting the white matter of the brain, predominantly [4,54–58]. In contrast, the signs of inflammation in the CSF are marginal, only.

4.3. Infectious Inflammations in the CNS with Predominance of Lymphocytes in CSF

On the other hand, inflammation induced by invasion of pathogens usually manifests itself directly in the CSF. Therefore, we can observe increased BCB permeability with a higher influx of immunocompetent cells and proteins into the CSF (Figures 2 and 3). There is substantial demand for glucose and oxygen as immunocompetent cells are activated. This finally leads to the development of anaerobic metabolism in the CSF [8–10,12,14].

Lymphocytic pleiocytosis and hyperproteinorhachia are typical in patients with thick-borne encephalitis and central neuroborreliosis (Figures 2–4). We found in general higher percentage of neutrophils in CSF in the early stages of tick-borne encephalitis in agreement with many authors (Figure 5) [30,34,36,38,39]. Some authors reported that the predominance of neutrophils can be confused with CSF pattern found in bacterial meningitis [34,39]. To avoid this misconduct our suggestion is to assess the energy status of CSF using KEB values. Whereas in patients with purulent inflammation induced by extracellular bacteria we found 99.1% of cases of strongly anaerobic CSF (KEB < 10.0) and 0.9% of moderately anaerobic CSF (20.0 > KEB > 10.0), in patients with tick-borne encephalitis we found 28.2% of aerobic CSF (KEB > 28.0) and 71.8% of slightly anaerobic CSF (28.0 > KEB > 20.0) (Figure 7). This is fully consistent with our previous already published results [8,9,12,14,17].

4.4. Purulent Inflammation in the CNS

Almost all samples of CSF of our patients with purulent inflammation in the CNS were characterized with high BCB permeability, large number of neutrophils and strong anaerobic metabolism in CSF (Figures 2, 3, 5 and 7). These findings are in accord with the mechanism of this inflammation type. Purulent inflammation is the only inflammatory response, which cellular substrate are the cells of innate immunity, neutrophils. This type of inflammation is characterized by an oxidative burst of these cells with increased production of reactive oxygen species (ROS) [22–28]. The production of ROS results in significant oxygen consumption and the intensive development of anaerobic metabolism [8–10,12,14,15,17].

4.5. Infectious Inflammation with Cytologically Proven "Serous" Inflammation and Energy Proven "Purulent Inflammation"

We separately evaluated a small group of cases with cytologically proven "serous" inflammation and energy proven "purulent inflammation". These included one patient with cryptococcal meningitis, one patient with neurotuberculosis, one patient with neurolisteriosis, and three patients with neuroborreliosis with an atypical CSF laboratory picture. These cases are very similar with regards to mononuclear pleiocytosis, strong anaerobic metabolism in the CSF compartment (KEB < 10.0) and very high BCB permeability (Table 1 and Figures 2–4, 6 and 7). Bicanic and Harrison (2005) describe the stimulation of the innate immune response through the interaction of cryptococcal mannoproteins with Toll-like receptors expressed on innate immunity cells [49]. This is followed by the activation of macrophages and their oxidative burst, which is manifested by strong anaerobic metabolism in the CSF. The similar mechanism is induced by intracellular bacteria, i.e., *Mycobacterium tuberculosis* and *Listeria monocytogenes* [62–64]. Our patient cohort comprised 54 confirmed cases of central neuroborreliosis. However, three of these cases showed a strikingly different CSF pattern. The high BCB permeability and strong anaerobic metabolism in the CSF compartment of these patients were more consistent with the results in patients with neurotuberculosis, neurolisteriosis, and cryptococcal meningitis (Table 1). Thus, in patients with central neuroborreliosis, a rare intensive inflammation with an oxidative burst of macrophages might also be found.

For this reason, we excluded these three cases from our group of patients with central neuroborreliosis.

4.6. Non-Infectious Inflammatory Response in the CSF of Patients with Malignant Infiltration of Meninges

Some authors described hyperproteinorhachia, pleiocytosis with lymphocyte predominance, and hypoglycorrhachia in the CSF of patients with malignant infiltration of meninges [51,53,59–61]. Our results are consistent with these findings. Marked similarity of the CSF findings in patients with neuroinfection with intracellular bacteria and yeasts allow us to speculate that an identical intensive inflammatory response with oxidative burst of macrophages is induced by tumor proliferation, in this case (Figures 2, 4, 6 and 7).

4.7. AST Catalytic Activity in CSF for Assessment of CNS Parenchyma Damage

We evidenced the catalytic activity of AST in CSF as a reliable parameter to assess CNS parenchyma damage in our recent studies [8,9,18]. In this study, we found that the level of AST is correlating with the intensity of the inflammatory response expressed as anaerobic metabolism in CSF. The normal level of catalytic activity of AST in CSF (<18.0 IU/L) corresponds to samples with a predominance of aerobic, slightly anaerobic and moderately anaerobic metabolism in patients with normal CSF results, patients with multiple sclerosis or tick-borne encephalitis, respectively. Elevation of AST in CSF (>18.0 IU/L) correlated with strongly anaerobic metabolism in CSF in patients with purulent inflammation induced by extracellular bacteria and oxidative burst of macrophages induced by either intracellular bacteria or yeasts or the presence of tumor (Table 1 and Figures 7 and 8).

We have recently published the significance of AST catalytic activity evaluation in CSF of patients after CNS hemorrhage [18]. Very promising results are also observed in patients with neurodegenerative CNS involvement in the long term. This could be another useful target for the measurement of this easily available and inexpensive parameter in CSF in clinical practice.

5. Conclusions

We consider basic CSF analysis as a solid framework for both rapid differentiation of the type of local inflammatory response in the CNS and for optimization of subsequent CSF investigation.

Inflammatory reactions in the cerebrospinal fluid are classified according to the predominant involvement of components of innate or adaptive immunity. Innate immunity activation is revealed by purulent inflammation usually induced by the presence extracellular bacteria in CNS. Reliable signs of this inflammation are extremely high numbers of neutrophils and strong anaerobic metabolism in CSF (KEB < 10.0).

Adaptive immunity activation is characterized by the presence of lymphocytes in the CSF. The significant presence of these immunocompetent cells is evident in other subgroups of our patients. Whereas aerobic (KEB > 28.0) and slight anaerobic metabolism (28.0 > KEB > 20.0) are significantly predominant in the CSF of patients with multiple sclerosis, tick-born encephalitis and central neuroborreliosis, CSF of patients with inflammation with oxidative burst of macrophages in the CNS induced by intracellular bacteria, yeasts and tumor is characterized by a predominantly strong anaerobic metabolism (KEB < 10.0).

Inflammatory response with a predominance of lymphocytes and a predominance of aerobic (multiple sclerosis) or slightly anaerobic metabolism (tick-born encephalitis and central neuroborreliosis) in the CSF is called serous inflammation. This type of inflammation is usually associated with low or slightly increased BCB permeability and absence of CNS tissue destruction. In contrast, intense inflammation with oxidative burst of neutrophils (purulent inflammation) or macrophages is associated with increased BCB permeability and destruction of CNS tissue is proven by increased catalytic activity of AST in the CSF (>18.0 IU/L).

Author Contributions: P.K. conceptualization; data curation; funding acquisition; investigation; methodology; project administration; resources; validation; visualization; writing—original draft. K.H. conceptualization; data curation; formal analysis; writing—review and editing. J.S. conceptualization; investigation; resources; writing—review and editing. P.V. conceptualization; investigation; resources; writing—review and editing. T.R. conceptualization; investigation; resources; writing—review and editing. E.H. conceptualization; investigation; writing—review and editing. J.K. conceptualization; supervision; validation; writing—review and editing. All authors have read and agreed to the published version of the manuscript.

Funding: The Internal Grants of the Krajská zdravotní, a.s. in Ústí nad Labem, Czech Republic "IGA-KZ-2021-1-2"; Charles University in Prague, Faculty of Medicine in Hradec Králové, Czech Republic, Cooperatio Program, research area IMMU.

Institutional Review Board Statement: This study was approved by the local Ethics Committee of the Masaryk Hospital Ústí nad Labem [reference number: 305/19].

Informed Consent Statement: Not applicable.

Data Availability Statement: All data used are with the author.

Acknowledgments: We thank Gregory Jeffrey Evans for critical proofreading of the manuscript.

Conflicts of Interest: The authors declare that they have no conflict of interest.

References

1. Solár, P.; Zamani, A.; Kubíčková, L.; Dubový, P.; Joukal, M. Choroid plexus and the blood–cerebrospinal fluid barrier in disease. *Fluids Barriers CNS* **2020**, *17*, 35. [CrossRef] [PubMed]
2. Hladky, B.; Barrand, M.A. Fluid and ion transfer across the blood-brain and blood-cerebrospinal fluid barriers: A comparative account of mechanisms and roles. *Fluids Barriers CNS* **2016**, *13*, 19. [CrossRef]
3. Spector, R.; Keep, R.F.; Snodgrass, S.R.; Smith, Q.R.; Johanson, C.E. A balanced view of choroid plexus structure and function: Focus on adult humans. *Exp. Neurol.* **2015**, *267*, 78–86. [CrossRef]
4. Giovannoni, G. Cerebrospinal fluid analysis. *Handb. Clin. Neurol.* **2014**, *122*, 681–702. [PubMed]
5. Damkier, H.H.; Brown, P.D.; Praetorius, J. Cerebrospinal Fluid Secretion by the Choroid Plexus. *Physiol. Rev.* **2013**, *93*, 1847–1892. [CrossRef] [PubMed]
6. Chodobski, A.; Zink, B.J.; Szmydynger-Chodobska, J. Blood–Brain Barrier Pathophysiology in Traumatic Brain Injury. *Transl. Stroke Res.* **2011**, *2*, 492–516. [CrossRef]
7. Gloor, S.M.; Wachtel, M.; Bolliger, M.F.; Ishihara, H.; Landmann, R.; Frei, K. Molecular and cellular permeability control at the blood–brain barrier. *Brain Res. Rev.* **2001**, *36*, 258–264. [CrossRef]
8. Kelbich, P.; Vachata, P.; Maly, V.; Novotny, T.; Spicka, J.; Matuchova, I.; Radovnicky, T.; Stanek, I.; Kubalik, J.; Karpjuk, O.; et al. Neutrophils in Extravascular Body Fluids: Cytological-Energy Analysis Enables Rapid, Reliable and Inexpensive Detection of Purulent Inflammation and Tissue Damage. *Life* **2022**, *12*, 160. [CrossRef]
9. Kelbich, P.; Hejčl, A.; Krejsek, J.; Radovnický, T.; Matuchová, I.; Lodin, J.; Špička, J.; Sameš, M.; Procházka, J.; Hanuljaková, E.; et al. Development of the Cerebrospinal Fluid in Early Stage after Hemorrhage in the Central Nervous System. *Life* **2021**, *11*, 300. [CrossRef]
10. Sobek, O.; Dušková, J. Laboratorní vyšetření likvoru. In *Spinální Neurologie*, 1st ed.; Štětkářová, I., Ed.; Prague: Maxdorf, Germany, 2019; pp. 57–81.
11. Zeman, D. *Praktický Průvodce Laboratorním Vyšetřením Likvoru*, 1st ed.; Univerzita Palackého: Olomouc, Czech Republic, 2018; pp. 30–32.
12. Kelbich, P.; Hejčl, A.; Staněk, I.; Svítilová, E.; Hanuljaková, E.; Sameš, M. Principles of the cytological-energy analysis of the extravascular body fluids. *Biochem. Mol. Biol. J.* **2017**, *3*, 6.
13. Mrázová, K.; Zeman, D.; Bořecká, K.; Ženková, J.; Brož, P.; Mareš, J.; Hanzalová, J.; Král, V.; Krbková, L. Recommendation to analysis of cerebrospinal fluid, Klin. *Biochem. Metab.* **2017**, *25*, 43–47.
14. Kelbich, P.; Hejčl, A.; Krulichová, I.S.; Procházka, J.; Hanuljaková, E.; Peruthová, J.; Koudelková, M.; Sameš, M.; Krejsek, J. Coefficient of energy balance, a new parameter for basic investigation of the cerebrospinal fluid. *Clin. Chem. Lab. Med. (CCLM)* **2014**, *52*, 1009–1017. [CrossRef] [PubMed]
15. Bořecká, K.; Adam, P.; Sobek, O.; Hajduková, L.; Lánská, V.; Nekola, P. Coefficient of Energy Balance: Effective Tool for Early Differential Diagnosis of CNS Diseases. *BioMed Res. Int.* **2013**, *2013*, 745943. [CrossRef]
16. Sobek, O.; Adam, P.; Koudelková, M.; Štourač, P.; Mareš, J. The algorithm of CSF examination according to the recommen-dation of the Committee of CSF and Neuroimmunology of the Czech Neurological Society. *Ceska A Slov. Neurol. A Neurochir.* **2012**, *75*, 159–163.
17. Kelbich, P.; Slavík, S.; Jasanská, J.; Adam, P.; Hanuljaková, E.; Jermanová, K.; Repková, E.; Šimečková, M.; Procházková, J.; Gajdošová, R.; et al. Evaluations of the energy relations in the CSF compartment by investigation of selected parameters of the glucose metabolism in the CSF. *Klin. Biochem. Metab.* **1998**, *6*, 213–225.
18. Kelbich, P.; Radovnický, T.; Selke-Krulichová, I.; Lodin, J.; Matuchová, I.; Sameš, M.; Procházka, J.; Krejsek, J.; Hanuljaková, E.; Hejčl, A. Can aspartate aminotransferase in the cerebrospinal fluid be a reliable predictive parameter? *Brain Sci.* **2020**, *10*, 698. [CrossRef]
19. Seehusen, D.A.; Reeves, M.M.; Fomin, D.A. Cerebrospinal Fluid Analysis. *Am. Fam. Physician* **2003**, *68*, 1103–1108.
20. Adam, P.; Táborský, L.; Sobek, O.; Hildebrand, T.; Kelbich, P.; Průcha, M.; Hyánek, J. Cerebrospinal fluid. *Adv. Clin. Chem.* **2001**, *36*, 1–62.
21. Teng, T.-S.; Ji, A.-L.; Ji, X.-Y.; Li, Y.-Z. Neutrophils and Immunity: From Bactericidal Action to Being Conquered. *J. Immunol. Res.* **2017**, *2017*, 9671604. [CrossRef]
22. Klebanoff, S.J.; Kettle, A.J.; Rosen, H.; Winterbourn, C.C.; Nauseef, W.M. Myeloperoxidase: A front-line defender against phagocyted microorganisms. *J. Leukoc. Biol.* **2013**, *93*, 185–198. [CrossRef]
23. Thomas, D.C. The phagocyte respiratory burst: Historical perspectives and recent advances. *Immunol. Lett.* **2017**, *192*, 88–96. [CrossRef] [PubMed]
24. O'Neill, L.A.; Kishton, R.J.; Rathmell, J. A guide to immunometabolism for immunologists. *Nat. Rev. Immunol.* **2016**, *16*, 553–565. [CrossRef]
25. Segal, A.W. How Neutrophils Kill Microbes. *Annu. Rev. Immunol.* **2005**, *23*, 197–223. [CrossRef] [PubMed]
26. Dahlgren, C.; Karlsson, A. Respiratory burst in human neutrophils. *J. Immunol. Methods* **1999**, *232*, 3–14. [CrossRef]
27. Wilson, E.; Olcott, M.C.; Bell, R.M.; Merrill, A.H., Jr.; Lambeth, J.D. Inhibition of the oxidative burst in human neutrophils by sphingoid long-chain bases. *J. Biol. Chem.* **1986**, *261*, 12616–12623. [CrossRef]
28. Borregaard, N.; Herlin, T. Energy Metabolism of Human Neutrophils during Phagocytosis. *J. Clin. Investig.* **1982**, *70*, 550–557. [CrossRef] [PubMed]

29. Pietikäinen, A.; Maksimow, M.; Kauko, T.; Hurme, S.; Salmi, M.; Hytönen, J. Cerebrospinal fluid cytokines in *Lyme neuroborreliosis*. *J. Neuroinflamm.* **2016**, *13*, 273. [CrossRef]
30. Bogovic, P.; Strle, F. Tick-borne encephalitis: A review of epidemiology, clinical characteristics, and management. *World J. Clin. Cases* **2015**, *16*, 430–441. [CrossRef]
31. Koedel, U.; Fingerle, V.; Pfister, H.-W. Lyme neuroborreliosis-epidemiology, diagnosis and management. *Nat. Rev. Neurol.* **2015**, *11*, 446–456. [CrossRef]
32. Djukic, M.; Schmidt-Samoa, C.; Lange, P.; Spreer, A.; Neubieser, K.; Eiffert, H.; Nau, R.; Schmidt, H. Cerebrospinal fluid findings in adults with acute *Lyme neuroborreliosis*. *J. Neurol.* **2011**, *259*, 630–636. [CrossRef]
33. van Burgel, N.D.; Bakels, F.; Kroes, A.C.M.; van Dam, A.P. Discriminating Lyme Neuroborreliosis from other Neuroin-flammatory Diseases by Levels of CXCL13 in Cerebrospinal Fluid. *J. Clin. Microbiol.* **2011**, *49*, 2027–2030. [CrossRef] [PubMed]
34. Kaiser, R. Tick-Borne Encephalitis. *Infect. Dis. Clin. N. Am.* **2008**, *22*, 561–575. [CrossRef] [PubMed]
35. Kaiser, R. Neuroborreliosis. *J. Neurol.* **1998**, *245*, 247–255. [CrossRef] [PubMed]
36. Lindquist, L.; Vapalahti, O. Tick-borne encephalitis. *Lancet* **2008**, *371*, 1861–1871. [CrossRef]
37. Oschmann, P.; Dorndorf, W.; Hornig, C.; Schäfer, C.; Wellensiek, H.J.; Pflughaupt, K.W. Stages and syndromes of neurobor-reliosis. *J. Neurol.* **1998**, *245*, 262–272. [CrossRef]
38. Holzmann, H. Diagnosis of tick-borne encephalitis. *Vaccine* **2003**, *21*, S36–S40. [CrossRef]
39. Dumpis, U.; Crook, D.; Oksi, J. Tick-Borne Encephalitis. *Clin. Infect. Dis.* **1999**, *28*, 882–890. [CrossRef]
40. Garcia-Monco, J.C.; Benach, J.L. Lyme Neuroborreliosis. *Ann. Neurol.* **1995**, *37*, 691–702. [CrossRef]
41. Tumani, H.; Nolker, G.; Reiber, H. Relevance of cerebrospinal fluid variables for early diagnosis of neuroborreliosis. *Neurology* **1995**, *45*, 1663–1670. [CrossRef]
42. Fisher, K.M.; Montrief, T.; Ramzy, M.; Koyfman, A.; Long, B. Cryptococcal meningitis: A review for emergency clinicians. *Intern. Emerg. Med.* **2021**, *16*, 1031–1042. [CrossRef]
43. Li, M.; Liu, J.; Deng, X.; Gan, Q.; Wang, Y.; Xu, X.; Jiang, Y.; Peng, F. Triple therapy combined with ventriculoperitoneal shunts can improve neurological function and shorten hospitalization time in non-HIV cryptococcal meningitis patients with in-creased intracranial pressure. *BMC Infect Dis.* **2020**, *20*, 844. [CrossRef] [PubMed]
44. Pereira, M.E.V.D.C.; Gonzalez, D.E.; Roberto, F.B.; Foresto, R.D.; Kirsztajn, G.M.; Júnior, M.D.S.D. Listeria monocytogenes meningoencephalitis in a patient with Systemic Lupus Erythematosus. *J. Bras. Nefrol.* **2020**, *42*, 375–379. [CrossRef] [PubMed]
45. Natrajan, M.; Daniel, B.D.; Grace, G.A. Tuberculous meningitis in children: Clinical management & outcome. *Indian J. Med. Res.* **2019**, *150*, 117–130. [CrossRef]
46. Heemskerk, A.D., Donovan, J.; Thu, D.D.A.; Marais, S.; Chaidir, L.; Dung, V.T.M.; Centner, C.M.; Ha, V.T.N.; Annisa, J.; Dian, S.; et al. Improving the microbiological diagnosis of tuberculous meningitis: A prospective, international, multicentre comparison of conventional and modified Ziehl–Neelsen stain, GeneXpert, and culture of cerebrospinal fluid. *J. Infect.* **2018**, *77*, 509–515. [CrossRef]
47. Shi, T.Y.; Zhang, Y.F.; Shi, X.H.; Wen, X.H.; Dong, X.; Meng, J.; Li, H.Y.; Yuan, X.X.; Zheng, Y.; Lu, Y.W. A rare case of me-ningoencephalitis by *Listeria monocytogenes* in systemic lupus erythematosus: Case report and review. *Clin. Rheumatol.* **2018**, *37*, 271–275. [CrossRef]
48. Philip, N.; William, T.; William, D.V. Diagnosis of tuberculous meningitis: Challenges and promises. *Malays. J. Pathol.* **2015**, *37*, 1–9.
49. Bicanic, T.; Harrison, T.S. Cryptococcal meningitis. *Br. Med. Bull.* **2005**, *72*, 99–118. [CrossRef]
50. Mink, S.; List, W.; Reimann, P.; Fraunberger, P. CSF-interleukin 6 for early diagnosis of ventriculitis in a broad intensive care setting. *Clin. Chem. Lab. Med. (CCLM)* **2022**, *60*, e129–e131. [CrossRef]
51. Behari, S.; Kumar, A.; Sardhara, J.C.; Singh, G.; Kanjilal, S.; Maurya, V.P. Malignant Meningitis Associated with Hydrocephalus. *Neurol. India* **2021**, *69*, 443. [CrossRef]
52. Wesenhagen, K.E.J.; Teunissen, C.E.; Visser, P.J.; Tijms, B.M. Cerebrospinal fluid proteomics and biological heterogeneity in Alzheimer's disease: A literature review. *Crit. Rev. Clin. Lab. Sci.* **2019**, *57*, 86–98. [CrossRef]
53. Chamberlain, M.C. Neoplastic meningitis. *Oncologist* **2008**, *13*, 967–977. [CrossRef] [PubMed]
54. O'Connor, K.C.; Bar-Or, A.; Hafler, D.A. The Neuroimmunology of Multiple Sclerosis: Possible Roles of T and B Lymphocytes in Immunopathogenesis. *J. Clin. Immunol.* **2001**, *21*, 81–92. [CrossRef] [PubMed]
55. Noseworthy, J.H.; Lucchinetti, C.; Rodriguez, M.; Weinshenker, B.G. Multiple sclerosis. *N. Engl. J. Med.* **2000**, *343*, 938–952. [CrossRef]
56. Magliozzi, R.; Cross, A.H. Can CSF biomarkers predict future MS disease activity and severity? *Mult. Scler.* **2020**, *26*, 582–590. [CrossRef]
57. Gajofatto, A.; Calabrese, M.; Benedetti, M.D.; Monaco, S. Clinical, MRI, and CSF Markers of Disability Progression in Multiple Sclerosis. *Dis. Markers* **2013**, *35*, 687–699. [CrossRef] [PubMed]
58. Chabas, D.; Ness, J.; Belman, A.; Yeh, E.A.; Kuntz, N.L.; Gorman, M.P.; Strober, J.B.; De Kouchkovsky, I.; McCulloch, C.; Chitnis, T.; et al. Younger children with MS have a distinct CSF inflammatory profile at disease onset. *Neurology* **2010**, *74*, 399–405. [CrossRef] [PubMed]
59. Wang, N.; Bertalan, M.S.; Brastianos, P.K. Leptomeningeal metastasis from systemic cancer: Review and update on management. *Cancer* **2018**, *124*, 21–35. [CrossRef]

60. Adams, M.; Doherty, C.; O'Kane, A.; Hall, S.; Forbes, R.B.; Herron, B.; McNaboe, E.J. Malignant meningitis secondary to oesophageal adenocarcinoma presenting with sensorineural hearing loss: A series of three cases and discussion of the literature. *Eur. Arch. Otorhinolaryngol.* **2016**, *273*, 2481–2486. [CrossRef]
61. Roth, P.; Weller, M. Management of neoplastic meningitis. *Chin. Clin. Oncol.* **2015**, *4*, 26. [CrossRef]
62. Remer, K.A.; Reimer, T.; Brcic, M.; Jungi, T.W. Evidence for involvement of peptidoglycan in the triggering of an oxidative burst by *Listeria monocytogenes* in phagocytes. *Clin. Exp. Immunol.* **2005**, *140*, 73–80. [CrossRef]
63. Piddington, D.L.; Fang, F.C.; Laessig, T.; Cooper, A.M.; Orme, I.M.; Buchmeier, N.A. Cu, Zn superoxide dismutase of Mycobacterium tuberculosis contributes to survival in activated macrophages that are generating an oxidative burst. *Infect. Immun.* **2001**, *69*, 4980–4987. [CrossRef] [PubMed]
64. Kuhn, M.; Goebel, W. Responses by murine macrophages infected with Listeria monocytogenes crucial for the development of immunity to this pathogen. *Immunol. Rev.* **1997**, *158*, 57–93. [CrossRef] [PubMed]

current issues in molecular biology

MDPI

Review

Optic Neuritis in Multiple Sclerosis—A Review of Molecular Mechanisms Involved in the Degenerative Process

Manuela Andreea Ciapă [1], Delia Lidia Șalaru [2,3,*], Cristian Stătescu [2,3], Radu Andy Sascău [2,3] and Camelia Margareta Bogdănici [4,5]

1 Emergency Hospital Dimitrie Castroian, 735100 Huși, Romania
2 Cardiology Clinic, Institute of Cardiovascular Diseases, 700503 Iași, Romania
3 Department of Internal Medicine, University of Medicine and Pharmacy "Grigore T. Popa", 700115 Iași, Romania
4 Department of Surgical Specialties (II), University of Medicine and Pharmacy "Grigore T. Popa", 700115 Iași, Romania
5 Ophthalmology Clinic, Saint Spiridon Hospital, Iași 700111, Romania
* Correspondence: deliasalaru@gmail.com

Abstract: Multiple sclerosis is a central nervous system inflammatory demyelinating disease with a wide range of clinical symptoms, ocular involvement being frequently marked by the presence of optic neuritis (ON). The emergence and progression of ON in multiple sclerosis is based on various pathophysiological mechanisms, disease progression being secondary to inflammation, demyelination, or axonal degeneration. Early identification of changes associated with axonal degeneration or further investigation of the molecular processes underlying remyelination are current concerns of researchers in the field in view of the associated therapeutic potential. This article aims to review and summarize the scientific literature related to the main molecular mechanisms involved in defining ON as well as to analyze existing data in the literature on remyelination strategies in ON and their impact on long-term prognosis.

Keywords: inflammation; demyelination; remyelination; axonal degeneration; molecular mechanisms

1. Background

Multiple sclerosis (MS) is a demyelinating and neurodegenerative disease of the central nervous system (CNS), influenced by both genetic, (auto)immune, and environmental factors [1,2]. Paresthesia, motor deficit, autonomic spinal cord symptoms, visual symptoms, ataxia, exhaustion, disorientation, lack of sleep, discomfort, and depression are among the most prevalent symptoms. Structural and functional abnormalities in the visual system are targeted in most patients with MS, typically at the earliest stages of the disease, defining a hallmark feature of MS, namely optic neuritis (ON). The evolution of the clinical picture of patients with MS is extremely variable and heterogeneous in terms of locations and extensions of brain and spinal cord lesions [3]. ON is an inflammatory injury of the optic nerve that leads to visual disability. Unilateral visual acuity diminution, visual field loss, color vision deficiencies, diminished contrast, and brightness perception are frequent clinical manifestations of ON [4]. Recurrence of acute episodes of ON as well as chronic axonal injury causing structural changes over time are responsible for optic pathway damage [5].

ON is ubiquitous in the evolution of MS, up to 70% of patients with MS having an acute episode of ON during their course [6]. For 15–20% of patients with MS, the diagnosis of an acute episode of ON requires additional investigations that subsequently identify the underlying pathology [7]. In the first 6 months after diagnosis of MS, targeting an episode of ON induces a significant change in measurement of retinal nerve fiber layer (RNFL) thickness (a drop down to 20 μm) [8,9]. More and more studies in the field are addressed to retinal measurements, identified in multiple researches as markers of neurodegeneration, with retinal damage already demonstrated 6 months after ON [10]. Calabia et al. [11] concluded on a similar clinical study that ON should not be regarded as a potential factor of clinical impairment in patients with MS.

Clinical studies have demonstrated that ON and MS associate the same characteristics of inflammatory demyelination, the substrate being perivascular infiltrates that induce a significant cellular response that secondarily causes myelin damage in the nerve parenchyma. On the other hand, ON and MS associate distinct pathophysiological mechanisms that support CNS immune involvement [3].

There is a growing interest in depicting intimate mechanisms of MS, starting with inflammation, demyelination, axonal degeneration and the possibility of remyelination, and the study of optic nerve pathology offers a promising perspective of understanding and, further on, extrapolating the physiopathological mechanisms in MS. Several clinical studies in the field give a leading role to inflammation and neurodegeneration in the development of central nervous system damage [12,13]. Injury to the optic nerve also causes optic neuropathy, an entity with neurodegenerative substrate that causes visual acuity impairment over time [14]. Several studies in the field have shown that neurodegeneration occurs early in patients with ON [15].

We conducted a search using PubMed and SCIENCE DIRECT in July 2022, using the terms and phrases, "optic neuritis", "multiple sclerosis", "inflammation", "molecular mechanisms", "axonal degeneration", "biomarkers" and "therapeutic targets" under different word associations. We focused on studies related to ON in MS (published between 1970 and July 2022), with an emphasis on future directions in research and treatment, and we explore the potential implications for improved management of disease progression.

2. Pathophysiology of Optic Neuritis, a Projection of MS Pathomechanism

In terms of MS pathophysiology, it is recognized that oligodendrocytes are responsible for myelination as well as for maintaining saltatory conduction to facilitate effective transmission of a nerve impulse down the axon in the CNS [5]. Damage to myelin (demyelination) and nerve fibers (axonal degeneration) in the CNS is the ultimate cause of MS. Immune cells are largely believed to assault myelinated axons in the CNS, resulting in demyelination and axonal degeneration [7]. Activated autoreactive T cells, myelin-specific T cells, B cells, plasma cells, dendritic cells, and macrophages, for example, can enhance macrophage recruitment by releasing different cytokines and chemokines [16]. Within the CNS, infiltrating inflammatory cells activate and interact with other immune cells and neuronal cells, resulting in oligodendroglial cell death-mediated demyelination, glial cell activation (including microglia and astrocytes), and axonal degeneration [17,18].

The structure of the anterior visual pathway is complex in which the retinal ganglion cells play a central role by positioning the nuclei at the level of the ganglion cell layer. Axons of the RNFL that are unmyelinated enter the optic nerve. Its path is through the optic canal to the level of the optic chiasm where the separation of the nasal fibers takes place. The synapse of most of the fibers takes place at the level of the lateral geniculate nucleus [19]. The role of immune mechanisms in the development and progression of inflammatory lesions of the optic nerve resides in understanding the anatomy and associated physiological mechanisms. The lamina cribosa separates the retina from the scleral wall of the eye socket, and is defined as a fibrous plaque composed of a dense network of collagen fibers. The nerve fibers within the lamina cribrosa are non-myelinated. The location of oligodendrocytes in the posterior compartment explains the inflammatory status of the optic nerve during ON, as retinal inflammation is not typical of this ocular disorder [20].

2.1. Inflammatory Phase

The main inflammatory cells that are activated in an early stage of the inflammatory process in the brain are microglia, macrophages, and peripheral T lymphocytes. Activated T cells mature and expand clonally before dividing into effector cells and migrating through the bloodstream to breach the blood–brain barrier (BBB). Endothelial cells in the CNS microvasculature contain adhesion molecules, which activated T cells can attach to and penetrate [3,18]. The release of cytokines and other proinflammatory mediators aggravates the inflammatory environment, attracting more immune cells to the CNS and eventually leading to demyelination [3,21,22]. Using a range of experimental animal models, the immunological processes underlying demyelination of the optic nerve secondary to the inflammatory process may be easily investigated [4]. The pathophysiological processes mentioned above are mediated by a variety of molecules with intrinsic action that potentiate the associated pro-inflammatory status [23].

The pathophysiological mechanisms involved in MS are based on the "inside-out" and "outside-in" theories, which have been intensively studied in the literature [24]. The first entity is based on the existence of a subsidiary primary degenerative process that determines in a secondary plan the activation of autoimmune mechanisms [25]. The "outside-in theory" of MS has been proposed, as opposed to the "inside-out hypothesis", according to which there is an autoimmune substrate that allows CD4+ T lymphocytes attack against myelin [25]. Antigen-presenting cells (APCs) reawaken autoreactive effector CD4 T cells in the CNS and attract more T cells and macrophages to develop the inflammatory lesion [26,27] (Figure 1).

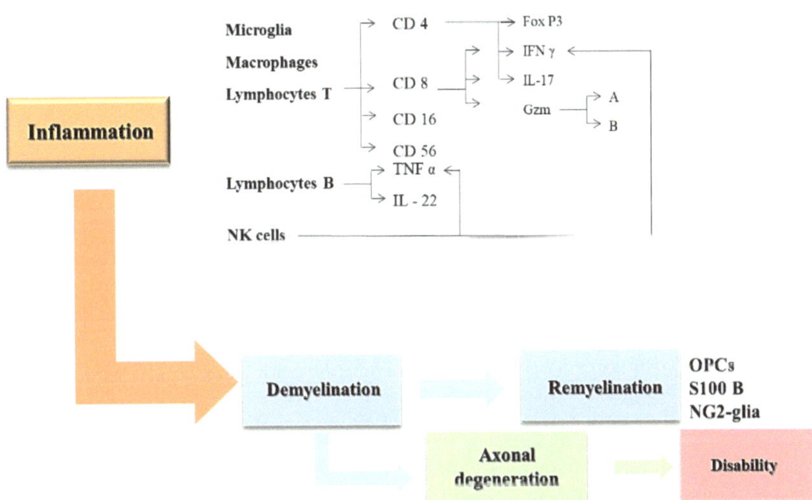

Figure 1. "Outside-in" theory (details in the text)-cells and processes involved.

CD4 T cells are identified in the cerebrospinal fluid (CSF) of MS patients and deep inside CNS lesions [26,28]. The activation of CD4 T lymphocytes is controlled by DR2 (DRB-1501/DQ6) is a major histocompatibility complex (MHC) class II locus [28]. Recent clinical studies in the field certified that Tr1 CD4+ regulatory populations are now recognized to control autoimmune T cell activity. Furthermore, reducing CD4 T cells would have little effect on CD8 T cells, which make up the bulk of CNS-resident T cells in patients and may play a critical role in the illness once CD4 T cells have started it [26]. CD4 T cells that secrete interferon gamma (IFNg) and interleukin-17 (IL-17) are thought to be the pathogenic initiators of MS.

CD4 T cells were originally divided into two functionally different types in the late 1980s: IFNg-producing Th1 cells that remove external infections and IL-4-producing Th2 cells that trigger allergic reactions [29,30]. Following that, researchers discovered CD4+ Th17 cells, which play a key role in autoimmunity. Tumor necrotic factor alpha (TNFα) promotes inflammation by activating STAT3 and IL-22 promotes inflammation by activating STAT3. They also have lower levels of IL-10, an anti-inflammatory cytokine [31].

CD8 T lymphocytes have an important role in MS in humans. CD8 T cells make up the bulk of T cells in the CNS perivascular infiltrate and at the periphery of CNS lesions in MS, unlike experimental autoimmune encephalomyelitis (EAE) [32]. The density of CD8+ T cells is 50 times higher than CD4+ T cells due to perivascular cells located at the periphery of active demyelinating plaques in patients with progressive MS. However, this ratio is not supported by CSF analysis where the ratio is at most 6:1 or by peripheral blood analysis where the ratio is much lower at only 2:1 [22]. CD8 T cells are also often seen in disease-related cortical plaques [33,34]. Some CD8+ T cell subtypes associate oligoclonal growth, thus being an indirect response of oligoclonal cell amplification to specific antigen responses [35].

CD8 T lymphocytes detect peptides of endogenous intracellular proteins given in the context of MHC class I molecules and destroy cells through a cell-contact-mediated mechanism involving granzyme A (GzmA) and granzyme B (GzmB) activities. While MHC class I is expressed ubiquitously and constitutively on all cells, MHC class I and class II expression is increased in oligodendrocytes, astrocytes, and neurons in patients with disease activity [36]. Antigen-presenting microglial cells have the ability to cross present foreign antigens on their MHC class I molecules, presumably resulting in the increased frequency of myelin-reactive CD8 T cells seen in MS patients [37].

IFNg is secreted by these myelin-reactive CD8 T cells, which destroy cells that express endogenously generated myelin. Because effector CD8 T cells' intracellular lytic granules are oriented toward adjacent axons in immunohistochemical investigation of postmortem CNS tissue slices, their cytotoxic action may play a key role in axonal injury. The presence of lesional CD8 T lymphocytes in close proximity to neurons has been linked to axonal damage [38]. In the setting of MS, at least two subgroups of CD4+ regulatory T (T-regs) cells have been discovered and examined. T-regs are a subset of regulatory T cells that express the transcription factor Forkhead box protein 3 (FoxP3) as well as a slew of inhibitory immune checkpoint surface molecules that help them suppress in vitro T cell proliferation via a cell-contact-mediated mechanism [39]. The Tr1 regulatory CD4+ T cell is a second kind of CD4+ regulatory T cell that controls cell proliferation predominantly through the release of IL-10 [40].

FoxP3+ Tregs, which account for fewer than 4% of circulating CD4 T cells, are known as "professional" suppressor cells because they prevent the activation of other cell types via a cell-to-cell contact mechanism [26]. Teff cells produced from patients is, in fact, immune to Treg-mediated repression [41]. According to published research, MS patients have both a deficiency in Tregs and a resistance to Treg suppression by Teff cells [26].

CD46, which substantially promotes IL-10, was used to stimulate CD4 T cells, and it was shown that MS CD4 T cells express less IL-10 than healthy CD4 T cells [26]. Because the expression of IL-10 and CD46 is increased in patients who react to IFNb treatment compared to cells from patients who do not respond, the ability of CD4 T cells to release IL-10 is related with lower disease activity in MS [42]. Il-10 secretion by non-pathogenic Th17 cells has also been observed to increase [43].

Natural killer (NK) cells release both pro-inflammatory (IFNg, TNFa) and anti-inflammatory (IL-4, IL-10) cytokines, and they' ve been linked to illness [26]. Although CD56 and CD16 cells, which account for 90% of NK cells in peripheral circulation, are cytotoxic right away, they are found in considerably lower numbers in tissue. CD56 bright cells, on the other hand, predominate in tissues, where they largely release cytokines and develop cytotoxic activity with time. Despite the fact that NK cells have been discovered in MS patients' demyelinating lesions, the majority of data suggests that NK cells play an immunoregulatory role in MS [32]. Immunomodulatory and immunosuppressive therapies increase CD56-bright NK cells, increases in NK frequency correlate with treatment response [44], decreased NK frequency has been linked to relapse [45], and in vitro NK functional activity increases during remission [26]. Untreated MS patients' CD56-bright NK cells show a lower capacity to limit the proliferation of autologous activated T cells, which might be related to CD56 bright NK cell malfunction as well as the discovery that MS CD4 T cells are less susceptible to NK cell regulation [46]. This "NK resistance" by patient-derived T cells has been attributed to increased T cell production of the NK-inhibitory ligand HLA-E or lower CD155 expression on patient-derived T cells [47].

The presence of oligoclonal bands (OCBs) in the CSF, which are found in 95% of MS patients and are caused by clonally enlarged Ig-secreting cells, is a hallmark observation in the disease [48]. It was found that CSF OCB antibodies from four MS patients have specificity for a variety of ubiquitous intracellular proteins that are produced as debris during tissue breakdown. Although antibodies to myelin lipids in the CSF have been linked to severe MS, anti-lipid antibodies are also seen in systemic lupus erythematosus and Grave' s illnesses [26].

MS patients' brain parenchyma, meninges, and CSF contain clonally enlarged B lymphocytes, which are more common in the CNS early in the illness [49,50]. Increased B cell frequency in the CSF is linked to a faster course of the illness [51]. B cells in the CNS might have a role in MS by secreting chemokines/cytokines and presenting antigen to T cells, in addition to their possible capacity to make autoantibodies [26]. In lymph-node-like follicles located in the meninges, which are typically close to cortical lesions, B lymphocytes can cross the blood-brain barrier and become long-term CNS residents [52]. The presence of these follicle-like structures shows that B cells expand and differentiate into plasmablasts and plasma cells within the CNS itself [53].

Anti-CD20 also lowers the number of T cells in the blood and CSF by 20% and 50%, respectively [45], and the remaining T cells' ability to release IL-17 and IFNg [26]. Anti CD20 has a quick start of benefit because it eliminates a pro-inflammatory B cell fraction that induces T cell activation through antigen presentation or cytokine release [26].

2.2. MS Triad: Demyelination, Axonal Degeneration, and Remyelination

MS is defined by a progressive inflammatory status associated with demyelination and autoimmune neurodegeneration in the CNS. Numerous studies published in the literature demonstrate the concern of researchers in the field in understanding the pathophysiological mechanisms underlying the chronic evolution and irreversible disability [26]. Clinical studies published to date attribute the disabling outcome to persistent chronic inflammation, ongoing demyelination and failure to remyelinate, the latter two being major factors associated with a poor neurological prognosis. These 3 main pathophysiological pillars have been recognized as the building blocks of this pathophysiological triad in MS [54].

2.2.1. Demyelination and Axonal Loss

The persistence of a pro-inflammatory status causes axon loss over time secondary to demyelination. Axonal function is directly affected by the direct action of inflammatory cytokines, enzymes and nitric oxide, which are produced by activated immune cells. Remission of inflammatory processes may result in remyelination of surviving axons, although most EAE phenotypes are characterized by neuronal cell death due to associated inflammatory stress. Paraclinical targeting of the RNFL is a marker of irreversible axonal injury [3]. T-cells interfere with the action of antibodies in the CNS contributing to the supplementation of demyelination secondary to inflammatory processes in EAE. The same effect is obtained by injecting the antibody into the brain with human complement. [3].

2.2.2. Animal Models Used to Study Remyelination

Endogenous remyelination ensures nerve conduction and prevents neurodegeneration, being a complex process involving various pathophysiological processes and representing a promising therapeutic strategy for the future [55]. The central role has been assigned to oligodendrocyte progenitor cells (aOPCs), which thus acquires potential therapeutic value. These cells mediate a variety of pathophysiological processes, including activation, migration, proliferation, or differentiation [56]. It has been shown that only mature aOPCs-derived from neonatal OPCs contributes to the remyelination process. These cells have the ability to reconstitute themselves and not to be replaced by neural stem cells [57,58].

The literature includes several clinical studies on animal models based on which remyelination has been studied. These animal models allow histopathological identification of the presence of remyelination processes, as the myelin state formed is thinner and shorter compared to that at the time of myelination [59,60]. Franklin et al. [61] highlights a number of factors that prevent remyelination in MS patients, such as altered aOPCs, a lack of pro-regenerative factors, or an excess of inhibitory factors or errors in aOPCs-mediated pathophysiological processes.

Experimental Autoimmune Encephalomyelitis

Experimental autoimmune encephalomyelitis is known as the animal model of MS and is frequently used for research purposes to further investigate pathophysiological mechanisms [16]. It is a CNS autoimmune illness that is deliberately generated in susceptible species such as rats and primates by vaccination with CNS-specific antigens, peptides derived from these antigens, or CNS tissue homogenates. Transfer of encephalitogenic CD4+ T cells from draining lymph nodes of animals vaccinated for active EAE induction into syngeneic animals can also cause the illness. However, the validity of EAE as an MS model has been called into question [62]. Several molecular and cellular processes of MS pathogenesis have been revealed in EAE research [63–65].

Demyelinating Illness Caused by the Virus Theiler' s Murine Encephalitis

Theiler' s murine encephalitis virus-induced demyelinating disease (TMEV-IDD) is a model frequently used in clinical trials in patients with various demyelinating diseases, including MS [66–68]. TMEV is a positive-stranded RNA virus from the Picornaviridae family (genus Cardiovirus). Between days 5 and 10 after injection, the TO subgroup of TMEV causes acute encephalitis. TMEV-IDD is of special relevance because it represents a hypothetical situation in people in which a virus is the primary contributor for CNS inflammation and demyelination.

Importantly, the clinical manifestations of TMEV-IDD are comparable to those seen in individuals with progressive MS, including stiffness, incontinence, extremity weakness, and, finally, paralysis [68]. Intrathecal antibody production has been seen in this model, which is similar to the oligoclonal bands detected in the CSF of MS patients [69]. The general objection against this model is that a non-human virus was utilized to simulate a human disease. Surprisingly, it was recently found that a human-TMEV recombinant virus might produce Vilyuisk encephalitis, a kind of encephalomyelitis [68]. Additional viruses, such as murine hepatitis virus, canine distemper virus, coronaviruses, and several retroviruses, are also being utilized in experimental animals to induce MS-like demyelinating illness [69–72].

The Role of Cuprizone or Other Toxins

Demyelination in mice caused by the copper chelator cuprizone is a useful tool for MS research [63–65]. Cuprizone consumption by mice results in early oligodendrocytes (ODC) mortality, activation of microglia/macrophages, and subsequent reversible demyelination [73]. This model is beneficial for researching demyelination and remyelination, as well as their relationship to axonal loss [74]. It is extremely important for the progression of type III and type IV MS lesions, where alterations in ODC appear to represent the key events in disease pathogenesis. In addition to cuprizone, additional toxins, such as ethidium bromide and lysolecithin, are employed to induce demyelination in experimental mice [74].

The Role of Lysophospholipid Lysophosphatidylcholine (LPC, Lysolecithin)

It has been used for decades to produce demyelination in animal models of multiple sclerosis. A recent investigation of LPC damage and homeostasis processes discovered that LPC nonspecifically altered myelin lipids and swiftly caused cell membrane permeability; LPC injury in mice was phenocopied by other lipid disrupting agents. A subsequent increase in LPC five days following the injection into white matter implies that the brain possesses mechanisms to buffer LPC, and albumin buffering greatly reduced LPC damage in culture [75]. LPC application was compared to agarose-gel loaded LPC (AL-LPC) in mouse optic nerve behind the globe via a small surgery in an attempt to research new processes of demyelination and to assess new medicines. Agarose loading was employed to extend the length of LPC exposure and thereby accomplish long-term demyelination.

Visual evoked potentials (VEPs) recordings revealed a large increase in the latency of the P1 wave and a decrease in the amplitude of the P1N1 wave at the lesion locations, as well as severe demyelination and axonal damage. The optimized model demonstrated that both AL-LPC and LPC groups had extended demyelination, axonal degeneration, and retinal ganglion cell (RGC) loss; however, these diseases were more widespread in the AL-LPC group [76]. Furthermore, the therapeutic potential of many medicines has piqued the interest of researchers, beginning with animal models of generated demyelinating diseases. Among the key factors known to limit CNS regeneration are myelin associated inhibitory factors such as NogoA [77], myelin associated glycoprotein (MAG) [78], and oligodendrocyte myelin glycoprotein (OMgp) [79]. These elements connect to a common receptor known as Nogo receptor 1 (NgR1) [80]. A wide range of cells express this receptor, including neurons, OPCs, astrocytes, microglia, macrophages, dendritic cells, and neural precursor cells. Although the physiological implications of Nogo-A/NgR interaction among glial cells are unclear, Nogo-A expressed on oligodendrocytes may interact with NgR produced by reactive astrocytes and microglia/macrophages in active demyelinating lesions of MS [81].

2.2.3. Axonal and Neuronal Degeneration

By secreting IFNg and IL-17, pathogenic CD8 T cells may also contribute to the disease [82]. In a BBB model using human cells and in mice models, these IFNg-, IL-17, and GzmB-producing effector CD8 T cells may also experience increased endothelial transmigration [83]. As a result, CD8 T cells may not only induce oligodendrocyte mortality and neuronal injury once within the CNS, but they may also amplify IFNg- and IL-17-mediated disease [26].

After demyelination, what happens to the axon? Axonal degeneration and morphological alterations of axonal organelles, such as axoplasmic reticulum (AR)-like structures, were observed to precede morphological abnormalities of myelin in EAE animals. It was discovered that morphological alterations in myelin, as well as morphological changes in axonal organelles, cause axonal degeneration. Although further research is needed, it appears to be a strong link between twisted axons and axonal degeneration [16].

In EAE and acute human MS lesions, axonal degeneration with localized axonal swellings and mitochondrial abnormalities are prominent. It has been suggested that intra-axonal mitochondrial disease in localized axonal degeneration might be the first ultrastructural indicator of damage, occurring before axon shape changes. Axonal degeneration has been linked to mitochondrial failure in several investigations of autopsied human MS brains and in vitro models. Axonal diseases were also seen in myelin-associated glycoprotein-2,3-cyclic nucleotide 3-phosphodiesterase-null animals, demonstrating that oligodendrocyte–axon interactions are necessary for structural and functional modulation between myelin and axons.

A growing body of data implies that axonal degeneration in MS and EAE is triggered by axonal AR and mitochondrial dysfunction, which is followed by an increase in axonal Ca^{2+} levels produced by AR and mitochondria. Axoplasmic reticulum Ca^{2+} release produced subsequent degeneration of spinal neurons [84]. Furthermore, it was discovered that in EAE spinal cords, the intensity of a mitochondrial fission-related protein, Drp1/Dlp1, rose, whereas the intensity of a mitochondrial fusion-related protein (MFN) dropped [16].

Reduced adenosine triphosphate synthesis in demyelinated upper motor neuron axon segments disrupts ion homeostasis, causes Ca^{2+} mediated axonal degeneration, and contributes to MS patients' increasing neurological impairment [16]. Glutamate excitotoxicity is one neurodegenerative process thought to be implicated in MS pathogenesis [85]. Because RGCs have a high density of dendritic glutamate receptors, they are especially sensitive to elevated glutamate levels in the retina [86]. Over-stimulation of ionotropic glutamate receptors is thought to lead to prolonged intracellular calcium increases capable of activating downstream pathways leading to cell death, and their over-stimulation is thought to lead to prolonged intracellular calcium increases capable of activating downstream pathways leading to cell death [87]. It was found that ultrastructural alterations in RGC axons of the optic nerve, as well as elongation of nodes of Ranvier, were observed at the outset of illness [85].

A loss in visual acuity and changes in the optic nerve cytoskeleton (as evidenced by modifications in actin treadmilling and expression of its regulatory proteins) occur during the induction phase of autoimmune optic neuritis (AON), as well as RGC degeneration, which may be replicated by intravitreal glutamate injection. Sühs et al. [88] demonstrated that intravenous administration of the NMDA receptor blocker MK-801 during the induction phase of AON causes activation of NMDA receptors before the onset of demyelinating optic nerve lesions associated with the inflammatory status associated. Another group of investigators emphasizes the beneficial role of the retinal calcium increase during the induction phase, which potentiates the aforementioned effect, contributing to the restoration of visual integrity, the resumption of optic nerve actin dynamics as well as RGCs neuroprotection [89]. This is backed up by the fact that the retinal calcium level rises during AON at the same time. This points to the NMDA receptor as the most likely possibility, which leads us back to the "inside-out" theory [85] (Figure 2).

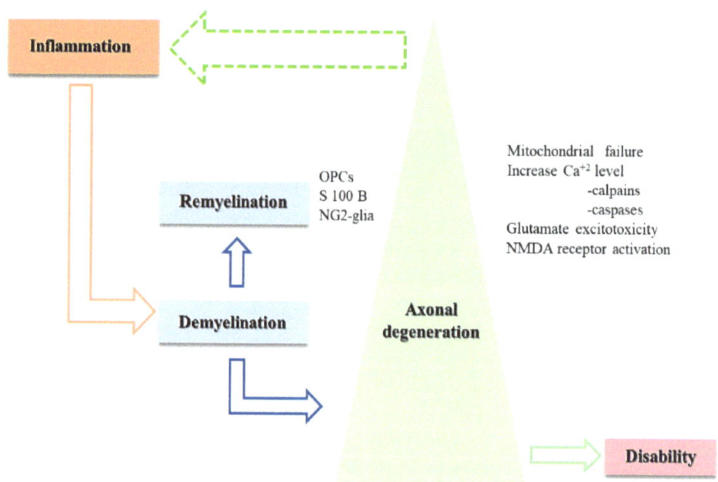

Figure 2. "Inside-out" theory (details in the text)–the green dotted arrow represents a possible temporal, but non-causal relationship.

Disturbances in the actin cytoskeletal dynamics of the optic nerve seen throughout the course of AON may have consequences for RGC degeneration since growing data indicates that actin is both a sensor and a mediator of apoptosis. F-actin disintegration is caused by both NMDA receptor activation [90] and increased intracellular calcium, resulting in actin network instability.

Calcium-dependent proteases, such as calpains and caspases, are activated by significant increases in intracellular calcium, further destabilizing the actin cytoskeleton. The actin-severing protein gelsolin is one such calcium-activated protease [91]. At the same time, calpain/caspase cleaves gelsolin [92], making the cell more sensitive to NMDA receptor activation as an anti-apoptotic agent [93]. A functional role in apoptotic signaling is also played by fractin, a calpain/caspase-cleaved actin monomer product that accumulates after activation of apoptosis [94]. Furthermore, the reorganization of nodes of Ranvier might be influenced by changes in actin network dynamics [85].

Gelsolin levels may be affected by NMDA receptor activation as well as other disease-related variables that are currently unknown. In contrast, while gelsolin protects cells against apoptosis [93] its expression might be up-regulated in response to glutamate-mediated stress, although for unknown reasons [85]. The early degeneration shown in this model, which occurs before the demyelination and inflammatory infiltration that define optic neuritis, contradicts the traditional belief that secondary RGC degeneration results from axonal injury in the demyelinated optic nerve [85].

Early AON retinal events might cause anterograde alterations in actin cytoskeletal dynamics in the optic nerve, which are most likely mediated by calcium build-up and activation of actin-regulatory proteases. NMDA receptor manipulation might be a therapeutically viable method for retinal neuroprotection in autoimmune neuro-inflammatory diseases.

2.2.4. Remyelination in Optic Neuritis

Immune-modulatory networks are activated, limiting inflammation, and initiating repair, resulting in at least partial remyelination and clinical remission [26]. S100B, a protein generated predominantly by astrocytes, has been shown to help with relapsing–remitting EAE. Administration of pentamidine isothionate (PTM) to EAE-induced mice abolishes S100B activity causing in a secondary plan improvement of preclinical scores, increase of remission rate and decrease of activity of some molecules present in the brain, such as IFNg, TNFa, or NOS activity. When comparing EAE animals treated with PTM to EAE mice not treated with medication, the number of CD68+ cells and demyelinating lesions were lower in PTM-treated EAE mice. Overall, this research implies that the severity of EAE is reduced by targeting neurotoxic mediators released by astrocytes [95].

MS pathophysiology is characterized by demyelination. NG2-glia are oligodendrocyte progenitors that can develop into adult oligodendrocytes and hence may help individuals with MS remyelinate [95]. The phenotypic heterogeneity of NG2-glia in relation to their ontogenic origin was investigated, as well as whether EAE causes a clonal NG2-glial response. They discovered that NG2-glia from single progenitors are distributed clonally across the grey and white matter [95].

The proliferative oligodendrocyte progenitor cell has been reported as the most effective remyelinating cell in animal experiments for successfully repairing demyelinating lesions, particularly those of the optic nerve [96]. The existence of a comparable population of oligodendrocyte progenitor cells in normal adult human white matter, as well as in acute and chronic MS lesions, may be the source of oligodendrocyte proliferation after demyelinating lesions in humans [97]. Although the presence of oligodendrocyte progenitor cells impacts the eventual number of oligodendrocytes in a demyelinating lesion, it does not appear that the quantity of oligodendrocytes is the sole component required for effective remyelination [98]. Some oligodendrocytes in acute MS lesions may reveal mild, early pathologic abnormalities, indicating that their myelinating capacity has been reduced without overt cell death [99]. Endogenous remyelination after ON appears to be most prominent in optic nerve lesions that develop early in the course of MS, and when significant remyelination occurs, it usually becomes morphologically apparent at least 1 month after the initial insult, a time interval that corresponds to clinical recovery after isolated typical ON [100]. Shadow plaques, which are made up of sparsely myelinated axons, are hypothesized to be the result of remyelination following a single bout of acute demyelination [98].

Recurrent demyelinating optic nerve damage in the same region of white matter, on the other hand, may impair those reparative processes, resulting in permanently demyelinated axons and failure of remyelination [100]. This discovery explains why remyelination is seen early in the course of MS but not in typical chronic MS lesions, which are more likely to have had several, temporally different bouts of demyelination [101]. While beneficial, endogenous remyelination in ON and MS in general has limits [98]. When compared to normal axons, remyelinated axons have thinner myelin sheaths and shorter internodal lengths [102]. Remyelinated axons, on the other hand, have poor axonal conduction velocities [103]. Finally, lack of full remyelination is a major reason in the persistence of visual impairment after ON [98].

Jäkle et al. [104] performed an autopsy study on human brains from patients with MS and from unaffected controls, demonstrating both a reduced presence of ODC in shadowing lesions as well as changes in gene expression between areas of normal-appearing white matter of MS patients compared to a group of healthy subjects, raising the need for further clinical studies to understand the global cellular changes targeted in this category of patients. These results raise the observation that there are discrepancies between studies on animal models and those on humans, and that a comprehensive, potentially therapeutic approach is needed that addresses not only differentiation process [55,105,106].

The possibility of identifying therapeutic agents that offer neuroprotection to MS patients by potentiating remyelination has led to the emergence of various clinical trials—some ongoing, others completed—predominantly involving three types of agents: small molecules, hormones, and antibodies [107,108]. The most advanced clinical trials are hormone-based trials, most of which are Phase III clinical trials. Of all the incriminating agents, special attention is needed in the case of rHIgM22 (a remyelinating antibody) [109], which is currently the only agent acting on both OPCs and oligodendrocytes, leading to stimulation of acute and chronic myelination in preclinical models of demyelination [107,110].

The constant concern of researchers in the field to develop new molecules with remyelinating action has led to the emergence and conduct of multiple clinical trials whose interim results have already been presented in the literature. Thus, clemastine is an antihistamic agent acting on antimuscarinic receptors, with proven effects both in vitro and in vivo to date. It was tested in a Phase II randomized double-blind crossover placebo-controlled clinical trial (ReBUILD study), with the mechanism of action being the potentiation of OPC differentiation and proliferation. Preliminary results reported a shortening of P100 VEP latency by 1.7 ms/eye, indicating slightly faster neural transduction within the optic pathway but at the cost of fatigue as an adverse effect [111].

Olesosime is a cholesterol-like agent whose neuroprotective effect is exerted via mitochondrial metabolism. In vitro it induced maturation of OPCs and stimulation of myelin production. In the literature, there is a phase IB multicenter randomized double-blind placebo controlled clinical trial conducted to test the efficacy of this agent, but no superior results were observed compared to placebo [112–114]. In recent years, several phase II clinical trials have been conducted in which various therapeutic agents have been tested, such as bexarotene a retinoid x receptor γ (clinical trial in UK - EudraCT 2014–003145-99) [115,116], gold nanocrystals (stimulates ATP production by oxidizing nicotinamide adenine dinucleotide NADH to NAD+) [117,118], or domperidone (peripheral dopamine D2 receptor antagonist that stimulates prolactin secretion from the pituitary gland) [119,120] that stimulated remyelination by potentiating proliferation, differentiation, or maturation of OPCs, but they did not prove effective.

Opininumab is an anti-LINGO1 monoclonal antibody, which functions as a transmembrane protein at the OPCs and neuronal cell surface. Although the monoclonal antibody against LINGO1 has been shown to be effective in a phase I clinical trial, clinically significant results regarding visual acuity, VEP latency, or MRI measurements have not been demonstrated in several phase II clinical trials [121–124].

3. The "Big" Picture behind the MS Triad

Neuroimaging, CSF examination and VEP analysis are the main methods to establish the diagnosis of ON and assess the associated risk of developing MS.

3.1. MRI

ON is frequently the initial presentation of MS patients with no neurological history, especially demyelinating pathologies [125]. Neuroimaging is a central piece in the diagnostic and therapeutic puzzle. To date, clinical research in the field has not revealed the presence of molecules with a prognostic role for these patients, which has led to a shift of attention toward imaging explorations, especially MRI [126]. Structural imaging parameters quantified by MRI cannot distinguish between demyelination and axonal lesions produced within the central nervous system [127]. MRI targeting T2-hyperintense and gadolinium-enhancing of multiple lesions of the brain or spinal cord are arguments in favor of the present MS [128,129]. Within the first 20 days of visual acuity decline, 95% of patients with MS-associated ON show T1 gadolinium enhancement [130]. Existing clinical studies in the literature refute the existence of a correlation between the extent and severity of lesions identified on MRI and the rate of vision recovery [131].

Swanton et al. [132] demonstrated that the presence of spinal lesions has a disabling predictive value for patients who develop MS over time (72% risk) compared to those without identified lesions, where the risk of progression was estimated at 25% [125,133,134]. In addition to absence of lesions on MRI assessment, male sex, lack of typical symptoms and optic swelling are factors associated with a low risk of ON progression to MS [134].

Over time, patients with ON may associate subclinical demyelinating lesions in which the usual paraclinical evaluation (CSF and VEP analysis) does not reveal pathological changes, the definitive being the MRI imaging exploration. Lebrun et al. [135] demonstrated that patients without MRI lesions have a clinical conversion rate of 33% to clinically isolated syndrome in 5 years. The investigators have highlighted as associated risk factors VEPs abnormalities, youth, and gadolinium enhancement on follow-up MRI. McDonald criteria are widely used in patients at risk of progression to MS, the main radiological changes quantified being dissemination in space or time [125,136]. In a similar clinical study, Tintore et al. [137] confirms the prognostic role of MRI scanning in assessing the occurrence of MS, compared to the Poser criteria, with the new standards associating superior sensitivity and specificity.

Frohman et al. [8] investigated the role of MRI versus optical coherence tomography (OCT) and laser polarimetry methods in the assessment of RNFL thickness vs. brain measures and concluded that measurement of RNFL thickness and radius of the optic nerve are preferred in clinical studies due to identification of more pronounced differences between patients with MS and controls.

3.2. Visual Evoked Potentials Analysis

VEPs is part of the diagnostic work-up of patients with ON, including asymptomatic forms, being an alternative to MRI imaging exploration [138]. Clinical studies show that 65% of patients show changes in VEPs, which are a clinical reflection of demyelination in the afferent visual pathways [139]. The most common findings are increased latencies and reduced amplitudes and abnormal waveforms [140].

Prolonged latency measurements suggest subclinical demyelinating damage, while reduced wave amplitudes are the paraclinical expression of axonal degeneration and loss in MS patients [141]. The parameters obtained by measuring VEPs have predictive value as well, being indirect markers, directly proportional to the severity of MS [142,143].

Recent clinical studies in the field focused on the multifocal visual evoked potentials and its role in ON and MS [144]. The evaluation of these potentials allows obtaining anatomical data on the localization of particular lesions, thus facilitating the deciphering of pathophysiological mechanisms focused on the triad demyelination, atrophy and remyelination [145]. De Santiago et al. [146] evaluated multifocal VEPs from 15 patients with radiologically isolated syndrome and concluded that measuring signal-to-noise ratio increases the risk of identifying patients with a high risk of developing MS over time.

Multifocal VEP have therapeutic value, their evaluation being used in various clinical trials with remyelination therapies as end-points. Klistorner et al. [145] demonstrated that Opicinumab (a human monoclonal antibody) vs. placebo in patients with ON decreases the risk of long-term visual impairment after remission of the acute episode, having a satisfying safety and tolerability profile [123,124,147]. Both VEPs and multifocal VEP have proven diagnostic value in the clinical studies presented above, with the latter having superior sensitivity (95%) and specificity (90%) [148].

Klistorner et al. [149] also demonstrated that amplitude of waves measured by VEP correlates positively with RFNL thickness after an acute episode of ON, with the most significant structural changes in RFNL being at the temporal level. Laron et al. [150] demonstrated that multifocal potentials analysis provides superior prognostic data compared to Humphrey visual field and OCT in MS patients.

3.3. Cerebrospinal Fluid Examination

Cerebrospinal fluid (CSF) analysis has both diagnostic and therapeutic value, due to biomarkers with predictive value for the development of MS in patients with acute ON [151–154]. Research presented in the literature in recent years attests to the concern of researchers in identifying molecules with both a diagnostic and prognostic role, on the basis of which the disease activity or therapeutic response in patients with MS can be assessed [155].

Olesen et al. conducted a prospective study on 40 patients with ON of which 16 were diagnosed with MS during the 2.5-year follow-up period. The CSF analysis demonstrated that TNF-α, IL-10, CXCL13, and NF-L correlates positively with the diagnosis of MS, thus raising the hypothesis of the existence of inflammatory and neurodegenerative processes that started earlier [139]. Based on the potential biomarkers identified, the same investigators proposed two models to predict ON patients' risk of developing MS. Statistical analysis of the proposed models revealed an associated risk of up to 10% of developing MS after an ON episode and up to 15% for potential biomarkers.

IL-10 is a cytokine with an anti-inflammatory and immunosuppressive role that mediates a variety of pathophysiological processes in various inflammatory pathologies, not only MS [156]. Previous studies concluded that IL-10 correlates with higher IgG levels in patients with positive oligoclonal IgG bands [157]. IL-10 also interferes with pathophysiological mechanisms involved in MS, mediated by B cells [158]. The presence of a pleocytosis below 50 cells/mm^3 in the CSF is highly suggestive of an acute episode of ON in the context of MS [159,160].

The role of metabolomics in the onset and progression of MS has also been studied in recent years [161]. Thus, based on the hypothesis that metabolomics highlights a series of metabolic alterations encountered in patients with severe forms of MS, it' s role in the establishment of therapeutic profiles has been studied in order to assess the degree of response to the therapy administered [162,163]. This technique allows for the analysis of a variety of small molecules below 1500 Da found in various bodily fluids, such as CSF, serum, plasma, or urine [164].

Reinke et al. [165] analyzed the CSF from 15 patients with MS and 17 from a control group and concluded that patients from the first group had energy and phospholipid metabolism alterations, which led to increased levels of choline, myoinositol, and threonate on one hand and on the other hand decreased levels of 3-hydroxybutyrate, citrate, phenylalanine, 2-hydroxyisovalerate, and mannose. In a similar study, Lutz et al. [166] demonstrated that elevated lactate and reduced phenylalanine in CSF levels contribute to the maintenance of pro-inflammatory status in MS.

3.4. Optical Coherence Tomography

The optic nerve is the most "visible" part for investigation in the CNS, and the fact that visual function can be measured objectively makes ON an important model for research into CNS inflammatory disease. The comparison "the eye as a window to the brain" became accurate when, for example, ON was diagnosed by optical coherence tomography (OCT) [167].

OCT is a marker of CNS axonal loss. OCT highlights a series of imaging parameters based on which correlations are made between neuronal loss and the degree of associated visual dysfunction. Several prognostic markers have been proposed, one of the most widely used being a thinning of the RNFL and the GCL ganglion cell layer that assesses the dynamic evolution of MS patients [168]. Trip et al. reported a 33% reduction in peripapillary

RNFL thickness in eyes with a history of ON and incomplete recovery. There was a 27% reduction in the affected eyes compared to the unaffected fellow eyes [169].

Similar clinical results have been reported by Frohman et al. [127] who demonstrated reduction of RNFL in patients with recurrent ON as well as in those previously diagnosed with MS. The OCT measurements showed both axonal loss and retinal ganglion cell loss and are able to predict both visual recovery or impaired visual function [132,170].

Saidha et al. [171] demonstrated that OCT facilitates the identification of pathological changes at the retinal level, the objectification of some inner and outer nuclear layer pathology associated with an advanced degree of disability and therefore with an increased severity of MS. The role of OCT in assessing axonal integrity has previously been demonstrated by Burkholder et al. [172]. Based on the pathophysiological concept that the macula contains an increased density of neuronal structures, measurement of macular thickness and volume allows indirect assessment of its properties. The same group of investigators demonstrated that pre-papillary thinning of the RNFL and inner macular volume loss are common imaging findings in MS patients with no history of ON [172]. Scanning laser polarimetry can be used as an alternative to the imaging methods presented above, with reported results showing detection sensitivity lower than OCT of lesions at 1 month (65% vs. 54%) and similar at 3 months (58% vs. 60%) [173].

OCT also facilitates the differential diagnosis between ON and myelin oligodendrocyte glycoprotein antibody associated disorder (MOGAD). Thus, while pRFNL thickening is above 5 μm in all patients with MOGAD, in MS, only 54% of cases have this associated change [174].

3.5. Transorbital B-Mode Ultrasonography

Transorbital B-mode ultrasonography indirectly assesses the associated inflammatory status of patients with ON, associating a narrowing of the retrobulbar portion of the optic nerve in patients with recurrent ON [175]. Despite increased sensitivity and easy accessibility, further clinical studies are needed to identify imaging parameters with prognostic value for progression to MS [175].

4. New Therapeutic Targets

Over the past decades, researchers in the field have been constantly concerned with identifying new molecules to explain the pathophysiological mechanisms underlying the connection between ON and MS [176]. In the era of polymedicine, the identification of effective therapeutic molecules with a reduced degree of interaction with the medication of other pathologies (especially those with cardiological target) [177–179]. CSF analysis revealed the presence of central nervous system autoimmune markers such as glial fibrillary acidic protein-IgG, with diagnostic, therapeutic, and prognostic roles alike [180]. The identification of this biomarker in the CSF suggests the presence of an autoimmune pathology, often paraneoplastic, with a high chance of a favorable therapeutic response to immunotherapy [181].

New pathological antibodies, notably against aquaporin-4 and, more recently, myelin oligodendrocyte protein, represent topics of interest to researchers in the field. Discovery of IgG1 antibodies directed against astrocyte water channel protein aquaporin 4 (AQP4) are involved in the pathophysiological mechanisms of ON in MS [182]. Identification of these autoantibodies has been more frequently associated with disease recurrence or the presence of ON [183,184].

The discovery of these molecules has had associated therapeutic value, with a number of potential new drugs being developed, such as aquaporumab (non-pathogenic antibody blocker of AQP4-IgG binding) [185,186]. Sivelestat (neutrophil elastase inhibitor) [187–189] and eculizumab (complement inhibitor) complete the list of molecules under investigation in various clinical trials at the moment [185].

Sodium channel blockade have also been proposed as potential therapeutic targets due to their role in energy metabolism in neuroinflammatory diseases [190].

Digitalization and technological advances over the last decade have enabled the discovery of new immunosuppressive agents and the development of monoclonal antibodies which, when administered, induce a superior therapeutic response and thus improve patient prognosis [176]. Mesenchymal stem cell therapy is a promising research direction, with promising clinical results in small group clinical trials [191–193]. This therapy has an anti-inflammatory effect and potentiates remyelination, but it is limited in its use in terms of identifying the anatomical site of the lesion in the optic nerve or retina [194].

5. Conclusions

The molecular mechanisms underlying the onset and progression of ON in patients with MS are extremely varied, incompletely elucidated to date, and continue to represent research challenges. Further clinical studies are needed to establish whether axonal degeneration is a consequence of demyelination or an independent process. Advances in technology have led to the refinement of diagnostic methods in ON and thus to increased diagnostic accuracy. Detecting the onset of axonal degeneration would be essential in establishing therapeutic behavior. Additionally, the identification of molecular mechanisms that favor remyelination would be a second direction for the therapeutic approach.

Author Contributions: Conceptualization, M.A.C. and D.L.Ș.; methodology, C.S., R.A.S. and C.M.B.; validation, D.L.Ș., C.S. and R.A.S.; writing—original draft preparation, M.A.C. and D.L.Ș.; writing—review and editing, C.S., R.A.S. and C.M.B. All authors contributed equally to this manuscript. All authors have read and agreed to the published version of the manuscript.

Funding: This research received no external funding.

Institutional Review Board Statement: Not applicable.

Informed Consent Statement: Not applicable.

Data availability statement: Not applicable.

Conflicts of Interest: The authors declare no conflict of interest.

References

1. Handel, A.E.; Giovannoni, G.; Ebers, G.C.; Ramagopalan, S.V. Environmental Factors and Their Timing in Adult-Onset Multiple Sclerosis. *Nat. Rev. Neurol.* **2010**, *6*, 156–166. [CrossRef] [PubMed]
2. Gourraud, P.-A.; Harbo, H.F.; Hauser, S.L.; Baranzini, S.E. The Genetics of Multiple Sclerosis: An up-to-Date Review: The Genetics of Multiple Sclerosis. *Immunol. Rev.* **2012**, *248*, 87–103. [CrossRef] [PubMed]
3. Wu, G.; Parker Harp, C.; Shindler, K. Optic Neuritis: A Model for the Immuno-Pathogenesis of Central Nervous System Inflammatory Demyelinating Diseases. *Curr. Immunol. Rev.* **2015**, *11*, 85–92. [CrossRef] [PubMed]
4. Redler, Y.; Levy, M. Rodent Models of Optic Neuritis. *Front. Neurol.* **2020**, *11*, 580951. [CrossRef] [PubMed]
5. Baumann, N.; Pham-Dinh, D. Biology of Oligodendrocyte and Myelin in the Mammalian Central Nervous System. *Physiol. Rev.* **2001**, *81*, 871–927. [CrossRef]
6. Bando, Y. Roads to Formation of Normal Myelin Structure and Pathological Myelin Structure. In *Myelin: Advances in Experimental Medicine and Biology*; Sango, K., Yamauchi, J., Ogata, T., Susuki, K., Eds.; Springer: Singapore, 2019; Volume 1190, pp. 257–264, ISBN 978-981-329-635-0.
7. Denic, A.; Johnson, A.J.; Bieber, A.J.; Warrington, A.E.; Rodriguez, M.; Pirko, I. The Relevance of Animal Models in Multiple Sclerosis Research. *Pathophysiology* **2011**, *18*, 21–29. [CrossRef]
8. Frohman, E.M.; Dwyer, M.G.; Frohman, T.; Cox, J.L.; Salter, A.; Greenberg, B.M.; Hussein, S.; Conger, A.; Calabresi, P.; Balcer, L.J.; et al. Relationship of Optic Nerve and Brain Conventional and Non-Conventional MRI Measures and Retinal Nerve Fiber Layer Thickness, as Assessed by OCT and GDx: A Pilot Study. *J. Neurol. Sci.* **2009**, *282*, 96–105. [CrossRef]
9. Costello, F.; Hodge, W.; Pan, Y.I.; Eggenberger, E.; Coupland, S.; Kardon, R.H. Tracking Retinal Nerve Fiber Layer Loss after Optic Neuritis: A Prospective Study Using Optical Coherence Tomography. *Mult. Scler. Houndmills Basingstoke Engl.* **2008**, *14*, 893–905. [CrossRef]
10. Henderson, A.P.D.; Altmann, D.R.; Trip, A.S.; Kallis, C.; Jones, S.J.; Schlottmann, P.G.; Garway-Heath, D.F.; Plant, G.T.; Miller, D.H. A Serial Study of Retinal Changes Following Optic Neuritis with Sample Size Estimates for Acute Neuroprotection Trials. *Brain J. Neurol.* **2010**, *133*, 2592–2602. [CrossRef]
11. Calabia, J.; Torguet, P.; Garcia, I.; Martin, N.; Mate, G.; Marin, A.; Molina, C.; Valles, M. The Relationship between Renal Resistive Index, Arterial Stiffness, and Atherosclerotic Burden: The Link between Macrocirculation and Microcirculation. *J. Clin. Hypertens. Greenwich Conn* **2014**, *16*, 186–191. [CrossRef]

12. Preiningerova, J.L.; Grishko, A.; Sobisek, L.; Andelova, M.; Benova, B.; Kucerova, K.; Havrdova, E.K. Do Eyes with and without Optic Neuritis in Multiple Sclerosis Age Equally? *Neuropsychiatr. Dis. Treat.* **2018**, *14*, 2281–2285. [CrossRef]
13. Matthews, P.M.; Roncaroli, F.; Waldman, A.; Sormani, M.P.; De Stefano, N.; Giovannoni, G.; Reynolds, R. A Practical Review of the Neuropathology and Neuroimaging of Multiple Sclerosis. *Pract. Neurol.* **2016**, *16*, 279–287. [CrossRef] [PubMed]
14. Khalilpour, S.; Latifi, S.; Behnammanesh, G.; Majid, A.M.S.A.; Majid, A.S.A.; Tamayol, A. Ischemic Optic Neuropathy as a Model of Neurodegenerative Disorder: A Review of Pathogenic Mechanism of Axonal Degeneration and the Role of Neuroprotection. *J. Neurol. Sci.* **2017**, *375*, 430–441. [CrossRef]
15. Herold, S.; Kumar, P.; Wichert, S.P.; Kretzschmar, B.; Bähr, M.; Rossner, M.J.; Hein, K. Neurodegeneration in Autoimmune Optic Neuritis Is Associated with Altered APP Cleavage in Neurons and Up-Regulation of P53. *PLoS ONE* **2015**, *10*, e0138852. [CrossRef]
16. Bando, Y. Mechanism of Demyelination and Remyelination in Multiple Sclerosis. *Clin. Exp. Neuroimmunol.* **2020**, *11*, 14–21. [CrossRef]
17. Wagner, C.A.; Roqué, P.J.; Goverman, J.M. Pathogenic T Cell Cytokines in Multiple Sclerosis. *J. Exp. Med.* **2020**, *217*, e20190460. [CrossRef]
18. Noseworthy, J.H.; Lucchinetti, C.; Rodriguez, M.; Weinshenker, B.G. Multiple Sclerosis. *N. Engl. J. Med.* **2000**, *343*, 938–952. [CrossRef]
19. Britze, J.; Frederiksen, J.L. Optical Coherence Tomography in Multiple Sclerosis. *Eye Lond. Engl.* **2018**, *32*, 884–888. [CrossRef]
20. Lightman, S.; McDonald, W.I.; Bird, A.C.; Francis, D.A.; Hoskins, A.; Batchelor, J.R.; Halliday, A.M. Retinal Venous Sheathing in Optic Neuritis. Its Significance for the Pathogenesis of Multiple Sclerosis. *Brain J. Neurol.* **1987**, *110 Pt 2*, 405–414. [CrossRef]
21. Barnett, M.H.; Henderson, A.P.; Prineas, J.W. The Macrophage in MS: Just a Scavenger after All? Pathology and Pathogenesis of the Acute MS Lesion. *Mult. Scler. J.* **2006**, *12*, 121–132. [CrossRef]
22. Duffy, S.S.; Lees, J.G.; Moalem-Taylor, G. The Contribution of Immune and Glial Cell Types in Experimental Autoimmune Encephalomyelitis and Multiple Sclerosis. *Mult. Scler. Int.* **2014**, *2014*, 285245. [CrossRef]
23. Adam, C.A.; Șalaru, D.L.; Prisacariu, C.; Marcu, D.T.M.; Sascău, R.A.; Stătescu, C. Novel Biomarkers of Atherosclerotic Vascular Disease—Latest Insights in the Research Field. *Int. J. Mol. Sci.* **2022**, *23*, 4998. [CrossRef]
24. Frontiers | Editorial: "Inside-Out"s, vs. "Outside-In" Paradigms in Multiple Sclerosis Etiopathogenesis. Available online: https://www.frontiersin.org/articles/10.3389/fncel.2021.666529/full (accessed on 14 July 2022).
25. Morgan, B.P.; Gommerman, J.L.; Ramaglia, V. An "Outside-In" and "Inside-Out" Consideration of Complement in the Multiple Sclerosis Brain: Lessons From Development and Neurodegenerative Diseases. *Front. Cell. Neurosci.* **2021**, *14*, 600656. [CrossRef]
26. Baecher-Allan, C.; Kaskow, B.J.; Weiner, H.L. Multiple Sclerosis: Mechanisms and Immunotherapy. *Neuron* **2018**, *97*, 742–768. [CrossRef]
27. Malpas, S.C. Sympathetic Nervous System Overactivity and Its Role in the Development of Cardiovascular Disease. *Physiol. Rev.* **2010**, *90*, 513–557. [CrossRef]
28. Hemmer, B.; Pinilla, C.; Gran, B.; Vergelli, M.; Ling, N.; Conlon, P.; McFarland, H.F.; Houghten, R.; Martin, R. Contribution of Individual Amino Acids Within MHC Molecule or Antigenic Peptide to TCR Ligand Potency. *J. Immunol.* **2000**, *164*, 861–871. [CrossRef]
29. Tada, T.; Takemori, T.; Okumura, K.; Nonaka, M.; Tokuhisa, T. Two Distinct Types of Helper T Cells Involved in the Secondary Antibody Response: Independent and Synergistic Effects of Ia− and Ia+ Helper T Cells. *J. Exp. Med.* **1978**, *147*, 446–458. [CrossRef]
30. Tian, A.-Y.; Zhang, R.-W.; Shi, X.-G.; Yu, H.-M. Alteration of T Helper Cell Subsets in the Optic Nerve of Experimental Autoimmune Encephalomyelitis. *Int. J. Mol. Med.* **2010**, *25*, 869–874. [CrossRef]
31. Simsek, I.; Erdem, H.; Pay, S.; Sobaci, G.; Dinc, A. Optic Neuritis Occurring with Anti-tumour Necrosis Factor α Therapy. *Ann. Rheum. Dis.* **2007**, *66*, 1255–1258. [CrossRef]
32. Traugott, U. Characterization and Distribution of Lymphocyte Subpopulations in Multiple Sclerosis Plaques versus Autoimmune Demyelinating Lesions. *Semin. Immunopathol.* **1985**, *8*, 71–95. [CrossRef]
33. Hauser, T.H.; Pinto, D.S.; Josephson, M.E.; Zimetbaum, P. Safety and Feasibility of a Clinical Pathway for the Outpatient Initiation of Antiarrhythmic Medications in Patients with Atrial Fibrillation or Atrial Flutter. *Am. J. Cardiol.* **2003**, *91*, 1437–1441. [CrossRef]
34. Losy, J. Is MS an Inflammatory or Primary Degenerative Disease? *J. Neural Transm.* **2013**, *120*, 1459–1462. [CrossRef]
35. Jacobsen, M.; Cepok, S.; Quak, E.; Happel, M.; Gaber, R.; Ziegler, A.; Schock, S.; Oertel, W.H.; Sommer, N.; Hemmer, B. Oligoclonal Expansion of Memory CD8+ T Cells in Cerebrospinal Fluid from Multiple Sclerosis Patients. *Brain* **2002**, *125*, 538–550. [CrossRef]
36. Gobin, S.J.P.; Montagne, L.; Van Zutphen, M.; Van Der Valk, P.; Van Den Elsen, P.J.; De Groot, C.J.A. Upregulation of Transcription Factors Controlling MHC Expression in Multiple Sclerosis Lesions. *Glia* **2001**, *36*, 68–77. [CrossRef]
37. Zang, Y.C.Q.; Li, S.; Rivera, V.M.; Hong, J.; Robinson, R.R.; Breitbach, W.T.; Killian, J.; Zhang, J.Z. Increased $CD8^+$ Cytotoxic T Cell Responses to Myelin Basic Protein in Multiple Sclerosis. *J. Immunol.* **2004**, *172*, 5120–5127. [CrossRef]
38. Melzer, N.; Meuth, S.G.; Wiendl, H. $CD8^+$ T Cells and Neuronal Damage: Direct and Collateral Mechanisms of Cytotoxicity and Impaired Electrical Excitability. *FASEB J.* **2009**, *23*, 3659–3673. [CrossRef]
39. Lu, L.-F.; Rudensky, A. Molecular Orchestration of Differentiation and Function of Regulatory T Cells. *Genes Dev.* **2009**, *23*, 1270–1282. [CrossRef]
40. Gregori, S.; Goudy, K.S.; Roncarolo, M.G. The Cellular and Molecular Mechanisms of Immuno-Suppression by Human Type 1 Regulatory T Cells. *Front. Immunol.* **2012**, *3*, 30. [CrossRef]

41. Schneider, A.; Long, S.A.; Cerosaletti, K.; Ni, C.T.; Samuels, P.; Kita, M.; Buckner, J.H. In Active Relapsing-Remitting Multiple Sclerosis, Effector T Cell Resistance to Adaptive T_{regs} Involves IL-6–Mediated Signaling. *Sci. Transl. Med.* **2013**, *5*, 170ra15. [CrossRef]
42. Chiarini, M.; Serana, F.; Zanotti, C.; Capra, R.; Rasia, S.; Rottoli, M.; Rovaris, M.; Caputo, D.; Cavaletti, G.; Frigo, M.; et al. Modulation of the Central Memory and Tr1-like Regulatory T Cells in Multiple Sclerosis Patients Responsive to Interferon-Beta Therapy. *Mult. Scler. J.* **2012**, *18*, 788–798. [CrossRef]
43. Lee, H.-M.; Bautista, J.L.; Scott-Browne, J.; Mohan, J.F.; Hsieh, C.-S. A Broad Range of Self-Reactivity Drives Thymic Regulatory T Cell Selection to Limit Responses to Self. *Immunity* **2012**, *37*, 475–486. [CrossRef]
44. Bielekova, B.; Catalfamo, M.; Reichert-Scrivner, S.; Packer, A.; Cerna, M.; Waldmann, T.A.; McFarland, H.; Henkart, P.A.; Martin, R. Regulatory CD56 ^{bright} Natural Killer Cells Mediate Immunomodulatory Effects of IL-2Rα-Targeted Therapy (Daclizumab) in Multiple Sclerosis. *Proc. Natl. Acad. Sci. USA* **2006**, *103*, 5941–5946. [CrossRef]
45. Morandi, B.; Bramanti, P.; Bonaccorsi, I.; Montalto, E.; Oliveri, D.; Pezzino, G.; Navarra, M.; Ferlazzo, G. Role of Natural Killer Cells in the Pathogenesis and Progression of Multiple Sclerosis. *Pharmacol. Res.* **2008**, *57*, 1–5. [CrossRef]
46. Laroni, A.; Armentani, E.; Kerlero de Rosbo, N.; Ivaldi, F.; Marcenaro, E.; Sivori, S.; Gandhi, R.; Weiner, H.L.; Moretta, A.; Mancardi, G.L.; et al. Dysregulation of Regulatory CD56 Bright NK Cells/T Cells Interactions in Multiple Sclerosis. *J. Autoimmun.* **2016**, *72*, 8–18. [CrossRef]
47. Gross, C.C.; Schulte-Mecklenbeck, A.; Rünzi, A.; Kuhlmann, T.; Posevitz-Fejfár, A.; Schwab, N.; Schneider-Hohendorf, T.; Herich, S.; Held, K.; Konjević, M.; et al. Impaired NK-Mediated Regulation of T-Cell Activity in Multiple Sclerosis Is Reconstituted by IL-2 Receptor Modulation. *Proc. Natl. Acad. Sci. USA* **2016**, *113*, E2973–E2982. [CrossRef]
48. Heidelberger, M.; Kabat, E.A.; Mayer, M. A Further Study of the Cross Reaction between the Specific Polysaccharides of Types III and VIII Pneumococci in Horse Antisera. *J. Exp. Med.* **1942**, *75*, 35–47. [CrossRef]
49. Henderson, V.W.; Guthrie, J.R.; Dennerstein, L. Serum Lipids and Memory in a Population Based Cohort of Middle Age Women. *J. Neurol. Neurosurg. Psychiatry* **2003**, *74*, 1530–1535. [CrossRef]
50. Lovato, L.; Willis, S.N.; Rodig, S.J.; Caron, T.; Almendinger, S.E.; Howell, O.W.; Reynolds, R.; O' Connor, K.C.; Hafler, D.A. Related B Cell Clones Populate the Meninges and Parenchyma of Patients with Multiple Sclerosis. *Brain* **2011**, *134*, 534–541. [CrossRef]
51. Cepok, S. Patterns of Cerebrospinal Fluid Pathology Correlate with Disease Progression in Multiple Sclerosis. *Brain* **2001**, *124*, 2169–2176. [CrossRef]
52. Serafini, B.; Rosicarelli, B.; Magliozzi, R.; Stigliano, E.; Aloisi, F. Detection of Ectopic B-Cell Follicles with Germinal Centers in the Meninges of Patients with Secondary Progressive Multiple Sclerosis. *Brain Pathol.* **2004**, *14*, 164–174. [CrossRef]
53. Naismith, R.T.; Piccio, L.; Lyons, J.A.; Lauber, J.; Tutlam, N.T.; Parks, B.J.; Trinkaus, K.; Song, S.K.; Cross, A.H. Rituximab Add-on Therapy for Breakthrough Relapsing Multiple Sclerosis: A 52-Week Phase II Trial. *Neurology* **2010**, *74*, 1860–1867. [CrossRef]
54. Rai, N.K.; Singh, V.; Li, L.; Willard, B.; Tripathi, A.; Dutta, R. Comparative Proteomic Profiling Identifies Reciprocal Expression of Mitochondrial Proteins Between White and Gray Matter Lesions From Multiple Sclerosis Brains. *Front. Neurol.* **2021**, *12*, 779003.
55. Cunniffe, N.; Coles, A. Promoting Remyelination in Multiple Sclerosis. *J. Neurol.* **2021**, *268*, 30–44. [CrossRef]
56. Sampaio-Baptista, C.; Johansen-Berg, H. White Matter Plasticity in the Adult Brain. *Neuron* **2017**, *96*, 1239–1251. [CrossRef]
57. Ffrench-Constant, C.; Raff, M.C. Proliferating Bipotential Glial Progenitor Cells in Adult Rat Optic Nerve. *Nature* **1986**, *319*, 499–502. [CrossRef]
58. Psachoulia, K.; Jamen, F.; Young, K.M.; Richardson, W.D. Cell Cycle Dynamics of NG2 Cells in the Postnatal and Ageing Mouse Brain. *Neuron Glia Biol.* **2009**, *5*, 57–67. [CrossRef]
59. Zawadzka, M.; Rivers, L.E.; Fancy, S.P.J.; Zhao, C.; Tripathi, R.; Jamen, F.; Young, K.; Goncharevich, A.; Pohl, H.; Rizzi, M.; et al. CNS-Resident Glial Progenitor/Stem Cells Produce Schwann Cells as Well as Oligodendrocytes during Repair of CNS Demyelination. *Cell Stem Cell* **2010**, *6*, 578–590. [CrossRef]
60. Blakemore, W.F. Pattern of Remyelination in the CNS. *Nature* **1974**, *249*, 577–578. [CrossRef]
61. Franklin, R.J.M.; Ffrench-Constant, C. Regenerating CNS Myelin—From Mechanisms to Experimental Medicines. *Nat. Rev. Neurosci.* **2017**, *18*, 753–769. [CrossRef]
62. Baxter, A.G. The Origin and Application of Experimental Autoimmune Encephalomyelitis. *Nat. Rev. Immunol.* **2007**, *7*, 904–912. [CrossRef]
63. Constantinescu, C.S.; Farooqi, N.; O' Brien, K.; Gran, B. Experimental Autoimmune Encephalomyelitis (EAE) as a Model for Multiple Sclerosis (MS): EAE as Model for MS. *Br. J. Pharmacol.* **2011**, *164*, 1079–1106. [CrossRef]
64. Krishnamoorthy, G.; Wekerle, H. EAE: An Immunologist' s Magic Eye: FORUM. *Eur. J. Immunol.* **2009**, *39*, 2031–2035. [CrossRef]
65. Wekerle, H. Lessons from Multiple Sclerosis: Models, Concepts, Observations. *Ann. Rheum. Dis.* **2008**, *67*, iii56–iii60. [CrossRef]
66. Drescher, K.M. Being a Mouse in a Man' s World: What TMEV Has Taught Us about Human Disease. *Front. Biosci.* **2008**, *13*, 3775–3785. [CrossRef]
67. McCarthy, D.P.; Richards, M.H.; Miller, S.D. Mouse Models of Multiple Sclerosis: Experimental Autoimmune Encephalomyelitis and Theiler' s Virus-Induced Demyelinating Disease. In *Autoimmunity: Methods in Molecular Biology*; Perl, A., Ed.; Humana Press: Totowa, NJ, USA, 2012; Volume 900, pp. 381–401, ISBN 978-1-60761-719-8.
68. Lipton, H.L. Human Vilyuisk Encephalitis. *Rev. Med. Virol.* **2008**, *18*, 347–352. [CrossRef]
69. Pachner, A.R. Experimental Models of Multiple Sclerosis. *Curr. Opin. Neurol.* **2011**, *24*, 291–299. [CrossRef]

70. Lane, T.; Buchmeier, M. Murine Coronavirus Infection: A Paradigm for Virus-Induced Demyelinating Disease. *Trends Microbiol.* **1997**, *5*, 9–14. [CrossRef]
71. Matthews, A.; Weiss, S.; Paterson, Y. Murine Hepatitis Virus–A Model for Virus-Induced CNS Demyelination. *J. Neurovirol.* **2002**, *8*, 76–85. [CrossRef]
72. van der Star, B.J.; Vogel, D.Y.S.; Kipp, M.; Puentes, F.; Baker, D.; Amor, S. In Vitro and In Vivo Models of Multiple Sclerosis. *CNS Neurol. Disord.-Drug Targets* **2012**, *11*, 570–588. [CrossRef]
73. Hesse, A.; Wagner, M.; Held, J.; Brück, W.; Salinas-Riester, G.; Hao, Z.; Waisman, A.; Kuhlmann, T. In Toxic Demyelination Oligodendroglial Cell Death Occurs Early and Is FAS Independent. *Neurobiol. Dis.* **2010**, *37*, 362–369. [CrossRef]
74. Torkildsen, Ø.; Brunborg, L.A.; Myhr, K.-M.; Bø, L. The Cuprizone Model for Demyelination. *Acta Neurol. Scand.* **2008**, *117*, 72–76. [CrossRef] [PubMed]
75. Plemel, J.R.; Michaels, N.J.; Weishaupt, N.; Caprariello, A.V.; Keough, M.B.; Rogers, J.A.; Yukseloglu, A.; Lim, J.; Patel, V.V.; Rawji, K.S.; et al. Mechanisms of Lysophosphatidylcholine-Induced Demyelination: A Primary Lipid Disrupting Myelinopathy. *Glia* **2018**, *66*, 327–347. [CrossRef] [PubMed]
76. Dehghan, S.; Aref, E.; Raoufy, M.R.; Javan, M. An Optimized Animal Model of Lysolecithin Induced Demyelination in Optic Nerve; More Feasible, More Reproducible, Promising for Studying the Progressive Forms of Multiple Sclerosis. *J. Neurosci. Methods* **2021**, *352*, 109088. [CrossRef] [PubMed]
77. GrandPré, T.; Nakamura, F.; Vartanian, T.; Strittmatter, S.M. Identification of the Nogo Inhibitor of Axon Regeneration as a Reticulon Protein. *Nature* **2000**, *403*, 439–444. [CrossRef] [PubMed]
78. McKerracher, L.; David, S.; Jackson, D.L.; Kottis, V.; Dunn, R.J.; Braun, P.E. Identification of Myelin-Associated Glycoprotein as a Major Myelin-Derived Inhibitor of Neurite Growth. *Neuron* **1994**, *13*, 805–811. [CrossRef]
79. Wang, K.C.; Kim, J.A.; Sivasankaran, R.; Segal, R.; He, Z. P75 Interacts with the Nogo Receptor as a Co-Receptor for Nogo, MAG and OMgp. *Nature* **2002**, *420*, 74–78. [CrossRef]
80. Fournier, A.E.; GrandPre, T.; Strittmatter, S.M. Identification of a Receptor Mediating Nogo-66 Inhibition of Axonal Regeneration. *Nature* **2001**, *409*, 341–346. [CrossRef]
81. Satoh, J.-I.; Onoue, H.; Arima, K.; Yamamura, T. Nogo-A and Nogo Receptor Expression in Demyelinating Lesions of Multiple Sclerosis. *J. Neuropathol. Exp. Neurol.* **2005**, *64*, 129–138. [CrossRef]
82. Huber, G.; Schuster, F.; Raasch, W. Brain Renin-Angiotensin System in the Pathophysiology of Cardiovascular Diseases. *Pharmacol. Res.* **2017**, *125*, 72–90. [CrossRef]
83. Larochelle, C.; Lécuyer, M.-A.; Alvarez, J.I.; Charabati, M.; Saint Laurent, O.; Ghannam, S.; Kebir, H.; Flanagan, K.; Yednock, T.; Duquette, P.; et al. Melanoma Cell Adhesion Molecule-Positive CD8 T Lymphocytes Mediate Central Nervous System Inflammation: MCAM $^{+}$ CD8 in Neuroinflammation. *Ann. Neurol.* **2015**, *78*, 39–53. [CrossRef]
84. Stirling, D.P.; Cummins, K.; Wayne Chen, S.R.; Stys, P. Axoplasmic Reticulum Ca^{2+} Release Causes Secondary Degeneration of Spinal Axons: Intra-Axonal Ca^{2+} Stores. *Ann. Neurol.* **2014**, *75*, 220–229. [CrossRef]
85. Bojcevski, J.; Stojic, A.; Hoffmann, D.B.; Williams, S.K.; Müller, A.; Diem, R.; Fairless, R. Influence of Retinal NMDA Receptor Activity during Autoimmune Optic Neuritis. *J. Neurochem.* **2020**, *153*, 693–709. [CrossRef]
86. Aizenman, E.; Frosch, M.P.; Lipton, S.A. Responses Mediated by Excitatory Amino Acid Receptors in Solitary Retinal Ganglion Cells from Rat. *J. Physiol.* **1988**, *396*, 75–91. [CrossRef]
87. Choi, H.J.; Byun, M.S.; Yi, D.; Choe, Y.M.; Sohn, B.K.; Baek, H.W.; Lee, J.H.; Kim, H.J.; Han, J.Y.; Yoon, E.J.; et al. Association Between Serum Triglycerides and Cerebral Amyloidosis in Cognitively Normal Elderly. *Am. J. Geriatr. Psychiatry Off. J. Am. Assoc. Geriatr. Psychiatry* **2016**, *24*, 604–612. [CrossRef]
88. Sühs, K.-W.; Wegner, F.; Skripuletz, T.; Trebst, C.; Tayeb, S.B.; Raab, P.; Stangel, M. Heterogeneity of Clinical Features and Corresponding Antibodies in Seven Patients with Anti-NMDA Receptor Encephalitis. *Exp. Ther. Med.* **2015**, *10*, 1283–1292. [CrossRef]
89. Hoffmann, D.B.; Williams, S.K.; Jovana, B.; Müller, A.; Stadelmann, C.; Naidoo, V.; Bahr, B.A.; Diem, R.; Fairless, R. Calcium Influx and Calpain Activation Mediate Preclinical Retinal Neurodegeneration in Autoimmune Optic Neuritis. *J. Neuropathol. Exp. Neurol.* **2013**, *72*, 745–757. [CrossRef]
90. Halpain, S.; Hipolito, A.; Saffer, L. Regulation of F-Actin Stability in Dendritic Spines by Glutamate Receptors and Calcineurin. *J. Neurosci.* **1998**, *18*, 9835–9844. [CrossRef]
91. Yin, H.L.; Stossel, T.P. Control of Cytoplasmic Actin Gel–Sol Transformation by Gelsolin, a Calcium-Dependent Regulatory Protein. *Nature* **1979**, *281*, 583–586. [CrossRef]
92. Kothakota, S.; Azuma, T.; Reinhard, C.; Klippel, A.; Tang, J.; Chu, K.; McGarry, T.J.; Kirschner, M.W.; Koths, K.; Kwiatkowski, D.J.; et al. Caspase-3-Generated Fragment of Gelsolin: Effector of Morphological Change in Apoptosis. *Science* **1997**, *278*, 294–298. [CrossRef]
93. Harms, C.; Bösel, J.; Lautenschlager, M.; Harms, U.; Braun, J.S.; Hörtnagl, H.; Dirnagl, U.; Kwiatkowski, D.J.; Fink, K.; Endres, M. Neuronal Gelsolin Prevents Apoptosis by Enhancing Actin Depolymerization. *Mol. Cell. Neurosci.* **2004**, *25*, 69–82. [CrossRef]
94. Brown, S.B.; Bailey, K.; Savill, J. Actin Is Cleaved during Constitutive Apoptosis. *Biochem. J.* **1997**, *323*, 233–237. [CrossRef] [PubMed]
95. Wan, E.C.K. Cellular and Molecular Mechanisms in the Pathogenesis of Multiple Sclerosis. *Cells* **2020**, *9*, 2223. [CrossRef] [PubMed]

96. Carroll, W.M.; Jennings, A.R.; Mastaglia, F.L. The Origin of Remyelinating Oligodendrocytes in Antiserum-Mediated Demyelinative Optic Neuropathy. *Brain* **1990**, *113*, 953–973. [CrossRef] [PubMed]
97. Scolding, N. Oligodendrocyte Progenitors Are Present in the Normal Adult Human CNS and in the Lesions of Multiple Sclerosis. *Brain* **1998**, *121*, 2221–2228. [CrossRef]
98. Al-Louzi, O.; Saidha, S. Pathophysiology of Optic Neuritis. *Mult. Scler. Mech. View* **2016**, 281–309. [CrossRef]
99. Rodriguez, M.; Scheithauer, B.W.; Forbes, G.; Kelly, P.J. Oligodendrocyte Injury Is an Early Event in Lesions of Multiple Sclerosis. *Mayo Clin. Proc.* **1993**, *68*, 627–636. [CrossRef]
100. Prineas, J.W.; Barnard, R.O.; Kwon, E.E.; Sharer, L.R.; Cho, E.-S. Multiple Sclerosis: Remyelination of Nascent Lesions: Remyelination of Nascent Lesions. *Ann. Neurol.* **1993**, *33*, 137–151. [CrossRef]
101. Lucchinetti, C.F.; Brück, W.; Rodriguez, M.; Lassmann, H. Distinct Patterns of Multiple Sclerosis Pathology Indicates Heterogeneity in Pathogenesis. *Brain Pathol.* **1996**, *6*, 259–274. [CrossRef] [PubMed]
102. Hanafy, K.A.; Sloane, J.A. Regulation of Remyelination in Multiple Sclerosis. *FEBS Lett.* **2011**, *585*, 3821–3828. [CrossRef]
103. Wu, L.M.N.; Williams, A.; Delaney, A.; Sherman, D.L.; Brophy, P.J. Increasing Internodal Distance in Myelinated Nerves Accelerates Nerve Conduction to a Flat Maximum. *Curr. Biol.* **2012**, *22*, 1957–1961. [CrossRef]
104. Jäkel, S.; Agirre, E.; Mendanha Falcão, A.; van Bruggen, D.; Lee, K.W.; Knuesel, I.; Malhotra, D.; ffrench-Constant, C.; Williams, A.; Castelo-Branco, G. Altered Human Oligodendrocyte Heterogeneity in Multiple Sclerosis. *Nature* **2019**, *566*, 543–547. [CrossRef] [PubMed]
105. Bodini, B.; Veronese, M.; García-Lorenzo, D.; Battaglini, M.; Poirion, E.; Chardain, A.; Freeman, L.; Louapre, C.; Tchikviladze, M.; Papeix, C.; et al. Dynamic Imaging of Individual Remyelination Profiles in Multiple Sclerosis. *Ann. Neurol.* **2016**, *79*, 726–738. [CrossRef] [PubMed]
106. Patrikios, P.; Stadelmann, C.; Kutzelnigg, A.; Rauschka, H.; Schmidbauer, M.; Laursen, H.; Sorensen, P.S.; Brück, W.; Lucchinetti, C.; Lassmann, H. Remyelination Is Extensive in a Subset of Multiple Sclerosis Patients. *Brain J. Neurol.* **2006**, *129*, 3165–3172. [CrossRef] [PubMed]
107. Sutiwisesak, R.; Burns, T.C.; Rodriguez, M.; Warrington, A.E. Remyelination Therapies for Multiple Sclerosis: Optimizing Translation from Animal Models into Clinical Trials. *Expert Opin. Investig. Drugs* **2021**, *30*, 857–876. [CrossRef] [PubMed]
108. Hooijmans, C.R.; Hlavica, M.; Schuler, F.A.F.; Good, N.; Good, A.; Baumgartner, L.; Galeno, G.; Schneider, M.P.; Jung, T.; de Vries, R.; et al. Remyelination Promoting Therapies in Multiple Sclerosis Animal Models: A Systematic Review and Meta-Analysis. *Sci. Rep.* **2019**, *9*, 822. [CrossRef]
109. Zorina, Y.; Stricker, J.; Caggiano, A.O.; Button, D.C. Human IgM Antibody RHIgM22 Promotes Phagocytic Clearance of Myelin Debris by Microglia. *Sci. Rep.* **2018**, *8*, 9392. [CrossRef]
110. Eisen, A.; Greenberg, B.M.; Bowen, J.D.; Arnold, D.L.; Caggiano, A.O. A Double-Blind, Placebo-Controlled, Single Ascending-Dose Study of Remyelinating Antibody RHIgM22 in People with Multiple Sclerosis. *Mult. Scler. J.-Exp. Transl. Clin.* **2017**, *3*, 2055217317743097. [CrossRef]
111. Green, A.J.; Gelfand, J.M.; A Cree, B.; Bevan, C.; Boscardin, W.J.; Mei, F.; Inman, J.; Arnow, S.; Devereux, M.; Abounasr, A.; et al. Clemastine fumarate as a remyelinating therapy for multiple sclerosis (ReBUILD): A randomised, controlled, double-blind, crossover trial. *Lancet* **2017**, *390*, 2481–2489. [CrossRef]
112. Pelletier, J.; Ranjeva, J.-P.; Tourbah, A.; Edan, G.; Barillot, C.; Le Lamer, S.; Audoin, B.; Rico, A.; Crespy, L.; Rid-ley, B.; et al. *Results of a Phase 1b Study to Confirm Safety and Tolerability of Olesoxime in Multiple Sclerosis Patients*; American Academy of Neurology: Minneapolis, MN, USA, 2015.
113. Magalon, K.; Zimmer, C.; Cayre, M.; Khaldi, J.; Bourbon, C.; Robles, I.; Tardif, G.; Viola, A.; Pruss, R.M.; Bordet, T.; et al. Olesoxime accelerates myelination and promotes repair in models of demyelination. *Ann. Neurol.* **2011**, *71*, 213–226. [CrossRef]
114. Bordet, T.; Berna, P.; Abitbol, J.-L.; Pruss, R.M. Olesoxime (TRO19622): A Novel Mitochondrial-Targeted Neuroprotective Compound. *Pharmaceuticals* **2010**, *3*, 345–368. [CrossRef]
115. Chiang, A.C.A.; Seua, A.V.; Singhmar, P.; Arroyo, L.D.; Mahalingam, R.; Hu, J.; Kavelaars, A.; Heijnen, C.J. Bexarotene normalizes chemotherapy-induced myelin decompaction and reverses cognitive and sensorimotor deficits in mice. *Acta Neuropathol. Commun.* **2020**, *8*, 193. [CrossRef] [PubMed]
116. A Randomised Placebo-Controlled Study of the Safety and Tolerability of a Retinoid-X Receptor Agonist' s Ability to Promote Remyelination in People with Relapsing-Remitting Multiple Sclerosis Already on Interferon-Beta Therapy: A Phase 2a Trial-AdisInsight. Available online: https://adisinsight.springer.com/trials/700259921 (accessed on 29 August 2022).
117. Shen, X.; Liu, W.; Gao, X.; Lu, Z.; Wu, X.; Gao, X. Mechanisms of Oxidase and Superoxide Dismutation-like Activities of Gold, Silver, Platinum, and Palladium, and Their Alloys: A General Way to the Activation of Molecular Oxygen. *J. Am. Chem. Soc.* **2015**, *137*, 15882–15891. [CrossRef] [PubMed]
118. Clene Nanomedicine VISIONARY-MS LTE: A Multi-Center, Open-Label Long-Term Extension Study Assessing the Safety, Efficacy, Tolerability, and Pharmacokinetics of CNM-Au8 In Patients With Stable Relapsing Multiple Sclerosis. 2022. Available online: https://clinicaltrials.gov/ (accessed on 20 August 2022).
119. Koch, M.W.; Liu, W.-Q.; Camara-Lemarroy, C.; Zhang, Y.; Pike, G.B.; Metz, L.; Yong, V.W. Domperidone-induced elevation of serum prolactin levels and immune response in multiple sclerosis. *J. Neuroimmunol.* **2019**, *334*, 576974. [CrossRef]
120. Zhornitsky, S.; Yong, V.W.; Weiss, S.; Metz, L.M. Prolactin in multiple sclerosis. *Mult. Scler. J.* **2012**, *19*, 15–23. [CrossRef]

121. Jepson, S.; Vought, B.; Gross, C.H.; Gan, L.; Austen, D.; Frantz, J.D.; Zwahlen, J.; Lowe, D.; Markland, W.; Krauss, R. LINGO-1, a Transmembrane Signaling Protein, Inhibits Oligodendrocyte Differentiation and Myelination through Intercellular Self-interactions. *J. Biol. Chem.* **2012**, *287*, 22184–22195. [CrossRef] [PubMed]
122. Tran, J.Q.; Rana, J.; Barkhof, F.; Melamed, I.; Gevorkyan, H.; Wattjes, M.P.; de Jong, R.; Brosofsky, K.; Ray, S.; Xu, L.; et al. Randomized phase I trials of the safety/tolerability of anti-LINGO-1 monoclonal antibody BIIB033. Neurol.-Neuroimmunol. *Neuroinflammation* **2014**, *1*, e18. [CrossRef]
123. Cadavid, D.; Balcer, L.; Galetta, S.; Aktas, O.; Ziemssen, T.; Vanopdenbosch, L.; Frederiksen, J.; Skeen, M.; Jaffe, G.J.; Butzkueven, H.; et al. Safety and efficacy of opicinumab in acute optic neuritis (RENEW): A randomised, placebo-controlled, phase 2 trial. *Lancet Neurol.* **2017**, *16*, 189–199. [CrossRef]
124. Cadavid, D.; Mellion, M.; Hupperts, R.; Edwards, K.R.; A Calabresi, P.; Drulović, J.; Giovannoni, G.; Hartung, H.-P.; Arnold, D.L.; Fisher, E.; et al. Safety and efficacy of opicinumab in patients with relapsing multiple sclerosis (SYNERGY): A randomised, placebo-controlled, phase 2 trial. *Lancet Neurol.* **2019**, *18*, 845–856. [CrossRef]
125. Kale, N. Optic Neuritis as an Early Sign of Multiple Sclerosis. *Eye Brain* **2016**, *8*, 195–202. [CrossRef]
126. Mamarabadi, M.; Razjouyan, H.; Mohammadi, F.; Moghaddasi, M. Assessment of Outcome Predictors after First Attack of Optic Neuritis. *Can. J. Neurol. Sci. J. Can. Sci. Neurol.* **2011**, *38*, 887–895. [CrossRef]
127. Frohman, E.; Costello, F.; Zivadinov, R.; Stuve, O.; Conger, A.; Winslow, H.; Trip, A.; Frohman, T.; Balcer, L. Optical Coherence Tomography in Multiple Sclerosis. *Lancet Neurol.* **2006**, *5*, 853–863. [CrossRef]
128. Thompson, A.J.; Banwell, B.L.; Barkhof, F.; Carroll, W.M.; Coetzee, T.; Comi, G.; Correale, J.; Fazekas, F.; Filippi, M.; Freedman, M.S.; et al. Diagnosis of Multiple Sclerosis: 2017 Revisions of the McDonald Criteria. *Lancet Neurol.* **2018**, *17*, 162–173. [CrossRef]
129. Bove, R.M.; Hauser, S.L. Diagnosing Multiple Sclerosis: Art and Science. *Lancet Neurol.* **2018**, *17*, 109–111. [CrossRef]
130. Kupersmith, M.J.; Alban, T.; Zeiffer, B.; Lefton, D. Contrast-Enhanced MRI in Acute Optic Neuritis: Relationship to Visual Performance. *Brain J. Neurol.* **2002**, *125*, 812–822. [CrossRef]
131. Bennett, J.L. Optic Neuritis. *Contin. Minneap. Minn* **2019**, *25*, 1236–1264. [CrossRef]
132. Swanton, J.K.; Fernando, K.T.; Dalton, C.M.; Miszkiel, K.A.; Altmann, D.R.; Plant, G.T.; Thompson, A.J.; Miller, D.H. Early MRI in Optic Neuritis: The Risk for Disability. *Neurology* **2009**, *72*, 542–550. [CrossRef] [PubMed]
133. Hoorbakht, H.; Bagherkashi, F. Optic Neuritis, Its Differential Diagnosis and Management. *Open Ophthalmol. J.* **2012**, *6*, 65–72. [CrossRef]
134. Optic Neuritis Study Group Multiple Sclerosis Risk after Optic Neuritis: Final Optic Neuritis Treatment Trial Follow-Up. *Arch. Neurol.* **2008**, *65*, 727–732. [CrossRef]
135. Lebrun, C.; Bensa, C.; Debouverie, M.; Wiertlevski, S.; Brassat, D.; de Seze, J.; Rumbach, L.; Pelletier, J.; Labauge, P.; Brochet, B.; et al. Association between Clinical Conversion to Multiple Sclerosis in Radiologically Isolated Syndrome and Magnetic Resonance Imaging, Cerebrospinal Fluid, and Visual Evoked Potential: Follow-up of 70 Patients. *Arch. Neurol.* **2009**, *66*, 841–846. [CrossRef]
136. Brownlee, W.J.; Miszkiel, K.A.; Tur, C.; Barkhof, F.; Miller, D.H.; Ciccarelli, O. Inclusion of Optic Nerve Involvement in Dissemination in Space Criteria for Multiple Sclerosis. *Neurology* **2018**, *91*, e1130–e1134. [CrossRef]
137. Tintoré, M.; Rovira, A.; Río, J.; Nos, C.; Grivé, E.; Sastre-Garriga, J.; Pericot, I.; Sánchez, E.; Comabella, M.; Montalban, X. New Diagnostic Criteria for Multiple Sclerosis: Application in First Demyelinating Episode. *Neurology* **2003**, *60*, 27–30. [CrossRef] [PubMed]
138. Petzold, A.; Wattjes, M.P.; Costello, F.; Flores-Rivera, J.; Fraser, C.L.; Fujihara, K.; Leavitt, J.; Marignier, R.; Paul, F.; Schippling, S.; et al. The Investigation of Acute Optic Neuritis: A Review and Proposed Protocol. *Nat. Rev. Neurol.* **2014**, *10*, 447–458. [CrossRef] [PubMed]
139. Chan, J.W. Recent Advances in Optic Neuritis Related to Multiple Sclerosis. *Acta Ophthalmol.* **2012**, *90*, 203–209. [CrossRef]
140. Zafeiropoulos, P.; Katsanos, A.; Kitsos, G.; Stefaniotou, M.; Asproudis, I. The Contribution of Multifocal Visual Evoked Potentials in Patients with Optic Neuritis and Multiple Sclerosis: A Review. *Doc. Ophthalmol. Adv. Ophthalmol.* **2021**, *142*, 283–292. [CrossRef] [PubMed]
141. Hood, D.C.; Odel, J.G.; Winn, B.J. The Multifocal Visual Evoked Potential. *J. Neuro-Ophthalmol. Off. J. N. Am. Neuro-Ophthalmol. Soc.* **2003**, *23*, 279–289. [CrossRef] [PubMed]
142. Fraser, C.; Klistorner, A.; Graham, S.; Garrick, R.; Billson, F.; Grigg, J. Multifocal Visual Evoked Potential Latency Analysis: Predicting Progression to Multiple Sclerosis. *Arch. Neurol.* **2006**, *63*, 847–850. [CrossRef]
143. Klistorner, A.; Arvind, H.; Nguyen, T.; Garrick, R.; Paine, M.; Graham, S.; Yiannikas, C. Fellow Eye Changes in Optic Neuritis Correlate with the Risk of Multiple Sclerosis. *Mult. Scler. Houndmills Basingstoke Engl.* **2009**, *15*, 928–932. [CrossRef] [PubMed]
144. Pihl-Jensen, G.; Schmidt, M.F.; Frederiksen, J.L. Multifocal Visual Evoked Potentials in Optic Neuritis and Multiple Sclerosis: A Review. *Clin. Neurophysiol. Off. J. Int. Fed. Clin. Neurophysiol.* **2017**, *128*, 1234–1245. [CrossRef]
145. Klistorner, A.; Fraser, C.; Garrick, R.; Graham, S.; Arvind, H. Correlation between Full-Field and Multifocal VEPs in Optic Neuritis. *Doc. Ophthalmol. Adv. Ophthalmol.* **2008**, *116*, 19–27. [CrossRef]
146. De Santiago, L.; Ortiz Del Castillo, M.; Blanco, R.; Barea, R.; Rodríguez-Ascariz, J.M.; Miguel-Jiménez, J.M.; Sánchez-Morla, E.M.; Boquete, L. A Signal-to-Noise-Ratio-Based Analysis of Multifocal Visual-Evoked Potentials in Multiple Sclerosis Risk Assessment. *Clin. Neurophysiol. Off. J. Int. Fed. Clin. Neurophysiol.* **2016**, *127*, 1574–1580. [CrossRef]

147. Petrillo, J.; Balcer, L.; Galetta, S.; Chai, Y.; Xu, L.; Cadavid, D. Initial Impairment and Recovery of Vision-Related Functioning in Participants With Acute Optic Neuritis From the RENEW Trial of Opicinumab. *J. Neuro-Ophthalmol. Off. J. N. Am. Neuro-Ophthalmol. Soc.* **2019**, *39*, 153–160. [CrossRef] [PubMed]
148. Grover, L.K.; Hood, D.C.; Ghadiali, Q.; Grippo, T.M.; Wenick, A.S.; Greenstein, V.C.; Behrens, M.M.; Odel, J.G. A Comparison of Multifocal and Conventional Visual Evoked Potential Techniques in Patients with Optic Neuritis/Multiple Sclerosis. *Doc. Ophthalmol. Adv. Ophthalmol.* **2008**, *117*, 121–128. [CrossRef] [PubMed]
149. Klistorner, A.; Arvind, H.; Nguyen, T.; Garrick, R.; Paine, M.; Graham, S.; O' Day, J.; Yiannikas, C. Multifocal VEP and OCT in Optic Neuritis: A Topographical Study of the Structure-Function Relationship. *Doc. Ophthalmol. Adv. Ophthalmol.* **2009**, *118*, 129–137. [CrossRef]
150. Laron, M.; Cheng, H.; Zhang, B.; Schiffman, J.S.; Tang, R.A.; Frishman, L.J. Comparison of Multifocal Visual Evoked Potential, Standard Automated Perimetry and Optical Coherence Tomography in Assessing Visual Pathway in Multiple Sclerosis Patients. *Mult. Scler. Houndmills Basingstoke Engl.* **2010**, *16*, 412–426. [CrossRef]
151. Olesen, M.N.; Soelberg, K.; Debrabant, B.; Nilsson, A.C.; Lillevang, S.T.; Grauslund, J.; Brandslund, I.; Madsen, J.S.; Paul, F.; Smith, T.J.; et al. Cerebrospinal Fluid Biomarkers for Predicting Development of Multiple Sclerosis in Acute Optic Neuritis: A Population-Based Prospective Cohort Study. *J. Neuroinflamm.* **2019**, *16*, 59. [CrossRef]
152. Ottervald, J.; Franzén, B.; Nilsson, K.; Andersson, L.I.; Khademi, M.; Eriksson, B.; Kjellström, S.; Marko-Varga, G.; Végvári, Á.; Harris, R.A.; et al. Multiple Sclerosis: Identification and Clinical Evaluation of Novel CSF Biomarkers. *J. Proteom.* **2010**, *73*, 1117–1132. [CrossRef]
153. Weinshenker, B.G.; Wingerchuk, D.M. Neuromyelitis Spectrum Disorders. *Mayo Clin. Proc.* **2017**, *92*, 663–679. [CrossRef] [PubMed]
154. Frederiksen, J.L.; Larsson, H.B.; Olesen, J. Correlation of Magnetic Resonance Imaging and CSF Findings in Patients with Acute Monosymptomatic Optic Neuritis. *Acta Neurol. Scand.* **1992**, *86*, 317–322. [CrossRef]
155. Tumani, H.; Hartung, H.-P.; Hemmer, B.; Teunissen, C.; Deisenhammer, F.; Giovannoni, G.; Zettl, U.K. Cerebrospinal Fluid Biomarkers in Multiple Sclerosis. *Neurobiol. Dis.* **2009**, *35*, 117–127. [CrossRef]
156. Uhlig, H.H. Monogenic Diseases Associated with Intestinal Inflammation: Implications for the Understanding of Inflammatory Bowel Disease. *Gut* **2013**, *62*, 1795–1805. [CrossRef]
157. Nakashima, I.; Fujihara, K.; Misu, T.; Okita, N.; Takase, S.; Itoyama, Y. Significant Correlation between IL-10 Levels and IgG Indices in the Cerebrospinal Fluid of Patients with Multiple Sclerosis. *J. Neuroimmunol.* **2000**, *111*, 64–67. [CrossRef]
158. Ries, S.; Hilgenberg, E.; Lampropoulou, V.; Shen, P.; Dang, V.D.; Wilantri, S.; Sakwa, I.; Fillatreau, S. B-Type Suppression: A Role Played by "Regulatory B Cells" or "Regulatory Plasma Cells"? *Eur. J. Immunol.* **2014**, *44*, 1251–1257. [CrossRef] [PubMed]
159. Jarius, S.; Ruprecht, K.; Kleiter, I.; Borisow, N.; Asgari, N.; Pitarokoili, K.; Pache, F.; Stich, O.; Beume, L.-A.; Hümmert, M.W.; et al. MOG-IgG in NMO and Related Disorders: A Multicenter Study of 50 Patients. Part 2: Epidemiology, Clinical Presentation, Radiological and Laboratory Features, Treatment Responses, and Long-Term Outcome. *J. Neuroinflamm.* **2016**, *13*, 280. [CrossRef]
160. Jarius, S.; Paul, F.; Franciotta, D.; Ruprecht, K.; Ringelstein, M.; Bergamaschi, R.; Rommer, P.; Kleiter, I.; Stich, O.; Reuss, R.; et al. Cerebrospinal Fluid Findings in Aquaporin-4 Antibody Positive Neuromyelitis Optica: Results from 211 Lumbar Punctures. *J. Neurol. Sci.* **2011**, *306*, 82–90. [CrossRef] [PubMed]
161. Andersen, S.L.; Briggs, F.B.S.; Winnike, J.H.; Natanzon, Y.; Maichle, S.; Knagge, K.J.; Newby, L.K.; Gregory, S.G. Metabolome-Based Signature of Disease Pathology in MS. *Mult. Scler. Relat. Disord.* **2019**, *31*, 12–21. [CrossRef]
162. Liu, Z.; Waters, J.; Rui, B. Metabolomics as a Promising Tool for Improving Understanding of Multiple Sclerosis: A Review of Recent Advances. *Biomed. J.* 2022, *in press*. [CrossRef]
163. Housley, W.J.; Pitt, D.; Hafler, D.A. Biomarkers in Multiple Sclerosis. *Clin. Immunol.* **2015**, *161*, 51–58. [CrossRef]
164. Wishart, D.S. Emerging Applications of Metabolomics in Drug Discovery and Precision Medicine. *Nat. Rev. Drug Discov.* **2016**, *15*, 473–484. [CrossRef]
165. Reinke, S.; Broadhurst, D.; Sykes, B.; Baker, G.; Catz, I.; Warren, K.; Power, C. Metabolomic Profiling in Multiple Sclerosis: Insights into Biomarkers and Pathogenesis. *Mult. Scler. J.* **2014**, *20*, 1396–1400. [CrossRef]
166. Lutz, N.W.; Viola, A.; Malikova, I.; Confort-Gouny, S.; Audoin, B.; Ranjeva, J.-P.; Pelletier, J.; Cozzone, P.J. Inflammatory Multiple-Sclerosis Plaques Generate Characteristic Metabolic Profiles in Cerebrospinal Fluid. *PLoS ONE* **2007**, *2*, e595. [CrossRef]
167. Jenkins, T.M.; Toosy, A.T. Optic Neuritis: The Eye as a Window to the Brain. *Curr. Opin. Neurol.* **2017**, *30*, 61–66. [CrossRef] [PubMed]
168. Iorga, R.E.; Moraru, A.; Ozturk, M.R.; Costin, D. The Role of Optical Coherence Tomography in Optic Neuropathies. *Rom. J. Ophthalmol.* **2018**, *62*, 3–14. [CrossRef]
169. Trip, S.A.; Schlottmann, P.G.; Jones, S.J.; Altmann, D.R.; Garway-Heath, D.F.; Thompson, A.J.; Plant, G.T.; Miller, D.H. Retinal Nerve Fiber Layer Axonal Loss and Visual Dysfunction in Optic Neuritis. *Ann. Neurol.* **2005**, *58*, 383–391. [CrossRef] [PubMed]
170. Costello, F.; Coupland, S.; Hodge, W.; Lorello, G.R.; Koroluk, J.; Pan, Y.I.; Freedman, M.S.; Zackon, D.H.; Kardon, R.H. Quantifying Axonal Loss after Optic Neuritis with Optical Coherence Tomography. *Ann. Neurol.* **2006**, *59*, 963–969. [CrossRef] [PubMed]
171. Saidha, S.; Syc, S.B.; Ibrahim, M.A.; Eckstein, C.; Warner, C.V.; Farrell, S.K.; Oakley, J.D.; Durbin, M.K.; Meyer, S.A.; Balcer, L.J.; et al. Primary Retinal Pathology in Multiple Sclerosis as Detected by Optical Coherence Tomography. *Brain* **2011**, *134*, 518–533. [CrossRef]

172. Burkholder, B.M.; Osborne, B.; Loguidice, M.J.; Bisker, E.; Frohman, T.C.; Conger, A.; Ratchford, J.N.; Warner, C.; Markowitz, C.E.; Jacobs, D.A.; et al. Macular Volume Determined by Optical Coherence Tomography as a Measure of Neuronal Loss in Multiple Sclerosis. *Arch. Neurol.* **2009**, *66*, 1366–1372. [CrossRef]
173. Kupersmith, M.J.; Mandel, G.; Anderson, S.; Meltzer, D.E.; Kardon, R. Baseline, One and Three Month Changes in the Peripapillary Retinal Nerve Fiber Layer in Acute Optic Neuritis: Relation to Baseline Vision and MRI. *J. Neurol. Sci.* **2011**, *308*, 117–123. [CrossRef]
174. Chen, J.J.; Sotirchos, E.S.; Henderson, A.D.; Vasileiou, E.S.; Flanagan, E.P.; Bhatti, M.T.; Jamali, S.; Eggenberger, E.R.; Dinome, M.; Frohman, L.P.; et al. OCT Retinal Nerve Fiber Layer Thickness Differentiates Acute Optic Neuritis from MOG Antibody-Associated Disease and Multiple Sclerosis. *Mult. Scler. Relat. Disord.* **2022**, *58*, 103525. [CrossRef]
175. Lochner, P.; Leone, M.A.; Coppo, L.; Nardone, R.; Zedde, M.L.; Cantello, R.; Brigo, F. B-Mode Transorbital Ultrasononography for the Diagnosis of Acute Optic Neuritis. A Systematic Review. *Clin. Neurophysiol. Off. J. Int. Fed. Clin. Neurophysiol.* **2016**, *127*, 803–809. [CrossRef]
176. Phuljhele, S.; Kedar, S.; Saxena, R. Approach to Optic Neuritis: An Update. *Indian J. Ophthalmol.* **2021**, *69*, 2266–2276. [CrossRef]
177. Wilhelm, H.; Schabet, M. The Diagnosis and Treatment of Optic Neuritis. *Dtsch. Ärztebl. Int.* **2015**, *112*, 616–626. [CrossRef] [PubMed]
178. Marcu, D.T.M.; Adam, C.A.; Dorobanțu, D.-M.; Șalaru, D.L.; Sascău, R.A.; Balasanian, M.O.; Macovei, L.; Arsenescu-Georgescu, C.; Stătescu, C. Beta-Blocker-Related Atrioventricular Conduction Disorders—A Single Tertiary Referral Center Experience. *Medicina* **2022**, *58*, 320. [CrossRef] [PubMed]
179. Marcu, D.T.M.; Arsenescu-Georgescu, C. Adverse Drug Reactions and Atrioventricular Conduction Disorders—A Female Gender Related Aproach. *Intern. Med.* **2021**, *18*, 15–29. [CrossRef]
180. Shan, F.; Long, Y.; Qiu, W. Autoimmune Glial Fibrillary Acidic Protein Astrocytopathy: A Review of the Literature. *Front. Immunol.* **2018**, *9*, 2802. [CrossRef]
181. Flanagan, E.P.; Hinson, S.R.; Lennon, V.A.; Fang, B.; Aksamit, A.J.; Morris, P.P.; Basal, E.; Honorat, J.A.; Alfugham, N.B.; Linnoila, J.J.; et al. Glial Fibrillary Acidic Protein Immunoglobulin G as Biomarker of Autoimmune Astrocytopathy: Analysis of 102 Patients. *Ann. Neurol.* **2017**, *81*, 298–309. [CrossRef]
182. Papadopoulos, M.C.; Verkman, A.S. Aquaporin 4 and Neuromyelitis Optica. *Lancet Neurol.* **2012**, *11*, 535–544. [CrossRef]
183. Lennon, V.A.; Kryzer, T.J.; Pittock, S.J.; Verkman, A.S.; Hinson, S.R. IgG Marker of Optic-Spinal Multiple Sclerosis Binds to the Aquaporin-4 Water Channel. *J. Exp. Med.* **2005**, *202*, 473–477. [CrossRef]
184. Collongues, N.; de Seze, J. Current and Future Treatment Approaches for Neuromyelitis Optica. *Ther. Adv. Neurol. Disord.* **2011**, *4*, 111–121. [CrossRef]
185. Tradtrantip, L.; Zhang, H.; Saadoun, S.; Phuan, P.-W.; Lam, C.; Papadopoulos, M.C.; Bennett, J.L.; Verkman, A.S. Anti-Aquaporin-4 Monoclonal Antibody Blocker Therapy for Neuromyelitis Optica. *Ann. Neurol.* **2012**, *71*, 314–322. [CrossRef]
186. Tradtrantip, L.; Zhang, H.; Anderson, M.O.; Saadoun, S.; Phuan, P.-W.; Papadopoulos, M.C.; Bennett, J.L.; Verkman, A.S. Small-Molecule Inhibitors of NMO-IgG Binding to Aquaporin-4 Reduce Astrocyte Cytotoxicity in Neuromyelitis Optica. *FASEB J. Off. Publ. Fed. Am. Soc. Exp. Biol.* **2012**, *26*, 2197–2208. [CrossRef]
187. Saadoun, S.; Waters, P.; MacDonald, C.; Bell, B.A.; Vincent, A.; Verkman, A.S.; Papadopoulos, M.C. Neutrophil Protease Inhibition Reduces Neuromyelitis Optica-Immunoglobulin G-Induced Damage in Mouse Brain. *Ann. Neurol.* **2012**, *71*, 323–333. [CrossRef] [PubMed]
188. Herges, K.; de Jong, B.A.; Kolkowitz, I.; Dunn, C.; Mandelbaum, G.; Ko, R.M.; Maini, A.; Han, M.H.; Killestein, J.; Polman, C.; et al. Protective Effect of an Elastase Inhibitor in a Neuromyelitis Optica-like Disease Driven by a Peptide of Myelin Oligodendroglial Glycoprotein. *Mult. Scler. Houndmills Basingstoke Engl.* **2012**, *18*, 398–408. [CrossRef] [PubMed]
189. Zhang, H.; Bennett, J.L.; Verkman, A.S. Ex Vivo Spinal Cord Slice Model of Neuromyelitis Optica Reveals Novel Immunopathogenic Mechanisms. *Ann. Neurol.* **2011**, *70*, 943–954. [CrossRef]
190. Smith, K.J. Sodium Channels and Multiple Sclerosis: Roles in Symptom Production, Damage and Therapy. *Brain Pathol.* **2007**, *17*, 230–242. [CrossRef] [PubMed]
191. da Silva-Junior, A.J.; Mesentier-Louro, L.A.; Nascimento-dos-Santos, G.; Teixeira-Pinheiro, L.C.; Vasques, J.F.; Chimeli-Ormonde, L.; Bodart-Santos, V.; de Carvalho, L.R.P.; Santiago, M.F.; Mendez-Otero, R. Human Mesenchymal Stem Cell Therapy Promotes Retinal Ganglion Cell Survival and Target Reconnection after Optic Nerve Crush in Adult Rats. *Stem Cell Res. Ther.* **2021**, *12*, 69. [CrossRef] [PubMed]
192. Labrador-Velandia, S.; Alonso-Alonso, M.L.; Alvarez-Sanchez, S.; González-Zamora, J.; Carretero-Barrio, I.; Pastor, J.C.; Fernandez-Bueno, I.; Srivastava, G.K. Mesenchymal Stem Cell Therapy in Retinal and Optic Nerve Diseases: An Update of Clinical Trials. *World J. Stem Cells* **2016**, *8*, 376–383. [CrossRef] [PubMed]
193. Nicoară, S.D.; Brie, I.; Jurj, A.; Sorițău, O. The Future of Stem Cells and Their Derivates in the Treatment of Glaucoma. A Critical Point of View. *Int. J. Mol. Sci.* **2021**, *22*, 11077. [CrossRef]
194. Aneesh, A.; Liu, A.; Moss, H.E.; Feinstein, D.; Ravindran, S.; Mathew, B.; Roth, S. Emerging Concepts in the Treatment of Optic Neuritis: Mesenchymal Stem Cell-Derived Extracellular Vesicles. *Stem Cell Res. Ther.* **2021**, *12*, 594. [CrossRef]

current issues in molecular biology

MDPI

Article

Pro-Inflammatory and Pro-Apoptotic Effects of the Non-Protein Amino Acid L-Azetidine-2-Carboxylic Acid in BV2 Microglial Cells

Jordan Allan Piper [1], Margo Iris Jansen [1], Sarah Thomas Broome [1], Kenneth J. Rodgers [2], Giuseppe Musumeci [3,4] and Alessandro Castorina [1,*]

[1] Laboratory of Cellular and Molecular Neuroscience (LCMN), School of Life Sciences, Faculty of Science, University of Technology Sydney, P.O. Box 123, Broadway, Sydney, NSW 2007, Australia
[2] Neurotoxin Research Group, School of Life Sciences, Faculty of Science, University of Technology Sydney, P.O. Box 123, Broadway, Sydney, NSW 2007, Australia
[3] Department of Biomedical and Biotechnological Sciences, Anatomy, Histology and Movement Science Section, School of Medicine, University of Catania, Via S. Sofia No. 87, 95123 Catania, Italy
[4] Research Center on Motor Activities (CRAM), University of Catania, Via S. Sofia No. 97, 95123 Catania, Italy
* Correspondence: alessandro.castorina@uts.edu.au

Abstract: L-Azetidine-2-carboxylic acid (AZE) is a toxic non-protein coding amino acid (npAA) that is highly abundant in sugar and table beets. Due to its structural similarity with the amino acid L-proline, AZE can evade the editing process during protein assembly in eukaryotic cells and be misincorporated into L-proline-rich proteins, potentially causing protein misfolding and other detrimental effects to cells. In this study, we sought to determine if AZE treatment triggered pro-inflammatory and pro-apoptotic responses in BV2 microglial cells. BV2 microglial cells exposed to AZE at increasing concentrations (0–2000 μM) at 0, 3, 6, 12 and 24 h were assayed for cell viability (MTT) and nitric oxide release (Griess assay). Annexin V-FITC/propidium iodide (PI) staining was used to assess apoptosis. Real-time qPCR, Western blot and immunocytochemistry were used to interrogate relevant pro- and anti-inflammatory and other molecular targets of cell survival response. AZE (at concentrations > 1000 μM) significantly reduced cell viability, increased BAX/Bcl2 ratio and caused cell death. Results were mirrored by a robust increase in nitric oxide release, percentage of activated/polarised cells and expression of pro-inflammatory markers (*IL-1β*, *IL-6*, *NOS2*, *CD68* and *MHC-2a*). Additionally, we found that AZE induced the expression of the extracellular matrix degrading enzyme matrix metalloproteinase 9 (*MMP-9*) and brain derived neurotrophic factor (*BDNF*), two critical regulators of microglial motility and structural plasticity. Collectively, these data indicate that AZE-induced toxicity is associated with increased pro-inflammatory activity and reduced survival in BV2 microglia. This evidence may prompt for an increased monitoring of AZE consumption by humans.

Keywords: L-azetidine-2-carboxylic acid; microglia; beets; multiple sclerosis; non-protein amino acid; neuroinflammation; environmental toxin

1. Introduction

In nature, in addition to the 20 canonical amino acids involved in protein assembly in eukaryotic cells, there are hundreds of plant-derived amino acids, namely non-protein amino acids (npAAs) [1]. In some cases a npAA can mimic a protein amino acid and replace it in a physiological process; including as a substrate in protein synthesis [1]. Some of these 'proteinogenic' npAAs are secreted by plants as deterrents against predation, as well as growth inhibitors for competing plants in a phenomenon known as allelopathy [2]. In part owing to their relatively low concentrations and their negligible nutritional value, npAAs have been often overlooked, although there is growing evidence suggesting that prolonged exposure or their undetected entry in the food chain may cause significant biochemical changes and pose a risk to human health [3,4].

L-Azetidine-2-carboxylic acid (AZE), firstly identified by Dr Rubenstein in table beets and sugar beets in 2006 [5], is a proteinogenic npAA potentially implicated in multiple sclerosis (MS) pathogenesis [6]. AZE shares high structural similarity with L-proline, a protein-coding amino acid that is abundant in collagen, keratin, hemoglobin and core myelin proteins [5]. Due to its ability to evade recognition by transfer RNAs, the impostor AZE evades the editing process and is erroneously misplaced in lieu of the authentic L-proline, causing structural changes to L-proline-containing proteins [6]. According to Rubenstein's initial theory [6], more recently supported by an interesting work from his colleagues [7], AZE misplacement increases the immunogenicity of certain myelin proteins, to likely initiate the autoimmune events leading to oligodendrogliopathy [8] and microgliosis [9], two known pathogenic features of MS.

In humans, myelination of the central nervous system (CNS) occurs during late gestational age and perinatal period, to then progressively reduce during early childhood development [10]. It is during this developmental stage that myelin, myelin-producing cells and other CNS cell types are more plastic, but also more susceptible to pathological changes [11]. In view of AZE ability to misincorporate into proteins and cause structural alterations, it is reasonable to hypothesise that the detrimental effects of AZE can extend beyond myelin or oligodendrocytes, and perhaps affect more broadly other cell populations within the CNS, including microglia.

Perturbations in protein assembly can lead to protein misfolding [12], and the accumulation of misfolded proteins triggers endoplasmic reticulum (ER)-stress [13]. However, the ER is equipped with highly specific signalling pathways called the unfolded protein response (UPR) to cope with the accumulation of unfolded or misfolded proteins [12].

Recently, UPR has been studied in myeloid cells, where it was demonstrated to act as a fundamental proteostatic pathway to coordinate inflammatory responses [14]. Microglia, the resident innate immune cell of the CNS, are responsible for the ongoing CNS surveillance, the release of pro-inflammatory factors and act as scavengers to clear cellular and toxic debris [15]. Depending on the nature of the insult/stimulus, microglial cells undergo dynamic morphological and functional changes ranging from quiescent/resting state to either polarised/activated pro-inflammatory or anti-inflammatory states [16]. Current evidence suggests that prolonged microglial polarisation may promote neuronal damage and aggravate oligodendroglial pathology, similar to what we see in neuroinflammatory diseases such as MS [17,18]. For such reasons, aberrantly activated microglia have also been implicated in the pathogenic cascade of a diverse range of neurodegenerative diseases, including demyelinating ones [18].

In the recent work by Sobel et al., [7], the authors provide evidence that AZE supplementation in rodents triggers the UPR in the CNS white matter, which is associated with the appearance of microglial nodules and the activation of pro-inflammatory signalling. However, whether this is due to a direct effect on microglia or it is secondary to oligodendrocyte or myelin damage remains to be established. To address this issue, using an in vitro model of AZE toxicity, we aimed at investigating the biological effects of AZE exposure in murine BV2 microglial cells.

2. Materials and Methods

2.1. Cell Culture and Treatments

The study was carried out using the murine microglial BV2 cell line. Cells were grown in Dulbecco's modified Eagle's medium (DMEM)/F12 and were supplemented with 10% heat-inactivated fetal bovine serum (FBS), 2 mM L-glutamine, 100 U/mL penicillin and 200 μg/mL streptomycin (Sigma–Aldrich, Castle Hill, NSW, Australia). Cells were seeded in T25 flasks at a density of 1×10^5 cells. Cells were maintained at 37 °C in a humidified atmosphere with 5% CO_2 in air. Cells were incubated until they reached 75–80% confluence before being used for experimental testing. Upon treatment, cell media was replaced with either fresh DMEM (for untreated controls), or media containing increasing concentrations of AZE (0–2000 μM; A0760, Sigma-Aldrich, Castle Hill, NSW, Australia). For this purpose, a 100 mM AZE stock solution was freshly prepared and diluted as required. Cells exposed or not to AZE were then placed in a CO_2 incubator for different time points, depending on the assay.

2.2. MTT Assay

To assess cell viability, we used the Cell Proliferation Kit I (MTT) following manufacturer's instructions (Cat #11465007001, Sigma-Aldrich, Castle Hill, NSW, Australia). Cells were seeded into 96-well plates at a concentration of 1×10^4 cells/well. DMEM containing 0.5 mg/mL 3-[4,5-dimethylthiazol-2-yl]-2,5-diphenyltetrazolium bromide (MTT) (Sigma–Aldrich) was added in each well. Following incubation for 4 h at 37 °C, medium was removed, and 100 µL of DMSO was added. Formazan formed by the cleavage of the yellow tetrazolium salt MTT was analysed using a spectrophotometer by measuring absorbance change at 550–600 nm using a microplate reader.

2.3. Griess Assay

Griess assay was performed as indicated in previous work [19]. The assay was specifically used to measure the relative abundance of nitric oxide (NO) released by BV2 microglia upon stimulation with AZE. Cells were seeded at 2×10^4 cells per well in a 96-well plate and incubated at 37 °C with 5% CO_2 until cells reached 80% confluence. Cells were treated with either control media or increasing concentrations of AZE (0, 125, 250, 500, 1000 and 2000 µM) for 0, 3, 6, 12 and 24 h. The supernatant was collected and placed into a new 96-well plate. A total of 100 µL of freshly prepared Griess reagent was then added to each well and incubated at room temperature for 15 min on a slow oscillation protected from light. Absorbance was measured at 540 nm using the TECAN infinite M1000-PRO ELISA reader. Optical density values from each group were recorded and reported as a percentage of control.

2.4. RNA Extraction and cDNA Synthesis

Total RNA was extracted from untreated BV2 cells (Ctrl) or cells exposed to 1000 µM AZE for 6 and 24 h, respectively. Briefly, cells were lysed using 1 mL TRI reagent (Sigma-Aldrich, Castle Hill, NSW, Australia) and 0.2 mL chloroform and precipitated with 0.5 mL 2-propanol (Sigma-Aldrich) [20]. Pellets were washed twice with 75% ethanol and air-dried. RNA concentrations were calculated using NanoDrop™ 2000 (ThermoFisher Scientific, Waltham, MA, USA). A total of 1 µg of total RNA were loaded in each cDNA synthesis reaction. cDNA synthesis was conducted using the T1000 thermal cycler (Bio-Rad, Gladesville, NSW, Australia) in a final volume of 20 µL. Each reaction contained 1 µg of RNA diluted in a volume of 11 µL, to which we added 9 µL of cDNA synthesis mix (Tetro cDNA synthesis kit; Bioline, Redfern, NSW, Australia). Samples were incubated at 45 °C for 40 min followed by 85 °C for 5 min. Finally, cDNA samples were diluted at a final concentration of 10 ng/mL in milliQ H_2O and stored at −20 °C until use.

2.5. Real Time Quantitative PCR Analysis

Real-time qPCR analyses were carried out as previously reported [20,21], with minor modifications. For each gene of interest, qPCRs were performed in a final volume of 10 µL, which comprised 3 µL cDNA, 0.4 µL milliQ H_2O, 5 µL of iTaq Universal SYBR green master mix (BioRad, Gladesville, NSW, Australia) and 0.8 µL of the corresponding forward and reverse primers (5 µM, Sigma-Aldrich, Castle Hill, NSW, Australia) to obtain a final primer concentration of 400 nM. The primers are described in Table 1. Reaction mixtures were loaded in Hard-Shell® 96-Well PCR Plates, and four genes of interest were tested in each run using the CFX96 Touch™ Real-Time PCR Detection System (Bio-Rad, Gladesville, NSW, Australia). Instrument settings were as follows: (1) 95 °C for 2 min, (2) 60 °C for 10 s, (3) 72 °C for 10 s, (4) plate read, (5) repeat step 2 to 4, for 45 cycles. For the melting curve analyses, settings were (1) 65 °C for 35 s, (2) plate read, (3) repeat step 1–2 for 60 times). To examine changes in expression, we analysed the mean fold change values of each sample, calculated using the ΔΔCt method, as previously described by Schmittgen and Livak [22]. PCR product specificity was evaluated by melting curve analysis, with each gene showing a single peak (data not shown).

Table 1. Oligonucleotide primers sequences used to amplify the genes of interest. Sequences were optimised for use in real-time qPCR studies and SYBR green technology, with predicted amplicons < 165 bp.

Gene	Forward Sequence 5′–3′ Reverse Sequence 3′–5′	Tm (°C)	Product Size	Accession No.
IL-1β	GCTACCTGTGTCTTTCCCGT CATCTCGGAGCCTGTAGTGC	59.68 60.25	164	NM_008361.4
Itgam	GAGCAGGGGTCATTCGCTAC GCTGGCTTAGATGCGATGGT	60.53 60.53	94	NM_001082960.1
Il-6	CCCCAATTTCCAATGCTCTCC CGCACTAGGTTTGCCGAGTA	59.24 60.11	141	NM_031168.2
Cd68	CTCCCACCACAAATGGCACT CTTGGACCTTGGACTAGGCG	60.54 60.11	95	NM_001291058.1
Mhc-2a	CAAGCTGTCTTATCTCACCTTCA ATCTCAGGTTCCCAGTGTTTCA	60.34 61.81	108	NM_010378.3
Mmp-9	ATCATAGAGGAAGCCCATTACAG TTTGACGTCCAGAGAAGAAGAAA	59.86 59.96	129	NM_013599.4
Nos2	TACCAAAGTGACCTGAAAGAGG TCATCTTGTATTGTTGGGCTGA	60.06 59.96	89	NM_010927.4
Il-10	GCATGGCCCAGAAATCAAGG GAGAAATCGATGACAGCGCC	59.54 59.42	91	NM_010548.2
Arg-1	ACAAGACAGGGCTCCTTTCAG TTAAAGCCACTGCCGTGTTC	59.93 59.05	105	NM_007482.3
Aif1	ACGTTCAGCTACTCTGACTTTC GTTGGCCTCTTGTGTTCTTTG	60.23 60.18	107	NM_001361501.1
Bdnf	CGAGTGGGTCACAGCGGCAG GCCCCTGCAGCCTTCCTTGG	60.04 59.97	160	NM_007540.4
S18	CCCTGAGAAGTTCCAGCACA GGTGAGGTCGATGTCTGCTT	59.60 59.75	145	NM_011296.2

2.6. Protein Extraction and Western Blot Analyses

Proteins from either untreated (Ctrl) or 1000 μM AZE-treated BV2 microglial cells at 6 and 24 h were extracted using radioimmunoprecipitation assay (RIPA) buffer (Sigma-Aldrich, Castle Hill, NSW, Australia) containing 1× Protease Inhibitor cocktail (cOmplete™, Mini, EDTA-free Protease Inhibitor Cocktail, Sigma-Aldrich, Castle Hill, NSW, Australia). Protein was quantified using the Bicinchoninic-Acid (BCA) Assay Protein Assay Kit (ThermoFisher Scientific, North Ryde, NSW, Australia) according to manufacturer's protocol and measured using the TECAN infinite M1000-PRO ELISA plate reader at 562 nm adsorbance.

Sample lysates were prepared by adding 3.75 μL of Laemmli Buffer (Bio-Rad, Gladesville, NSW, Australia) containing β-mercaptoethanol (Sigma-Aldrich, Castle Hill, NSW, Australia) mixture, (ratio 1:9 v/v) to 30 μg protein in a final volume of 15 μL. Samples were then heated for 10 min at 70 °C to denature proteins [23]. Proteins were then separated by SDS-polyacrylamide gel electrophoresis (SDS-PAGE) using 4–20% mini gels (Bio-Rad, Criterion 15-well Mini-Protean SFX), alongside with 5 μL of the molecular weight ladder/marker (BioRad Pre-stained HyperLadder Precision Plus Protein™; BioRad, Gladesville, NSW, Australia). Gels were transferred to a polyvinylidene fluoride (PVDF) membrane using the Trans-Blot Turbo instrument (BioRad). Once terminated, membranes were immediately placed in a container filled with TBS/0.1% Tween-20 (Sigma-Aldrich, Castle Hill, NSW, Australia) (TBST 1×) to wash out any residues during transfer. To block non-specific binding sites, membranes were blocked for 1 h in 5% dry non-fat skim milk in TBST with slow agitation (50–60 rpm).

Membranes were incubated with appropriately diluted primary antibodies in blocking buffer overnight at 4 °C with slow agitation. Primary antibodies used in this study and related dilutions are shown in Table 2. This was followed by incubation with host-specific secondary antibodies. Membranes were then placed in a container with 1 × TBST and washed rapidly three times, followed by three further 5 min washes. Finally, membranes were incubated in secondary antibody (HRP-conjugated goat anti-rabbit IgG; BioRad) for 1 h at room temperature, diluted in blocking buffer. The membranes were then washed once again as previously described to remove excess secondary antibody. Imaging was then performed on the Bio-Rad ChemiDoc MP Imaging System (BioRad). To detect bands, we utilized Clarity Western ECL Blotting Substrate (BioRad). Densitometric analyses of bands were computed using NIH ImageJ (https://imagej.nih.gov/ij/download/ (accessed on 14 October 2021)). Optical densities of target proteins were normalised to those of loading controls (GAPDH).

Table 2. Antibodies used in Western Blots.

Antibody	Source	Predicted Band Size	Dilution
Bcl2	ab182858, Abcam	26 kDa	1:2000
BAX	ab32503, Abcam	21 kDa	1:1000
Arg1	GTX109242, GeneTex	35 kDa	1:1000
BDNF	GTX132621, GeneTex	28 kDa	1:1000 (WB) 1:500 (IHC)
Iba1	GTX100042, GeneTex	17 kDa	1:500 (WB) 1:250 (IHC)
iNOS	GTX60599, GeneTex	32 kDa	1:1000
IL-6	GTX110527, GeneTex	24 kDa	1:1000 (WB)
GAPDH	VPA00187, Bio-Rad	37 kDa	1:2000
Goat anti Rabbit IgG HRP (Secondary)	STAR208P, Bio-Rad		1:10,000

WB = Western blot. IHC = Immunohistochemistry.

2.7. Flow Cytometry

Apoptosis and necrosis were detected by differential staining with annexin V (early and late apoptotic cells) and propidium iodide (PI) (necrotic cells only) using the Dead Cell Apoptosis Kit with Annexin V Alexa Fluor 488 and PI (#V13241; ThermoFisher Scientific), according to manufacturer's instructions. Briefly, BV2 cells were treated with 1000 μM of AZE for 24 h. Cells were washed in cold PBS, re-centrifuged and 1 × 10^6 cells were suspended in 1 × annexin-binding buffer. Cells were stained with Alexa Fluor 488 Annexin-V and propidium iodide (PI) for 15 min then analysed by flow cytometry. Unstained and single stained controls were used for compensation to correct for fluorescence photobleaching and gating (Supplementary Figure S1). FloJo software was used to analyse and curate flow cytometry data.

2.8. Immunocytochemistry

Sterile tissue culture coverslips (22 mm Ø, Sarstedt, SA, Australia) were coated with poly-L-lysine (100 μg/mL in sterile milliQ H_2O) (Sigma-Aldrich, Castle Hill, NSW, Australia) prior to cell culturing. Cells were cultured on coverslips at 1 × 10^4 cells in normal growth media or supplemented with AZE (1000 μM) for 6 or 24 h. Cells were then fixed with 4% filtered paraformaldehyde (PFA: 4% in PBS pH 7.4) (Sigma-Aldrich, Castle Hill, NSW, Australia) for 15 min at room temperature. Coverslips were then washed three times and permeabilised in PBS containing 0.25% Triton X-100 (Sigma-Aldrich, Castle Hill, NSW, Australia), followed 3× washes in PBS for 5 min [24]. Non-specific binding of antibodies was prevented by incubating coverslips with 1% BSA in PBST for 30 min. Once completed, the cells were incubated in diluted primary antibody (using 1% BSA in PBST) in a humidified chamber overnight at 4 °C (please see Table 2 for dilutions). The next day, the primary antibody was removed with 3× washes in PBS for 5 min. Cells were then incubated in the dark, with fluorophore-conjugated secondary antibodies (Alexa Fluor-488 or -594 anti-rabbit IgG) in 1% BSA in PBST overnight at 4 °C with gentle oscillation. Secondary antibody solution was then removed, and cells were washed again three times with PBS for 5 min in the dark. Cell nuclei were counterstained with 0.3 µg/mL DAPI for 1 min (DNA stain) (Cell Signalling Biotechnologies, Danvers, MA, USA) followed by a quick (1 min) rinsed with PBS. Finally, coverslips were mounted using a drop of mounting medium (Prolong Antifade Gold, Cell Signalling Biotechnologies) and sealed using nail polish to be stored in the dark at −20 °C before imaging.

2.9. Statistical Analysis

Statistical analyses were performed using GraphPad Prism software v9.3 (GraphPad Software, La Jolla, CA, USA). Pairwise comparisons were analysed by Student *t*-test. Comparisons between three or more groups were analysed by One-Way ANOVA followed by Sidak or Dunnett's post hoc test, as appropriate. *p*-values less than 0.05 were considered statistically significant.

3. Results

3.1. Dose–Response and Time Course Study of the Effects of AZE on Cell Morphology, Viability and Nitric Oxide (NO) Release

To determine if AZE exposure triggered gross phenotypic changes to BV2 microglia, we exposed cells to increasing concentrations of AZE (0, 500, 1000 and 2000 µM) at two different time intervals (12 and 24 h, respectively) and assessed cell morphology on a bright field microscope, using the embossing filter setting. The latter setting allows to discriminate microglial cells that acquire a flattened morphology (typical of activated / polarised BV2 cells). As shown in Figure 1A, BV2 cells exposed to increasing AZE concentration undergo considerable morphological changes in both, size, shape and overall appearance of cell somata and processes. Gross stereological assessment of cells displaying features of resting (small/raised somata) or polarised state (swollen/enlarged flat somata with rectracted processes) was performed in cells that were exposed to 1000 µM AZE for 12 and 24 h (Figure 1B). At time 0, only a small percentage of cells showed activated-like morphology (4.2% activated vs. 95.8% resting). After 12 h, there was already a remarkable increase in the percentage of activated microglia (33% activated vs. 67% resting), which was further increased after 24 h (54.2% activated vs. 45.8%).

Cell viability assessment using the MTT assay revealed a higher than expected reduction in nicotinamide adenine dinucleotide phosphate (NADPH)-dependent conversion of the yellow tetrazolium salt (3-(4,5-dimethylthiazol-2-yl)-2,5-diphenyltetrazolium bromide or MTT) to purple formazan crystals (Figure 1C), suggesting robust detrimental effects of AZE on BV2 cell metabolism. Time-course assessments demonstrated significant reduction in viability only at 2000 µM AZE (* $p < 0.05$ vs. Ctrl) after 6 h, whereas both 1000 and 2000 µM AZE significantly reduced viability at 12 h (*** $p < 0.001$ vs. Ctrl). Lastly, AZE concentrations from 125–2000 µM reduced viability after 24 h exposure to the npAA (*** $p < 0.001$ vs. Ctrl).

To examine if AZE treatment also influenced the release of nitric oxide (NO) in the supernatant (indicative of pro-inflammatory activity) we used the Griess reagent assay. Analyses of relative NO levels (shown as % of Ctrl) indicated that AZE, at the highest concentrations tested, significantly increased NO levels both at 6, 12 and 24 h (Figure 1D). Specifically, at 6 h, both 1000 and 2000 µM AZE reliably increase NO production (* $p < 0.05$ vs. Ctrl), whereas after 12 h, both 500, 1000 and 2000 µM AZE produced similar effects (** $p < 0.01$ vs. Ctrl at 500 and 1000 µM and * $p < 0.05$ vs. Ctrl at 2000 µM, respectively). A more robust increase in NO levels was seen after 24 h, with AZE significantly increasing NO at 500 and 1000 µM (* $p < 0.05$ vs. Ctrl) and 2000 µM (** $p < 0.01$ vs. Ctrl).

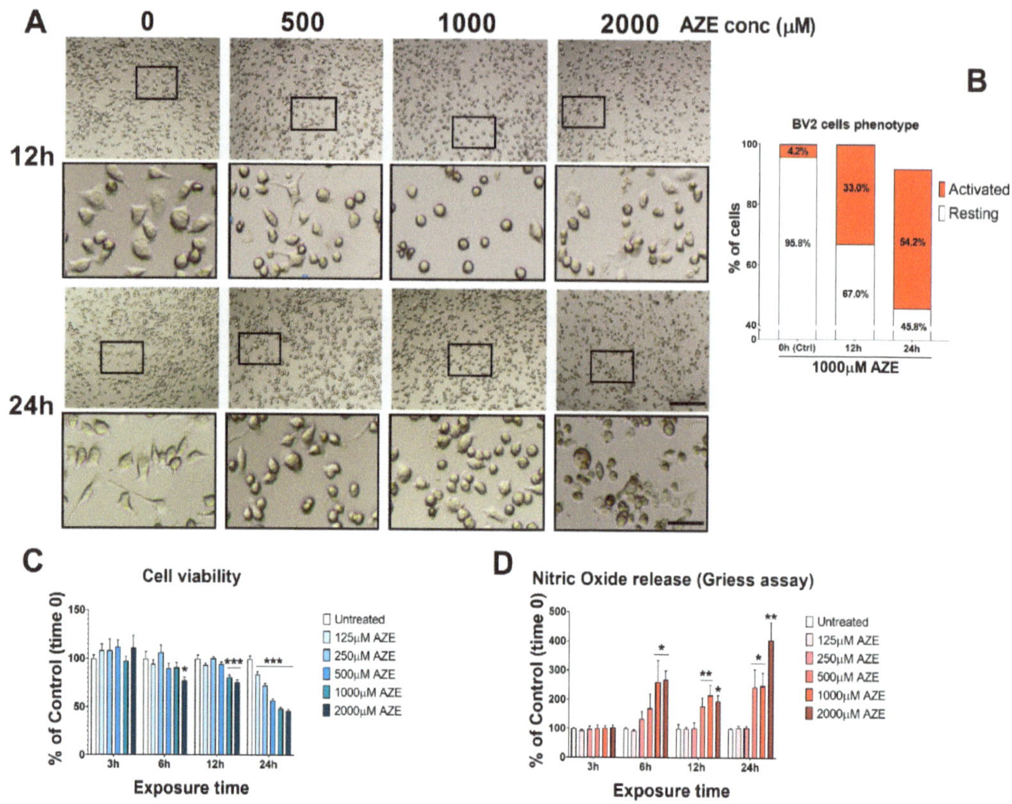

Figure 1. Dose–response effects of AZE exposure on BV2 microglial cell viability and inflammatory response. (**A**) Morphological changes seen in microglial BV2 cells following various AZE concentrations (0, 500, 1000, 2000 μM) after 12 and 24 h. Representative photomicrographs were taken using a bright field microscope with the embossing filter settings. Magnification = 10×, scale bar = 200 μm. Black squares indicate the ROI shown at higher magnification in insets. Insets below each photomicrograph show high magnification details of cellular morphology. Magnification = 40×, scale bar = 50 μm. (**B**) Phenotypic presentation of BV2 cells (Activated vs. Resting). % of cells of each phenotype was determined by counting the # of cells that showed signs of activation (flat and swollen) vs. the total number of cells per region of interest (ROI) and expressed as a percentage (n = 5 ROI × 3 batches of cells). (**C**) Cell viability, measured by MTT assay. Cells were treated with varying AZE concentrations (0, 125, 250, 500, 1000, 2000 μM) for 3, 6, 12 or 24 h. * $p < 0.05$ or *** $p < 0.001$, as determined by ANOVA followed by Dunnett's post hoc test. (**D**) Nitric oxide release, assessed using the Griess assay. Cells were treated as in C and NO levels were measured in culture media. Values are reported as the percentage NO release of untreated controls. Data reported as mean ± SEM. * $p < 0.05$, ** $p < 0.01$, as determined by ANOVA followed by Dunnett's post hoc test.

3.2. *Effects of AZE Exposure on Bcl2 and BAX Protein Expression in Murine BV2 Microglial Cells*

To investigate if AZE-driven reduction in cell viability was, at least in part, due to apoptosis, we determined the expression levels of the anti-apoptotic Bcl2 and pro-apoptotic BAX proteins by Western blot analyses. As indicated in Figure 2A, cells were either left untreated or exposed to 1000 μM AZE for 6 or 24 h.

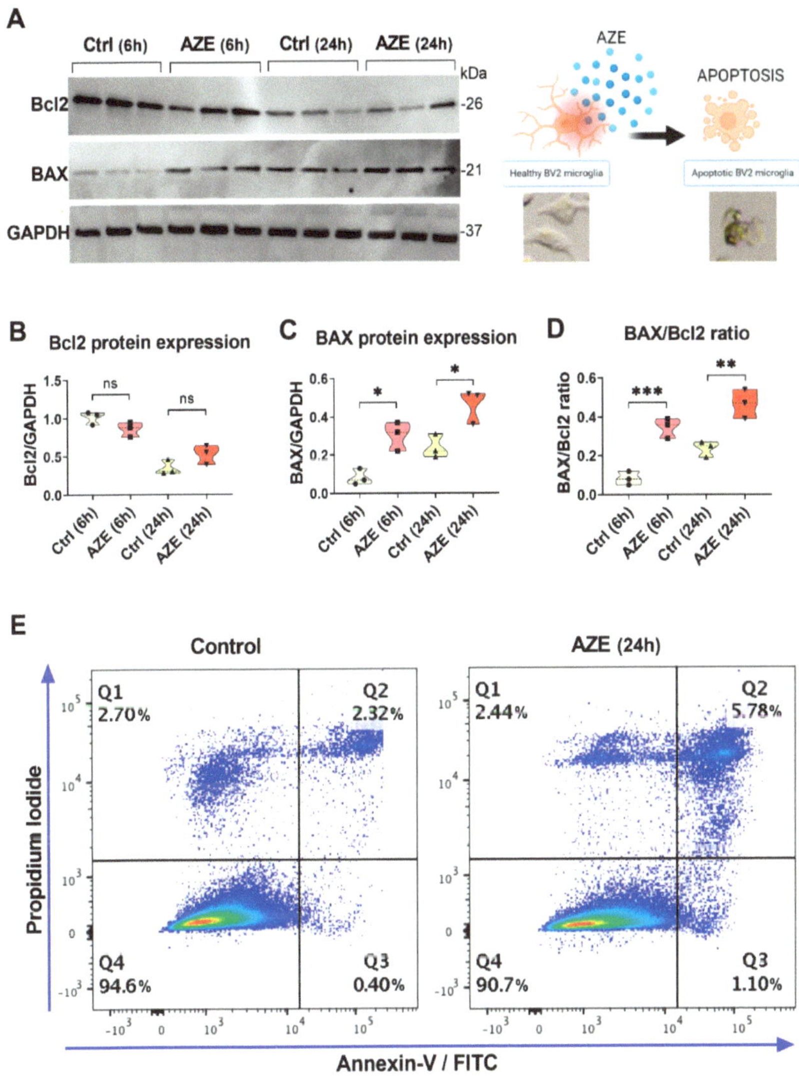

Figure 2. (**A**) Representative Western blots showing Bcl2 and BAX protein expression in BV2 cells cultured in the presence or not of AZE (1000 μM) for 6 or 24 h. GAPDH was used as loading control. (**B–D**) Violin plots depicting results from densitometric analyses of Bcl2 and BAX blots as well as BAX/Bcl2 ratios. Results shown are the mean ± SEM of two independent determinations, each run in triplicate. Ns = not significant. * $p < 0.05$, ** $p < 0.01$ or *** $p < 0.001$ vs. Ctrl at the corresponding time point, as determined by ANOVA and Sidak's post hoc test. (**E**) The incidence of apoptotic cells was examined by flow cytometry using Annexin V-FITC/PI staining. The experiment was repeated twice with overlapping results.

Bcl2 protein expression was not significantly affected by AZE treatment at any of time points tested ($p > 0.05$ vs. Ctrl; Figure 2B). In contrast, levels of the pro-apoptotic BAX protein were significantly increased both at 6 and 24 h (* $p < 0.05$ vs. Ctrl at the corresponding times; Figure 2C). We further analysed BAX/Bcl2 ratio, an indicator of apoptosis susceptibility in BV2 cells exposed to the same experimental conditions. We found that, already after 6 h after AZE exposure, the ratio was significantly increased (*** $p < 0.001$ vs. Ctrl (6 h)) and was still augmented at 24 h (** $p < 0.01$ vs. Ctrl (24 h); Figure 2D).

Finally, we conducted Annexin V-FITC/PI staining on BV2 cells exposed or not to 1000 µM AZE for 24 h. The experiment demonstrated a remarkable increase in the percentage of early apoptotic and necrotic or late apoptotic cells (about 5.8%) compared to the control group (2.3%) (Figure 2E).

3.3. Effects of AZE Exposure on the mRNA Expression of Pro- and Anti-Inflammatory Markers in Murine BV2 Microglial Cells

To explore whether AZE treatment alters the inflammatory profile of BV2 cells, we analysed the expression of a panel of pro- and anti-inflammatory markers by real-time quantitative polymerase chain reaction (qPCR).

As depicted in Figure 3A, AZE triggered a significant increase in interleukin-1β (*IL-1β*) gene expression both after 6 and 24 h (* $p < 0.05$ vs. Ctrl). In contrast, interleukin-6 (*IL-6*) gene induction was more prominent at 6 h (>15-fold of Ctrl, **** $p < 0.0001$ vs. Ctrl) vs. 24 h treatment (** $p < 0.01$ vs. Ctrl) (Figure 3B). *NOS2*, the gene encoding for inducible nitric oxide synthase (iNOS)—the enzyme that catalyses the production of NO—was only marginally increased after 6 h ($p > 0.05$) but was significant at 24 h (* $p < 0.05$; Figure 3C). The expression level of *Itgam*, the gene encoding for the macrophage marker CD11b, was not elevated in response to AZE ($p > 0.05$; Figure 3D). However, CD68 (aka microsialin)—another myeloid cell marker, was robustly induced after 6 h AZE exposure (>12-fold of Ctrl, **** $p < 0.0001$) and remained elevated at 24 h (** $p < 0.01$) (Figure 3E). Analyses of the expression of the major histocompatibility complex IIa (MHC-2a), which serves a critical role in the induction of immune responses through presentation of antigenic peptides to lymphocytes, was not induced at 6 h post-AZE treatment, but significantly up-regulated at 24 h (**** $p < 0.0001$; Figure 3F).

Expression of metalloproteinase-9 (MMP-9), an extracellular matrix degrading enzyme [25], was also robustly up-regulated by AZE treatment, but only at 24 h (* $p < 0.05$; Figure 3G).

Finally, we also interrogated two anti-inflammatory genes: interleukin-10 (IL-10) and arginase 1 (Arg1) [26]. Real-time qPCR revealed a significant up-regulation of the former at 6 h (* $p < 0.05$) but not at 24 h ($p > 0.05$) (Figure 3H), whereas the latter was significantly up-regulated only after 24 h (* $p < 0.05$).

3.4. Effects of AZE Exposure on IL-6 and Arg1 Protein Expression in Murine BV2 Microglial Cells

To confirm if the effects of AZE treatment on pro- and anti-inflammatory genes could also be appreciated at the protein level, we measured the protein expression of both IL-6 (pro-inflammatory) [27] and Arg1 (anti-inflammatory) [27] by Western blot.

In BV2 cells treated with AZE, IL-6 protein expression was heavily induced at 6 h (**** $p < 0.0001$ vs. Ctrl (6 h)); however, expression returned to baseline after 24 h ($p > 0.05$) (Figure 4A,B). In contrast, Arg1 expression was not affected after 6 h AZE ($p > 0.05$) but was remarkably increased at the 24 h time point (*** $p < 0.001$ vs. Ctrl) (Figure 4A,C).

3.5. Effects of AZE Treatment on the Gene and Protein Expression of the Pro-Inflammatory Marker Allograft Inflammatory Factor 1 (AIF1)/Ionized Calcium-Binding Adapter Molecule 1 (Iba1)

To better characterise AZE pro-inflammatory activities in BV2 microglia, cells were exposed to the same concentration of the npAA (1000 µM) for 6 or 24 h and the expression of *AIF1* (gene) and its protein product (Iba1) were interrogated using different experimental means.

Immunofluorescence revealed a remarkable enhancement in Iba1+ signal in BV2 cells exposed to AZE for 6 h; however, signal intensity returned to normal level by 24 h (Figure 5A). Similarly, *AIF1* transcripts were up-regulated after 6 h AZE (**** $p < 0.0001$ vs. Ctrl (6 h)), but almost returned to untreated levels within 24 h (Figure 5B). These results were corroborated by Western blots, showing significantly increased Iba1 protein levels at 6 h (*** $p < 0.001$), but not at 24 h ($p > 0.05$) (Figure 5C,D).

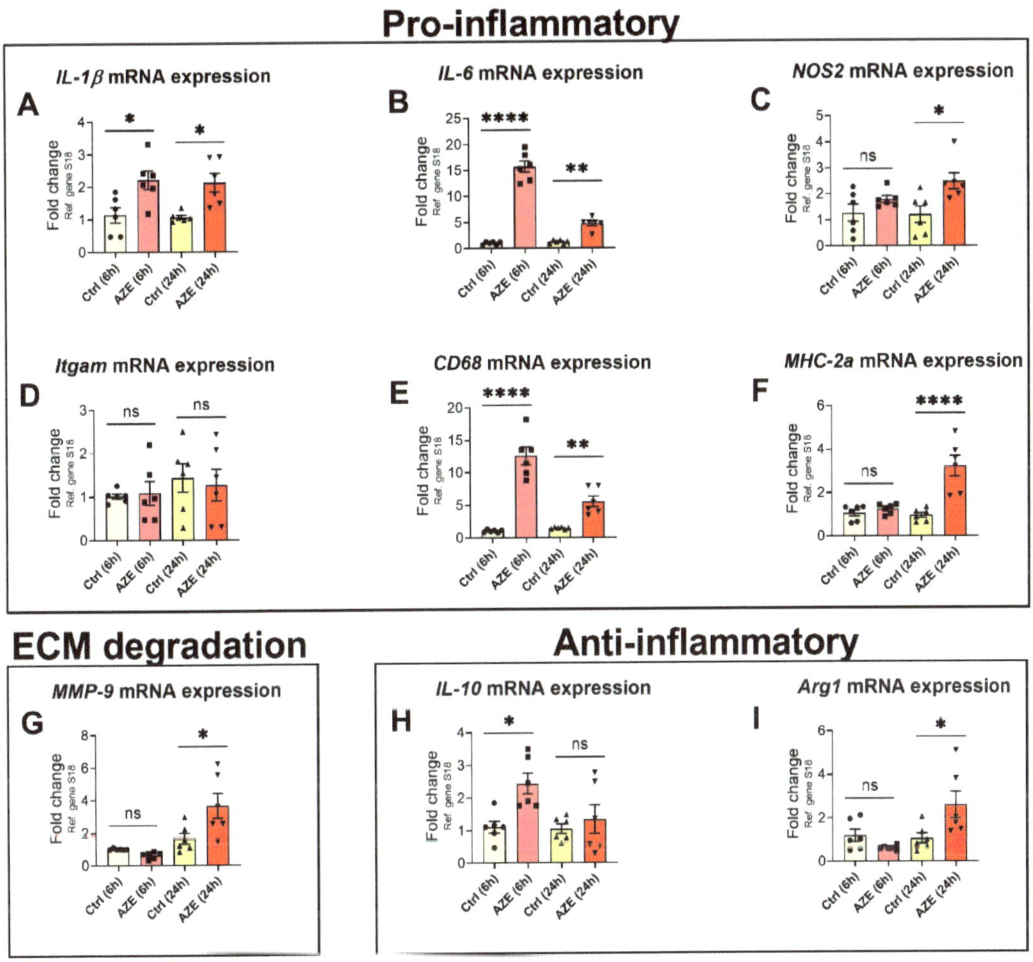

Figure 3. Gene expression of a panel of pro- and anti-inflammatory genes in BV2 microglial cells after 1000 μM AZE treatment for 6 and 24 h. Relative fold-changes were calculated using the ΔCt method after normalization to the S18 housekeeping gene. Box-and-whisker plots depict the differential expression of pro-inflammatory (**A–F**) *IL-1β, IL-6, NOS2, Itgam, CD68* and *MHC-2a*, (**G**) extracellular matrix (ECM) degradation *(MMP-9)* and (**H–I**) anti-inflammatory *IL-10* and *Arg1* transcripts. Results are presented as mean fold changes with respect to no treatment (Ctrl) ± SEM. Data represents n = 6 samples per group. * $p < 0.05$, ** $p < 0.01$ or **** $p < 0.0001$; as determined by ANOVA followed by Sidak's post hoc test. Ns = not significant.

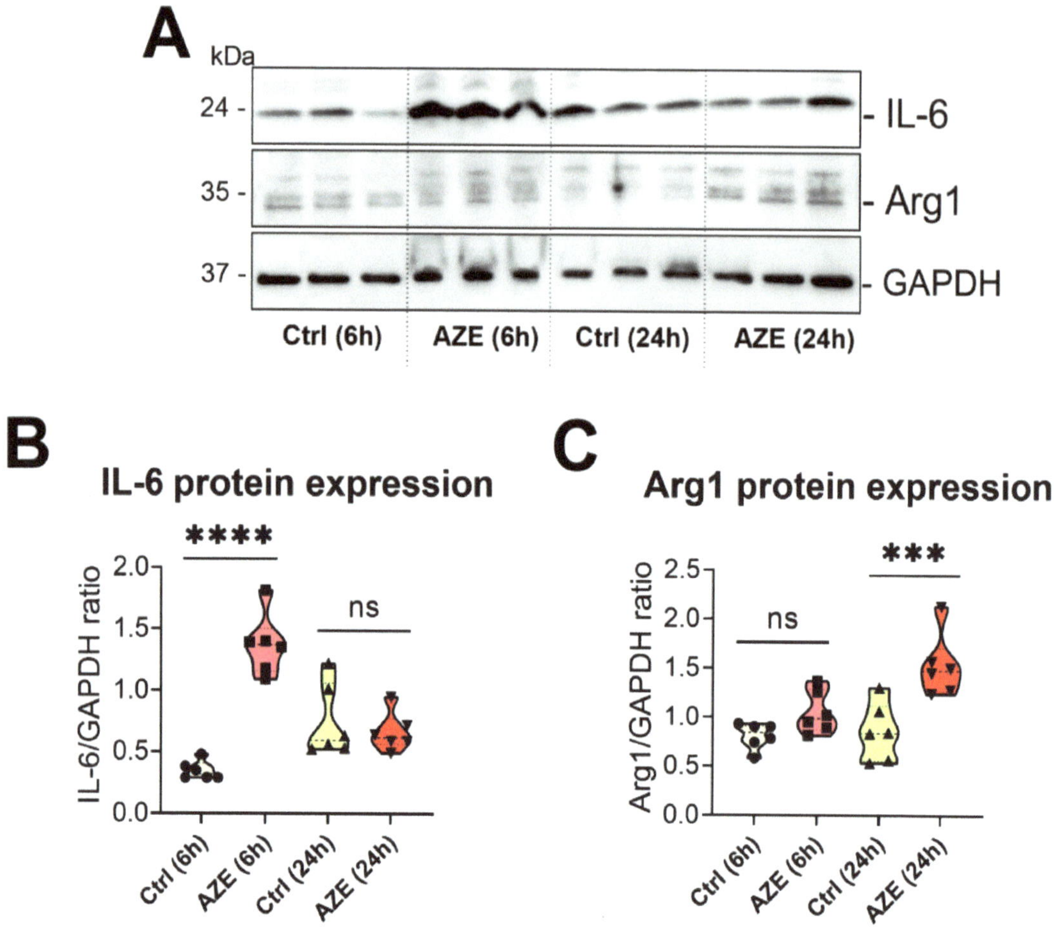

Figure 4. (**A**) Representative Western blots showing the protein expression of IL-6 and Arg1 in BV2 cells cultured or not in the presence of AZE (1000 μM) for 6 or 24 h. (**B**,**C**) Violin plots of bands densities demonstrating the effects of AZE on the expression of IL-6 and Arg1 at the indicated times. Data reported is the mean ± SEM, from two independent experiments using separate batches of cells (n = 6). GAPDH was used as loading control. Ns = not significant. *** $p < 0.001$ or **** $p < 0.0001$ vs. Ctrl at the indicated time, as determined by ANOVA followed by Sidak's post hoc test.

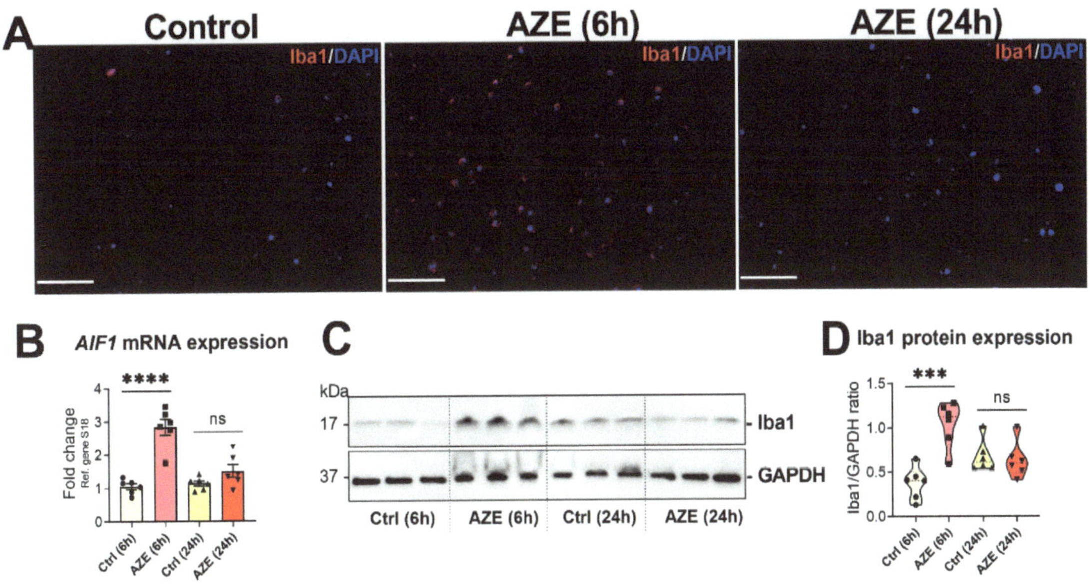

Figure 5. AZE treatment induces *AIF1*/Iba1 expression in BV2 cells. (**A**) Representative photomicrographs of Iba1+ staining in the BV2 microglial cell line. Cells were either left untreated or treated with AZE as indicated and then processed for immunocytochemistry (ICC) as detailed in Section 2. Red = Iba1+ cells (Alexa Fluor 594). DAPI = nuclei. Scale bar = 50 µm. (**B**) *AIF1* gene expression, as determined by real-time qPCR. Fold changes were calculated using the ΔCt method, with baseline expression set to 1. Data is the mean ± SEM (n = 6). **** $p < 0.0001$ vs. Ctrl at the indicated time points. (**C**,**D**) Western blot analyses of Iba protein expression and densitometric analyses of blots. Data reported is the mean ± SEM, from two independent experiments using separate batches of cells (n = 6). GAPDH was used as loading control. Ns = not significant. *** $p < 0.001$ or **** $p < 0.0001$ vs. Ctrl at the indicated time, as determined by ANOVA followed by Sidak's post hoc test.

3.6. Effects of AZE Treatment on the Gene and Protein Expression of Brain-Derived Neurotrophic Factor (BDNF)

BDNF is a neurotrophic factor known to play an important role in microglia inflammatory responses [28]. Here, we assessed BDNF mRNA and protein expression in cells exposed to 1000 µM AZE for 6 and 24 h.

ICC demonstrated a rapid increase in BDNF+ staining in cells after 6 h AZE (Figure 6A), which was attenuated at 24 h. Interestingly, BDNF mRNA expression was slightly (but not significantly) increased at 6 h post-AZE treatment ($p > 0.05$ vs. Ctrl (6 h)); however, the increase was significant at 24 h (* $p < 0.05$ vs. Ctrl (24 h)) (Figure 6B). At the protein level, BDNF expression was significantly increased at 6 h AZE (* $p < 0.05$), whereas the increased was no longer significant at 24 h (Figure 6C,D).

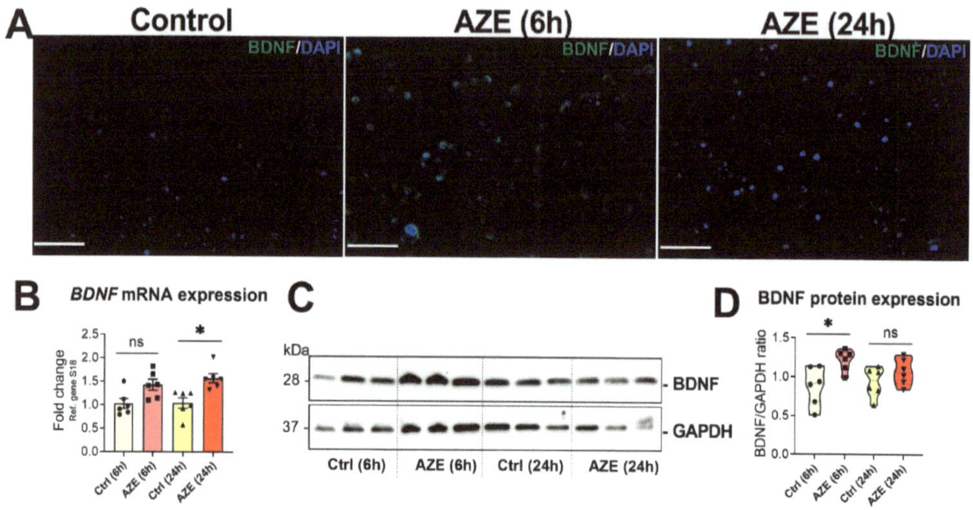

Figure 6. AZE treatment induces BDNF expression in BV2 cells. (**A**). Representative photomicrographs of BDNF+ staining in the BV2 microglial cell line. Cells were either left untreated or treated with AZE as indicated and then processed for immunocytochemistry (ICC) as detailed in Section 2. Red = BDNF+ cells (Alexa Fluor 488). DAPI = nuclei. Scale bar = 50 µm. (**B**). *BDNF* transcript levels, as determined by real-time qPCR. Fold changes were calculated using the ΔCt method. Data is the mean ± SEM (n = 6). * $p < 0.05$ vs. Ctrl at the indicated time points. (**C**,**D**) Western blot analyses of Iba protein expression and densitometric analyses of blots. Data reported is the mean ± SEM, from two independent experiments using separate batches of cells (n = 6). GAPDH was used as loading control. Ns = not significant. * $p < 0.05$ vs. Ctrl at the indicated time, as determined by ANOVA followed by Sidak's post hoc test.

4. Discussion

To the best of our knowledge, this is the first study portraying the pro-inflammatory and pro-apoptotic effects of acute AZE exposure in a microglial cell line.

Microglial cells are involved in several brain functions, and are recognised as "agents of the CNS" [29]. Their activities span from the clearing of cell debris after injury or pathogen attack (the well-known cell scavenging function) [30], going through the control of inflammatory responses [31], to latest reports highlighting microglial role in myelination [32]. Environmental factors able to disrupt the functionality of these cells may have a strong negative impact on CNS homeostasis, contributing to the onset of neurodegenerative diseases, including MS [33].

There is a growing body of work suggesting that certain npAAs produced by plants have the clear potential to adversely affect human health [1,34]. The exact pathogenic mechanisms are yet to be revealed; however, several theories have pinpointed the existence of geographical and historical links with the increased prevalence of CNS disorders among the population exposed to these toxins over a prolonged period of time [6,35,36], instigating researchers to conduct further investigations on this class of environmental risk factors.

Due to its similarity to L-proline, AZE is capable of entering cells, being charged onto the $tRNA^{Pro}$, where it can evade editing by aminoacyl-tRNA synthetase and be misincorporated into proline-containing proteins during protein assembly [37]. Since this mistaken incorporation is thought to be a random process dependent on the relative concentrations of AZE and proline, proline-rich proteins are more likely to contain AZE. Misincorporation of AZE is thought to alter the structural conformation of newly assembled proteins, resulting in protein misfolding and, consequently, ER-stress [38]. Sobel and collaborators have recently shown that administration of AZE to laboratory animals (especially young mice) triggers oligodendrocytes swelling, formation of microglial nodules and cell polarization [7], and providing essential proof-of-concept data to indicate that AZE consumption is associated with some degree of CNS pathogenicity. It is unclear though if AZE-induced protein misfolding is restricted to oligodendrocytes or it extends more globally to different CNS cell types, including microglia. In fact, whereas protein misfolding in oligodendrocytes could potentially activate neighbouring microglia—causing cell activation—it cannot be excluded that AZE may directly trigger an inflammatory response after it enters the cell. This idea is supported by emerging evidence providing a link between ER stress-mediated activation of the UPR in microglia and cell polarization [14] and previous evidence of cell death and mitochondrial dysfunction in SH-SY5Y neuronal-like cells [39].

In this study, using the BV2 microglial cell line, which shares several biochemical and transcriptional features with primary microglia [40,41], we aimed at determining if AZE in the culture media would trigger cell polarization and other detrimental effects. Our findings revealed that a relatively brief exposure to supraphysiological concentrations of AZE was capable of triggering a barrage of pro-inflammatory signals consistent with overt M1-like polarization. Cells acquired the typical morphology of activated microglia, with flattened and swollen somata and expressed high levels of pro-inflammatory mediators (*IL-1β*, *IL-6*, *NOS2*), the neurotrophic factor BDNF and other myeloid cell activation markers (*CD68*, *MHC-2a*, *MMP-9* and *AIF1*). In parallel, expression of the anti-inflammatory markers *IL-10* and *Arg1* were also increased. This an expected occurrence, likely due to the physiological attempt to regain homeostatic control over the inflammatory response by a subset of cells.

Unexpectedly, expression of *Itgam*—the gene encoding for the myeloid marker CD11b—was not affected by AZE. This is particularly interesting as CD11b induction occurs via a NO-dependent mechanism [42], and AZE reliably increased NO release as well as the expression of the *NOS2* gene. However, it should be noted that gene expression data returned largely variable results for this gene, likely due to individual batch effects. Alternatively, we cannot rule out that BV2 cells might require prolonged exposure to NO (>24 h) to effectively up-regulate *Itgam* gene expression, and such delayed response was not captured in our experimental setting.

In parallel with these studies, our investigations demonstrated that AZE treatment also triggered apoptotic cell death. Cell viability assays, flow cytometry and Western blotting all confirmed moderate cell loss at the highest concentrations of AZE. Annexin V/PI staining suggested mixed necrotic/apoptotic cell death; however, the increased expression of BAX protein levels and the gross microscopic observations of sparse cells with pyknotic nuclei points more towards apoptotic-like cell death. Additional observations to confirm whether AZE activates UPR-initiated cell death in BV2 microglia are warranted. Furthermore, if UPR is identified as the cause of AZE-mediated apoptosis, it would be interesting to determine whether this pathway leads the activation of the intrinsic or extrinsic apoptotic pathways, or both. In fact, there is evidence that ER-stress/UPR can also activate the extrinsic pathway via TRAIL receptor signalling [43] in addition to the intrinsic one [14].

AZE neurotoxicity, as well as its possible link with MS pathogenesis was initially hypothesized in 2008 by Rubenstein and coworkers in 2008 [6]. However, no direct links with other neurodegenerative conditions have been reported so far. Our findings showing that AZE triggers both apoptosis and inflammation support and extend the idea of a broader neuropathological mechanism underlying the toxic effects of this npAA. However, more mechanistic studies are warranted to ascertain how these pathogenic pathways are regulated and perhaps, can be reversed.

In conclusion, the present work provides novel evidence to indicate that AZE is both toxic and pro-inflammatory in BV2 microglia. The underlying mechanism still needs to be elucidated; however, published data supports a role for ER-stress and perhaps mitochondrial dysfunction as the two main pathogenic mechanisms. Understanding the detrimental activity of AZE and other npAAs is of great importance, as it may serve to raise awareness on the importance of monitoring consumption (or other means of exposure) to these potentially neurotoxic molecules.

Supplementary Materials: The following supporting information can be downloaded at: https://www.mdpi.com/article/10.3390/cimb44100308/s1, Figure S1: Gating of Annexin V-FITC/PI staining in flow cytometry.

Author Contributions: Conceptualization, A.C.; methodology, J.A.P., M.I.J. and S.T.B.; validation, J.A.P., M.I.J. and S.T.B.; formal analysis, J.A.P. and A.C.; investigation, J.A.P., M.I.J. and S.T.B.; resources, A.C.; data curation, J.A.P., M.I.J. and A.C.; writing—original draft preparation, J.A.P.; writing—review and editing, A.C., K.J.R. and G.M.; supervision, A.C.; project administration, A.C.; funding acquisition, A.C. and K.J.R. All authors have read and agreed to the published version of the manuscript.

Funding: This work was supported by grant funding from MS Australia (21-1-079) to A.C. and K.J.R.

Institutional Review Board Statement: Not applicable.

Informed Consent Statement: Not applicable.

Data Availability Statement: All data generated or analysed during this study are included in this published article.

Acknowledgments: We would like to acknowledge Kun Xiao for his technical support with flow cytometry. We would also like to express our scientific appreciation to Edward Rubenstein (deceased) for his past work and pioneering theory of MS pathogenesis, which was instrumental in the realization of this study.

Conflicts of Interest: The authors declare no conflict of interest.

References

1. Rodgers, K.J. Non-protein amino acids and neurodegeneration: The enemy within. *Exp. Neurol.* **2014**, *253*, 192–196. [CrossRef] [PubMed]
2. Soares, A.R.; Marchiosi, R.; Siqueira-Soares, R.D.C.; Barbosa de Lima, R.; Dantas dos Santos, W.; Ferrarese-Filho, O. The role of L-DOPA in plants. *Plant Signal. Behav.* **2014**, *9*, e28275. [CrossRef] [PubMed]
3. Rubenstein, E. Biologic effects of and clinical disorders caused by nonprotein amino acids. *Medicine* **2000**, *79*, 80–89. [CrossRef] [PubMed]
4. Rubenstein, E.; McLaughlin, T.; Winant, R.C.; Sanchez, A.; Eckart, M.; Krasinska, K.M.; Chien, A. Azetidine-2-carboxylic acid in the food chain. *Phytochemistry* **2009**, *70*, 100–104. [CrossRef]
5. Rubenstein, E.; Zhou, H.; Krasinska, K.M.; Chien, A.; Becker, C.H. Azetidine-2-carboxylic acid in garden beets (*Beta vulgaris*). *Phytochemistry* **2006**, *67*, 898–903. [CrossRef]
6. Rubenstein, E. Misincorporation of the proline analog azetidine-2-carboxylic acid in the pathogenesis of multiple sclerosis: A hypothesis. *J. Neuropathol. Exp. Neurol.* **2008**, *67*, 1035–1040. [CrossRef]
7. Sobel, R.A.; Albertelli, M.; Hinojoza, J.R.; Eaton, M.J.; Grimes, K.V.; Rubenstein, E. Azetidine-2-Carboxylic Acid-Induced Oligodendrogliopathy: Relevance to the Pathogenesis of Multiple Sclerosis. *J. Neuropathol. Exp. Neurol* **2022**, *81*, 414–433. [CrossRef]
8. Rone, M.B.; Cui, Q.-L.; Fang, J.; Wang, L.-C.; Zhang, J.; Khan, D.; Bedard, M.; Almazan, G.; Ludwin, S.K.; Jones, R.; et al. Oligodendrogliopathy in Multiple Sclerosis: Low Glycolytic Metabolic Rate Promotes Oligodendrocyte Survival. *J. Neurosci.* **2016**, *36*, 4698–4707. [CrossRef]
9. Marzan, D.E.; Brügger-Verdon, V.; West, B.L.; Liddelow, S.; Samanta, J.; Salzer, J.L. Activated microglia drive demyelination via CSF1R signaling. *Glia* **2021**, *69*, 1583–1604. [CrossRef]
10. Kinney, H.C.; Volpe, J.J. *Myelination Events, in Volpe's Neurology of the Newborn*; Elsevier: Amsterdam, The Netherlands, 2018; pp. 176–188.
11. Dikranian, K.; Cohen, R.; Mac Donald, C.; Pan, Y.; Brakefield, D.; Bayly, P.; Parsadanian, A. Mild traumatic brain injury to the infant mouse causes robust white matter axonal degeneration which precedes apoptotic death of cortical and thalamic neurons. *Exp. Neurol.* **2008**, *211*, 551–560. [CrossRef]
12. Zhang, K.; Kaufman, R.J. Protein folding in the endoplasmic reticulum and the unfolded protein response. *Handb. Exp. Pharmacol.* **2006**, *172*, 69–91.
13. Zhang, K.; Kaufman, R.J. The unfolded protein response: A stress signaling pathway critical for health and disease. *Neurology* **2006**, *66* (Suppl. 1), S102–S109. [CrossRef] [PubMed]
14. Fernández, D.; Geisse, A.; Bernales, J.I.; Lira, A.; Osorio, F. The Unfolded Protein Response in Immune Cells as an Emerging Regulator of Neuroinflammation. *Front. Aging Neurosci.* **2021**, *13*, 286. [CrossRef] [PubMed]
15. Colonna, M.; Butovsky, O. Microglia function in the central nervous system during health and neurodegeneration. *Annu. Rev. Immunol.* **2017**, *35*, 441–468. [CrossRef] [PubMed]

16. Boche, D.; Perry, V.H.; Nicoll, J.A. Review: Activation patterns of microglia and their identification in the human brain. *Neuropathol. Appl. Neurobiol.* **2013**, *39*, 3–18. [CrossRef] [PubMed]
17. Lull, M.E.; Block, M.L. Microglial activation and chronic neurodegeneration. *Neurotherapeutics* **2010**, *7*, 354–365. [CrossRef]
18. Howell, O.W.; Rundle, J.L.; Garg, A.; Komada, M.; Brophy, P.J.; Reynolds, R. Activated microglia mediate axoglial disruption that contributes to axonal injury in multiple sclerosis. *J. Neuropathol. Exp. Neurol.* **2010**, *69*, 1017–1033. [CrossRef]
19. Broome, S.T.; Fisher, T.; Faiz, A.; Keay, K.; Musumeci, G.; Al-Badri, G.; Castorina, A. Assessing the Anti-Inflammatory Activity of the Anxiolytic Drug Buspirone Using CRISPR-Cas9 Gene Editing in LPS-Stimulated BV-2 Microglial Cells. *Cells* **2021**, *10*, 1312. [CrossRef]
20. Giunta, S.; Castorina, A.; Adorno, A.; Mazzone, V.; Carnazza, M.L.; D'Agata, V. PACAP and VIP affect NF1 expression in rat malignant peripheral nerve sheath tumor (MPNST) cells. *Neuropeptides* **2010**, *44*, 45–51. [CrossRef]
21. Bucolo, C.; Leggio, G.M.; Maltese, A.; Castorina, A.; D'Agata, V.; Drago, F. Dopamine-3 receptor modulates intraocular pressure: Implications for glaucoma. *Biochem. Pharmacol.* **2012**, *83*, 680–686. [CrossRef]
22. Schmittgen, T.D.; Livak, K.J. Analyzing real-time PCR data by the comparative CT method. *Nat. Protoc.* **2008**, *3*, 1101–1108. [CrossRef] [PubMed]
23. Castorina, A.; Waschek, J.A.; Marzagalli, R.; Cardile, V.; Drago, F. PACAP interacts with PAC1 receptors to induce tissue plasminogen activator (tPA) expression and activity in schwann cell-like cultures. *PLoS ONE* **2015**, *10*, e0117799. [CrossRef] [PubMed]
24. Musumeci, G.; Castorina, A.; Magro, G.; Cardile, V.; Castorina, S.; Ribatti, D. Enhanced expression of CD31/platelet endothelial cell adhesion molecule 1 (PECAM1) correlates with hypoxia inducible factor 1 alpha (HIF-1alpha) in human glioblastoma multiforme. *Exp. Cell Res.* **2015**, *339*, 407–416. [CrossRef]
25. Artym, V.V.; Yamada, K.M.; Mueller, S.C. ECM degradation assays for analyzing local cell invasion. In *Extracellular Matrix Protocols*; Springer: Berlin/Heidelberg, Germany, 2009; pp. 211–219.
26. Miki, S.; Suzuki, J.-I.; Takashima, M.; Ishida, M.; Kokubo, H.; Yoshizumi, M. S-1-Propenylcysteine promotes IL-10-induced M2c macrophage polarization through prolonged activation of IL-10R/STAT3 signaling. *Sci. Rep.* **2021**, *11*, 22469. [CrossRef] [PubMed]
27. Broome, S.T.; Louangaphay, K.; Keay, K.A.; Leggio, G.M.; Musumeci, G.; Castorina, A. Dopamine: An immune transmitter. *Neural Regen. Res.* **2020**, *15*, 2173.
28. Ding, H.; Chen, J.; Su, M.; Lin, Z.; Zhan, H.; Yang, F.; Li, W.; Xie, J.; Huang, Y.; Liu, X.; et al. BDNF promotes activation of astrocytes and microglia contributing to neuroinflammation and mechanical allodynia in cyclophosphamide-induced cystitis. *J. Neuroinflamm.* **2020**, *17*, 19. [CrossRef]
29. Rodríguez-Gómez, J.A.; Kavanagh, E.; Engskog-Vlachos, P.; Engskog, M.K.; Herrera, A.J.; Espinosa-Oliva, A.M.; Joseph, B.; Hajji, N.; Venero, J.L.; Burguillos, M.A. Microglia: Agents of the CNS Pro-Inflammatory Response. *Cells* **2020**, *9*, 1717. [CrossRef]
30. Jansen, M.I.; Broome, S.T.; Castorina, A. Targeting the neurological comorbidities of multiple sclerosis: The beneficial effects of VIP and PACAP neuropeptides. *J. Integr. Neurosci.* **2022**, *21*, 33. [CrossRef]
31. Su, P.; Zhang, J.; Wang, D.; Zhao, F.; Cao, Z.; Aschner, M.; Luo, W. The role of autophagy in modulation of neuroinflammation in microglia. *Neuroscience* **2016**, *319*, 155–167. [CrossRef]
32. Lloyd, A.F.; Miron, V.E. The pro-remyelination properties of microglia in the central nervous system. *Nat. Rev. Neurol.* **2019**, *15*, 447–458. [CrossRef]
33. Li, Q.; Barres, B.A. Microglia and macrophages in brain homeostasis and disease. *Nat. Rev. Immunol.* **2018**, *18*, 225–242. [CrossRef] [PubMed]
34. Nunn, P.B.; Bell, E.A.; Watson, A.A.; Nash, R.J. Toxicity of non-protein amino acids to humans and domestic animals. *Nat. Prod. Commun* **2010**, *5*, 485–504. [CrossRef] [PubMed]
35. Main, B.J.; Bowling, L.C.; Padula, M.P.; Bishop, D.P.; Mitrovic, S.M.; Guillemin, G.J.; Rodgers, K.J. Detection of the suspected neurotoxin β-methylamino-l-alanine (BMAA) in cyanobacterial blooms from multiple water bodies in Eastern Australia. *Harmful Algae* **2018**, *74*, 10–18. [CrossRef]
36. Violi, J.P.; Mitrovic, S.M.; Colville, A.; Main, B.J.; Rodgers, K.J. Prevalence of β-methylamino-L-alanine (BMAA) and its isomers in freshwater cyanobacteria isolated from eastern Australia. *Ecotoxicol. Environ. Saf.* **2019**, *172*, 72–81. [CrossRef] [PubMed]
37. Song, Y.; Zhou, H.; Vo, M.-N.; Shi, Y.; Nawaz, M.H.; Vargas-Rodriguez, O.; Diedrich, J.K.; Yates, J.R.; Kishi, S.; Musier-Forsyth, K.; et al. Double mimicry evades tRNA synthetase editing by toxic vegetable-sourced non-proteinogenic amino acid. *Nat. Commun.* **2017**, *8*, 2281. [CrossRef] [PubMed]
38. Cheng, Z.; Teo, G.; Krueger, S.; Rock, T.M.; Koh, H.W.; Choi, H.; Vogel, C. Differential dynamics of the mammalian mRNA and protein expression response to misfolding stress. *Mol. Syst. Biol.* **2016**, *12*, 855. [CrossRef] [PubMed]
39. Samardzic, K.; Rodgers, K.J. Cell death and mitochondrial dysfunction induced by the dietary non-proteinogenic amino acid L-azetidine-2-carboxylic acid (Aze). *Amino Acids* **2019**, *51*, 1221–1232. [CrossRef]
40. Karunia, J.; Niaz, A.; Mandwie, M.; Broome, S.T.; Keay, K.A.; Waschek, J.A.; Al-Badri, G.; Castorina, A. PACAP and VIP Modulate LPS-Induced Microglial Activation and Trigger Distinct Phenotypic Changes in Murine BV2 Microglial Cells. *Int. J. Mol. Sci.* **2021**, *22*, 10947. [CrossRef]

41. Anja Henn, S.L.; Hedtjärn, M.; Schrattenholz, A.; Pörzgen, P.; Leist, M. The Suitability of BV2 Cells as Alternative Model System for Primary Microglia Cultures or for Animal Experiments Examining Brain Inflammation. *ALTEX Altern. Anim. Exp.* **2009**, *26*, 83–94.
42. Roy, A.; Fung, Y.K.; Liu, X.; Pahan, K. Up-regulation of microglial CD11b expression by nitric oxide. *J. Biol. Chem.* **2006**, *281*, 14971–14980. [CrossRef]
43. Stöhr, D.; Jeltsch, A.; Rehm, M. TRAIL receptor signaling: From the basics of canonical signal transduction toward its entanglement with ER stress and the unfolded protein response. *Int. Rev. Cell Mol. Biol.* **2020**, *351*, 57–99. [PubMed]

current issues in molecular biology

MDPI

Review

Multiple Sclerosis: Inflammatory and Neuroglial Aspects

Giulio Papiri [1], Giordano D'Andreamatteo [1], Gabriella Cacchiò [1], Sonila Alia [2], Mauro Silvestrini [3], Cristina Paci [1], Simona Luzzi [3] and Arianna Vignini [2,*]

1 Neurology Unit, Ospedale Provinciale "Madonna del Soccorso", 63074 San Benedetto del Tronto, Italy
2 Section of Biochemistry, Biology and Physics, Department of Clinical Sciences, Università Politecnica delle Marche, 60100 Ancona, Italy
3 Neurology Unit, Department of Experimental and Clinical Medicine, Università Politecnica delle Marche, 60100 Ancona, Italy
* Correspondence: a.vignini@univpm.it

Abstract: Multiple sclerosis (MS) represents the most common acquired demyelinating disorder of the central nervous system (CNS). Its pathogenesis, in parallel with the well-established role of mechanisms pertaining to autoimmunity, involves several key functions of immune, glial and nerve cells. The disease's natural history is complex, heterogeneous and may evolve over a relapsing-remitting (RRMS) or progressive (PPMS/SPMS) course. Acute inflammation, driven by infiltration of peripheral cells in the CNS, is thought to be the most relevant process during the earliest phases and in RRMS, while disruption in glial and neural cells of pathways pertaining to energy metabolism, survival cascades, synaptic and ionic homeostasis are thought to be mostly relevant in long-standing disease, such as in progressive forms. In this complex scenario, many mechanisms originally thought to be distinctive of neurodegenerative disorders are being increasingly recognized as crucial from the beginning of the disease. The present review aims at highlighting mechanisms in common between MS, autoimmune diseases and biology of neurodegenerative disorders. In fact, there is an unmet need to explore new targets that might be involved as master regulators of autoimmunity, inflammation and survival of nerve cells.

Keywords: multiple sclerosis; mitochondrial dysfunction; neurodegeneration; autoimmunity

1. Epidemiology, Etiology, Onset, Disease Course

Multiple sclerosis (MS) is a chronic demyelinating disorder of the central nervous system (CNS) characterized at its core by inflammation involving the gray and white matter of the CNS in a multifocal pattern. It results in demyelinating lesions, focal areas of inflammation characterized by myelin sheath damage surrounded by leukocyte infiltration (macrophages, mast cells, lymphocytes), blood–brain barrier (BBB) breakdown, but also complement and immunoglobulin deposition [1]. Within these areas, inflammation sustained by entry of peripheral cells coexists with damage to neural and synaptic elements while reactive glial elements are engaged in variable terms in cell debris clearance, myelin sheath repair and restoration of neuroaxonal functions [2]. MS is the most common among acquired demyelinating disorders and therefore is considered the most characteristic and prototypical. Symptomatic onset mostly occurs in the age range 20–40, although onset at younger or older ages is not infrequent [3]. The disease is most common in Caucasian populations dwelling in northern latitudes, while exhibiting a lower prevalence in populations dwelling in Africa and in Eastern Asia [4]. It has been observed that people migrating to countries with a lower prevalence appear to have some reduction in the risk of developing the disease [5].

Due to age distribution and prevalence, which is estimated to be as high as 100/100,000 in Western countries, it is regarded as the most frequent cause of non-traumatic disability among young people, affecting women more frequently than men [4].

Etiology of the disease is unknown and highly debated. Currently, the disease's mechanisms express themselves via a complex interaction between genetic susceptibility, hormonal factors, environmental stimuli and the neuroimmune axis, resulting in CNS directed autoimmunity.

As for environmental factors contributing to disease pathogenesis, a risk coming from low ultraviolet light exposure and low blood vitamin D has been suggested by the association with a higher prevalence in northern countries and reduced incidence in people migrating during adolescence from northern latitudes to warmer climate areas [6–8]. Other environmental factors thought to confer a greater susceptibility to develop the disease are smoking and obesity, hypothetically through their influence on inflammation and immune functions [9,10]. Among other lifestyle factors, it has been recently proposed that sleep deprivation at younger ages might increase the risk of developing MS later in life [11].

It is not yet clear whether sleep disorders might precede the disease; nonetheless, prolonged sleep deprivation has been found in experimental models to be mechanistically related to proinflammatory signaling axes within the CNS, such as microglial phagocytic activation, and to impact synaptic maintenance and myelination [12,13].

At variance from other autoimmune diseases, a single antigen either able to kickstart the disease process in humans or to transfer it to a recipient organism has not been defined, although the presence of a sustained antibody response against intracellular antigens is well established. In this regard oligoclonal bands, which are a cornerstone of MS diagnosis, despite being detectable in other diseases, are thought to derive mainly from production of autoantibodies against ubiquitous intracellular components [14].

Several pathogens have been proposed as triggers for disease onset, especially viruses from the *Herpesviridae* family, such as *Epstein–Barr virus* and *human herpes virus 6* [15–18]. In addition, viral DNA as well as antibodies, directed against viral antigens, have been isolated more frequently in plasma and cerebrospinal fluid (CSF) of subjects with the disease with respect to controls. However, evidence of causal association so far has been inconclusive [17,19]. Other viruses considered to have a relationship with the disease onset are *human endogenous retroviruses* (HERV), whose activation as transposable elements of the human genome might influence disease progression [20,21].

Several antigens might contemporarily contribute to disease onset or exacerbation. In this regard, infection from intracellular bacteria such as *Chlamydia pneumoniae* has been associated with MS onset [22], while contact with bacterial superantigens, such as toxins from *Staphylococcus aureus*, has been associated with disease onset and/or exacerbation [23].

Infections from other bacteria, such as *Spirochetes, Campylobacter, Mycoplasma, Chlamydia, Bartonella, Mycobacteria and Streptococcus,* have been linked to MS development, although to date these pathogens have not been directly isolated from CSF of patients [24]. Helminthic infections, on the other hand, have been reported as potentially protective against MS development [23]. Inflammation, once triggered, might progress through an asymptomatic phase where demyelinating lesions appear in a multiphasic, asynchronous pattern in non-contiguous sites, sometimes asymptomatically, thus configuring the phenomena of dissemination in time and space [25].

The prototypical clinical onset is constituted by acute neurological dysfunction, developing over hours or days, sustained by inflammation of discrete areas of the CNS, such as optic nerves as well as cerebral, brainstem or spinal sensorimotor pathways. Dysfunction coming from disease attacks usually resolves in a partial or complete manner. According to the current consensus definition, a single disease episode suggestive of MS, but not sufficient to fulfill criteria for dissemination in time and space, is termed clinically isolated syndrome (CIS) [26]. On the other hand, a condition where lesions suggestive of a demyelinating disease are present in the absence of clinical manifestations is termed radiological isolated syndrome (RIS) [27]. Over time, according to differences in lesion appearance, clinical manifestations and disability build-up, the disease might assume a relapsing-remitting (RRMS) or progressive course, which could be further distinguished between primarily (PPMS) or secondarily progressive (SPMS). While the former is characterized by repetition of brief episodes of neurologic dysfunction sustained by acute CNS inflammation and synchronous appearance of demyelinating lesions, in the latter, neurologic functioning, especially in motor systems, slowly decays over time regardless of the appearance of new demyelinating plaques. Progressive courses can be further distinguished into secondary or primary according to whether they have been preceded by a longstanding RRMS or not [28,29]. The occurrence of relapses and sustained progression of the disease are not mutually exclusive. Less frequently, a benign disease course, characterized by absence of relapses with conservation of neurologic functioning over decades, even without immunomodulatory therapy, has been described [30]. On the other hand, very aggressive courses, with high lesional loads, such as tumefactive MS [31] or a monophasic fulminant onset ab initio, have also been described [32].

2. Pathology: Demyelination

On a histologic basis, typical MS lesions consist of confluent foci of inflammatory myelin breakdown, centered on perivascular spaces close to cerebral venules and surrounded by reactive gliosis, which affect both white and gray matter of the brain and spinal cord. Aspects of parenchymal damage are combined with a varying degree of infiltration of blood-borne cells, such as $CD4^+$, $CD8^+$ lymphocytes and monocytes, entering through focal areas of BBB disruption. In addition, surrounding astroglial, microglial and oligodendroglial cells display a reactive phenotype [33,34].

Lesion types have been further subdivided into different patterns according to the major constituents of inflammatory infiltrates and CSF characteristics, potentially underlying nuances in their pathophysiology. Pattern I lesions display T cell and macrophage infiltration, while pattern II lesions show in addition antibody and complement deposition, suggesting a contribution of humoral mechanisms to disease pathology. Pattern III is characterized by distal oligodendrogliopathy with dysregulated myelin protein expression and oligodendrocyte apoptosis, which still occurs on an inflammatory background. A fourth pattern, which has been described in rarer cases, is characterized by oligodendrocyte degeneration occurring in the white matter surrounding plaques [35,36].

Lesions in the gray matter show more pronounced alterations in structure and numbers of synapses than their white matter counterparts [37]. Perivenular spaces, i.e., perivascular spaces surrounding venules, are thought to be a critical area of immune cell trafficking from peripheral organs, and demyelinating lesions are thought to originate from confluence of foci of inflammation surrounding these spaces [38].

Lesional activity has been characterized according to the relative preponderance of inflammation, tissue destruction and gliosis/repair processes. Active lesions are distinguished by increased permeability of the BBB and a significant infiltration of dendritic cells, B, $CD4^+$, $CD8^+$ T lymphocytes, mast cells, monocytes from the periphery, cytokine and adhesion molecule expression, coexisting with activated microglia. On the other hand, inactive lesions are characterized by a minor inflammatory component at their core, relatively preserved integrity of the BBB and presence of sparse phagocytes and microglia at the lesion border. Both active and inactive lesions exhibit neuroaxonal loss, whereas inactive ones might expand slowly over time [38]. Despite greater BBB integrity in chronic lesions, magnetic resonance imaging (MRI) studies in MS patients have detected impaired glymphatic flow, which appears to be more prominent in advanced disease [39].

In RRMS and PP/SPMS, both types of lesions coexist, albeit in different proportions. In fact, inactive lesions are thought to be the most common type of lesion in both forms, although active ones are more common in RRMS, underlying a direct pathophysiologic impact of acute inflammation. Progressive forms of the disease, on the other hand, show inactive slowly expanding lesions, while displaying aggregates of inflammatory cells resembling tertiary lymphoid follicles in leptomeningeal compartments combined with global CNS atrophy. Relative proportions of B, plasma cells and T cells also vary [33,40].

Both active and inactive lesions show histologic signs of impaired axonal transport, such as anterograde and retrograde axonal degeneration. These changes, albeit to a lesser degree, also occur in apparently normal gray and white matter in parallel with meningeal inflammation, microglial activation, gliosis and synaptic loss [41].

In addition to inflammation and axonal degeneration, other important features of MS pathology on a cellular level are alterations in synaptic morphology and numbers, iron deposition and mitochondrial changes. Iron deposition might take place in apparently normal white matter, in lesions, but also in basal nuclei [42].

Iron deposition begins in the earliest phases of the disease, increasing with age and is thought to contribute to oxidative stress and disability progression [43,44]. Mitochondria in MS are altered in numbers and distribution, displaying a reduced expression of components of the oxidative phosphorylation chain [45–47].

Functional aspects of mitochondrial impairment will be further discussed in the following sections given their critical relationship with neuroaxonal loss. Another important histologic feature of MS is the loss of glial cells and neurons, which might be operated by heterogeneous pathways [48]. Observations from autoptic studies and animal models suggest that mechanisms of cell death might express themselves through a continuous spectrum encompassing apoptosis, ferroptosis and also necroptosis [48–50].

Further enquiry is needed to elucidate details about the relevance of distinct mechanisms of cell death in MS over its natural history. The histopathological picture of MS also comprises remyelination, characterized by the formation of thin myelin sheaths around damaged axons, either sustained by activation of oligodendrocyte progenitor cells or by terminally differentiated oligodendrocytes [51,52]. These processes will be briefly described in the following sections.

3. Remyelination

Remyelination is a process which may be distinguished into repair of damaged myelin or de novo synthesis. It is thought to be operated in the CNS either by activation of terminally differentiated oligodendrocytes or by recruitment and migration of staminal precursors known as oligodendrocyte progenitor cells (OPCs) [53,54]. OPCs are also thought to be critical for tuning inflammation and angiogenesis; furthermore, they possess complex electrophysiological properties and are thought to form synapses with neurons [55,56].

It is well accepted that remyelination constitutes a continuous and ubiquitous process occurring within the CNS, although it is unclear whether it might be sufficient in restoring myelin function in lesioned areas. Some lesions, in fact, undergo an incomplete repair, characterized by formation of thin sheaths surrounding axons, especially at the lesion border [57]. These areas are defined as "shadow plaques" and are thought to be areas where the remyelination process has come to a halt [58]. It is not well known whether they are the result of single or repeated demyelinating processes, whether they are more prone to subsequent remyelination or whether they might harbor a quiescent recovery potential, but intriguingly, these areas are devoid of OPC elements and, therefore, myelin restoration is thought to be operated only by mature oligodendrocytes [59].

Remyelination declines with aging; it is regulated by synaptic activity but is also highly influenced by the secretory and signaling activity of astroglial elements, as well as by iron transport and phagocytic activity of macrophages and microglial cells [60,61]. Chronic inflammation might impair remyelination dynamics, yielding incomplete repair of damaged sheaths. In accordance with this hypothesis, it has been reported that in addition to shadow plaques, slowly expanding lesions, characteristic of progressive disease, possess a lower remyelination potential [62].

It is currently under debate whether in humans de novo myelination might be more effective in repairing injured structures in comparison to activation of differentiated oligodendrocytes. It has, however, been esteemed that only 0.3% of oligodendroglial elements are regenerated per year; therefore, activation of differentiated elements appears of crucial importance, as well as the mechanisms that might render this process more efficient [59]. Remyelination has also been shown to reverse the alteration in mitochondrial numbers observed in demyelinated axons, suggesting a potential in counteracting neuroaxonal loss [63]. On the whole, remyelination appears as a fundamental process in MS with the potential to preserve functioning of sensory and motor systems and, therefore, delaying and limiting disability.

Several biochemical cascades, involving lipid metabolism, cholesterol efflux, retinoid-X-receptor α dependent pathways, phagocytosis, but also epigenetic regulation through histone deacetylases, have been implied as potential mechanistic targets [64–67]. Among these, leucine-rich repeat and Ig domain-containing 1 (LINGO-1), a glycoprotein expressed by neurons, and OPCs, whose blockade has been shown to improve myelination in animal models of the disease, has been proposed as a promising target for remyelination [68]. Opicinumab, a monoclonal antibody targeting LINGO-1, has failed in trials to reach its efficacy endpoints, despite showing at the highest doses and in younger patients a small improvement in disability worthy of further research [69].

4. Pathogenesis: Immunologic Perspectives

4.1. Mechanisms Pertaining to T and B Lymphocytes

Pathogenesis has been mostly studied through animal models either involving immunization against CNS antigens, infection with neurotropic viruses or administration of neurotoxic/myelinotoxic compounds, such as lysolecithin or cuprizone [70].

The most commonly adopted models derive from parenteral administration of myelin-derived peptides, such as myelin basic protein (MBP), myelin oligodendrocytic glycoprotein (MOG) and proteolipid protein (PLP) complexed with adjuvants, which results in an inflammatory demyelinating disease of the CNS, termed experimental allergic encephalomyelitis (EAE). These models have allowed researchers to characterize in detail some pathogenetic aspects useful to extrapolate data for therapy development, although they do not allow reproduction of every aspect of the human disease, especially concerning its multiphasic clinical course [71]. Other animal models involve infection with neurotropic viruses, such as Theiler's encephalomyelitis virus (TMEV) [72].

Evidence from genomic studies suggests a critical role of loci involved in antigen presentation, such as HLA DRB1*15:0, in conferring susceptibility to the disease, while other HLA haplotypes, such as the A*02 and B*44, have been associated with a protective effect [5].

HLA genes can be distinguished into three classes: class I and class II HLA encode for major histocompatibility complex (MHC) proteins, which are crucial for antigen presentation, while class III HLA loci encode for molecules involved in the inflammatory cascade, such as complement proteins, tumor necrosis factors (TNFs), 21-hydroxylase and heat shock proteins [73,74].

MHC class I molecules (encoded by HLA-A, HLA-B and HLA-C loci), present intracellular self- or non-self-antigens to $CD8^+$ cytotoxic T cell receptors and killer cell immunoglobulin-like receptors (KIR) [75]. On the other hand, class II molecules (encoded by HLA-DP, HLA-DQ and HLA-DR) are expressed on the membrane of antigen-presenting cells (such as macrophages, B cells and dendritic cells) and serve the function of displaying short antigen peptides to $CD4^+$ helper T cells [76].

In addition to HLA loci, more than 200 non-MHC-coding genomic variants have been reported to confer susceptibility to MS, albeit with different effect sizes. In fact, many of these variants affect genes involved in immune system pathways, such as interleukin 2 receptor subunit α (IL-2RA), but also intronic and intragenic sequences related to splicing and quantitative gene expression [77]. Daclizumab, which inhibits IL2RA, has shown high clinical efficacy in preventing MS relapses, although it has been withdrawn for hyperacute hepatotoxicity [78].

As for effector mechanisms, in accordance with autoptic data, pathogenesis shows great similarities to T-cell-mediated diseases; therefore, a central role has been theorized for $CD4^+$ and $CD8^+$ lymphocytes [79,80]. The former, when primed towards their proinflammatory T_{h1} and T_{h17} phenotypes, are thought to be important directors of the immune response towards the CNS [38], while the latter, primed to their cytotoxic phenotypes, are the predominant cell type, under a quantitative perspective, surrounding demyelinated axons [33,81,82].

Many currently approved therapies for MS modulate various aspects of T cell function, including response to activating stimuli, functional polarization, egress from lymph nodes, migration and CNS entrance [83]. Glatiramer acetate is thought to modulate T helper cell polarization toward a Th_2 phenotype, dampening CNS-directed inflammation [84].

In addition, recent studies on distinct immune system cell subtypes in MS highlight the role of several regulatory subpopulations of the innate and adaptive immune system in balancing disease severity, such as forkhead box protein 3 (FOXP3) positive $CD4^+$ cells, Tr1-positive CD4 cells [5], $CD56^{bright}$ NK cells [85]. Subsets of anti-inflammatory $CD8^+$ cells have been described, but to date a single surface antigen combination conferring this functional phenotype has not been defined [85–87].

In recent decades, evidence from animal and clinical studies supported an important role for B cells, given their role in tuning T cell function, antigen presentation, autoantibody production and also in leptomeningeal lymphoid follicle formation [40]. A similar role is shared with dendritic cells, which orchestrate T cell activation through similar processes [88]. B cells comprise a heterogeneous host of naïve, memory and effector subpopulations also including tolerogenic and anti-inflammatory subsets, collectively termed as B_{regs}, characterized by production of IL-10, IL-35 and TGF-β [89].

In clinical studies, B cell-directed anti-CD20 antibodies (especially ocrelizumab) have shown significant benefits and have been approved in both RRMS and PPMS, where they possess lesser efficacy [90]. Their long-lived therapeutic effects might derive from their ability to blunt proliferation of proinflammatory clones such as mature naïve B cells and memory B cells with a parallel stimulation of regulatory populations, such as IL-10-producing B cells, including autoreactive regulatory clones [5,91]. Another very important target for B cell physiology, closely related to MS, is constituted by Bruton tyrosine kinase (BTK), a master regulator of B-cell activation, whose expression is not exclusive to B cells since it has also been detected in myeloid T cells and osteoclasts. It is considered as a "rheostat" of proinflammatory signaling and a regulator of autoreactive cells [92]. Besides tuning B cell receptor (BCR) activation, BTK takes part in signaling of toll-like and Fc receptors, modulating the inflammatory response; therefore, its excessive activity has been related to autoimmunity [93,94]. In addition to its effects on immune activation and inflammation cascades, a recent in vivo study on cultured cerebellar slices interestingly shows that BTK activity is upregulated after lysophosphatidylcholine and metronidazole-induced demyelination, while its inhibition might hasten myelin repair, suggesting complex effects on the CNS [93].

The observed effectiveness, in both animal models and human subjects, of BTK inhibitors in several autoimmune diseases further strengthens the hypothesis that regulation of this cascade might be of therapeutic value [95]. Currently, two brain-penetrant BTK inhibitors, evobrutinib and tolebrutnib, are being assessed with regard to their effectiveness in preventing MS relapses and in reducing disease activity [94].

Several studies have observed a shift in energy metabolism affecting lymphocytes, macrophages and dendritic cells towards aerobic glycolysis (the so-called Warburg effect) in association with dysfunctional oxidative phosphorylation in T lymphocytes [96,97]. It is not known whether this process, termed "metabolic reprogramming", might be the cause or a consequence of aberrant immune activation.

4.2. Mechanisms Pertaining to Innate Immunity

Given the predominance of immune-mediated mechanisms in animal models and the clinical responses associated with immune modulators, several efforts have been made to elucidate the relationship between specific cytokines and disease phenotypes, but also between effector mechanisms of the innate immune system, such as the kinin or complement cascade, and MS pathogenesis. Among cytokines, Th_1 and Th_{17} cytokines are considered pivotal proinflammatory signals, while IL-10, IL-27, IL-35 and especially type I interferons have been associated with disease amelioration [5,98].

TNF-α blockade has been shown to trigger significant disease exacerbation [99,100], while immunomodulation via interferon β (IFN-β) has shown significant clinical efficacy in preventing disease relapses [101]. IFN-β is thought to target antigen presentation processes, modulate cytokine secretion, T cell polarization and MHC molecule expression, although recent studies have also suggested that the activity of the cGAS-STING pathway, a critical regulator of endogenous type I IFN production, might constitute an important determinant of the effectiveness of interferon therapy [98,102,103].

The cGAS-STING pathway, in brief, is considered an intracellular "damage-sensing" cascade involved in innate immunity that is primarily activated by binding of cGAS (cyclic GMP-AMP synthase) to exogenous/endogenous double-stranded DNA fragments outside of the cell nucleus [104]. It has been suggested that its activity might be altered during infections but also in several brain inflammatory disorders [98]. cGAS activation produces 2′5′-cyclic adenosine monophosphate guanosine monophosphate (2′5′-cGAMP), which activates tank-binding kinase 1 (TBK1) and IκB kinase (IKK), inducing STING (stimulator of interferon genes) oligomerization [105–107]. STING activation leads to phosphorylation and activation of interferon regulatory factor 3 (IRF3) and nuclear factor kappa-light-chain-enhancer of activated B cells (NF-κB), which upregulate the type I interferon response, upregulating expression of interferon regulated genes, in turn regulating the synthesis of TNF-α, IL-1β and IL-6, but also of the STING protein [106]. It has been recently observed that RRMS patients might exhibit in peripheral blood mononuclear cells a downregulated activity of the cGAS-STING/IFN-β-axis, while also displaying a reduced expression of interferon regulated genes [103]. It has been therefore suggested that interferon therapy might be mostly effective in patients with a downregulated endogenous response, perhaps in addition to pharmacological modulation of STING activity [105].

Among other soluble signals of innate immunity, studies in EAE models have highlighted a role for bradykinin (BK) in modulating cytokine secretion and CNS lesion development [108]. BK type 1 receptor (B1) activation is thought to mediate BBB breakdown and increased vascular permeability, favoring inflammation [109]. In EAE models, enalapril administration has been shown to increase plasma BK concentration and reduce clinical and pathological severity, while B1 receptor blockade counteracted the protective effects of enalapril [110]. In human studies, increased B1 receptor expression has been detected in T lymphocytes isolated from peripheral blood of MS patients with respect to control subjects, suggesting a potential role in CNS inflammation [111]. As for the complement system, autoptic studies have shown involvement in myelin phagocytosis within acute lesions, but also persistent deposition in chronic lesions in PPMS as well as in gray matter lesions [112]. The complement system might play a complex role in disease pathogenesis since its effects are not limited to debris clearance, but also to processes related to survival cascades. Evidence from cell models has shown that astrocytes secrete complement proteins when stimulated by proinflammatory stimuli as TNF α, IL-1β and IL-8 [113], while sublytic levels of C5b-C9 proteins might drive antiapoptotic responses in oligodendroglial elements [114]. The complement system is also thought to play an important role in removal and maintenance of synaptic structures [115,116]. Evidence from plasma and CSF biomarker studies shows a trend towards increased concentration of complement components, such as C1q, C3 and C4 in RRMS, SPMS and PPMS, as well as an increase in endogenous inhibitors, such as factor H, suggesting heightened complement activity in all forms of the disease [117,118].

These observations might therefore constitute a rationale for assessing complement regulation as a therapeutic target; in a small series of patients, eculizumab, a C5 inhibitor, has recently shown a discrete tolerability in a small series of MS patients, with no severe adverse drug reactions nor disease relapses, supporting further clinical assessment [119].

Data from experimental models suggest that no single antigen or effector cell type might be sufficient to summarize every pathogenetic aspect of MS, whose immunopathogenesis is multifactorial and underlies an interaction, in the periphery and in the CNS, between proinflammatory stimuli, specific subtypes of immune cells and host-specific factors. Among host-specific factors, polygenic susceptibility, hormonal influences, epigenomic regulation, gut microbiome signals and environmental factors (including pollutants and smoking) might shape disease activity [120].

It has been proposed that the gut microbiome may alter the MS immunopathological framework at least by a dual mechanism. In fact, gut dysbiosis, i.e., imbalance between tolerogenic and proinflammatory commensals, might promote inflammation in remote sites, while molecular mimicry between gut antigens and CNS epitopes might select autoreactive cell clones. Gut microbes produce metabolites that also directly target the CNS. It was observed that dietary tryptophan may be metabolized through the serotonin, indole and kynurenine pathways into components that act as aryl hydrocarbon receptor agonists [121] and exert anti-inflammatory actions mediated by astrocytes [122]. The effectiveness, in preclinical models, of the immunomodulatory drug laquinimod, which however failed to reach significant clinical endpoints [123], is thought to derive from its effect on glial aryl hydrocarbon receptors [124]. In addition, dimethylfumarate, a drug approved to treat RRMS, has been found to reduce bacterial production of neurotoxic phenol and indole catabolites of phenylalanine and tryptophan [125].

Under this perspective, the efficacy of the so-called "immune reconstituting" therapies, such as cladribine, alemtuzumab and bone marrow transplantation, might depend not only on quenching of acute inflammation, but also on reconfiguring the immune repertoire to a point that allows previously suppressed cells to emerge and affect immunologic processing in distant sites [126,127]. Ocrelizumab, despite requiring maintenance therapy, could be considered, due to its long-lived effects, as a drug with a profile of action closely comparable to immune reconstituting therapies [128].

On the whole, acute inflammation, which is preponderant in RRMS, is considered highly dependent on the entrance in the CNS of pathogenic autoreactive cells from the periphery and might lead over time to formation of persistent meningeal tertiary lymphoid structures [129]. In accordance with this hypothesis, it has been observed that therapies targeting infiltration of autoreactive cells in the CNS, such as natalizumab, an anti-very late antigen 4 (VLA4) monoclonal antibody, are far more effective in RRMS [130,131], while they might induce devastating disease rebounds after a prolonged discontinuation [132].

In addition, another recently discovered layer of regulation of inflammatory activity is represented by endogenous transposable elements, such as *human endogenous retroviruses*, whose activation has been linked to both disease relapses and progression [21,23]. Recently, temelimab, a monoclonal antibody directed against the HERV-W envelope protein, has shown discrete tolerability in small MS cohorts and promising effects on radiological markers [133].

Despite the abundance of data highlighting the predominance of mechanisms pertaining to the innate and adaptive immune system in sustaining acute attacks, several signaling pathways pertaining to astrocytic, oligodendrocytic and microglial elements appear of primary importance in poising disease activity and determining neuron survival from the earliest phases [134].

5. Pathogenesis: A CNS-Centered Perspective

5.1. Role of Glial Cells

In MS, in analogy with other neurologic diseases, the degree of neurologic dysfunction and disability relates to the extension of damage to several functionally distinct circuits, which are composed of high-order networks of neuronal and glial cells. Glial cells are specialized elements that sustain neurons through several processes. For instance, astrocytes tune the surrounding microenvironment including pH, water and ion content according to neuronal metabolic demands, but also scavenge free radicals and participate directly in synaptic transmission [135]. Microglia are mesenchymal-derived immunocompetent cells whose principal functions are considered clearing cell debris through phagocytosis and coordinating inflammatory responses within the CNS [136], whereas oligodendrocytes, which reside exclusively in the CNS, are neuronal lineage cells specialized in myelin synthesis, maintenance and repair [137].

On the whole, glial cells are highly plastic and specialized elements that might alter their phenotype, integrating various electrical and molecular stimuli, including those produced by an inflammatory environment. Their signals directly tune the immune response within the CNS and vascular/BBB permeability, but also functional properties of neural cells. They secrete chemokines and cytokines, might change their morphology according to the surrounding microenvironment and their signals pose a significant influence on neuronal survival and functioning of the tripartite synapse [138]. Several efforts have been made to define functionally distinct subsets of astrocytes or microglial cells with either a neuroprotective or neurotoxic phenotype, although the heterogeneity of activation states and phenotypes of glial cells suggests the existence of a continuous spectrum, rather than distinct subcategories [139]. Therefore, the interplay between the immune system, glial cells and neurons might shape disease progression precociously, triggering processes that might follow a divergent direction from acute inflammation [34]. Hence, acute and chronic inflammation constitute stressors that might recruit, in the long run, signaling pathways tied to responses to neurotoxic insults such as protein misfolding, loss of membrane integrity and nucleic acid damage, yielding profound biochemical changes on a cellular level that ultimately impact on ion homeostasis (especially calcium and iron), growth-factor signaling, remyelination and cell survival cascades [140]. Such processes are all mechanistically tied to mitochondrial oxidative phosphorylation, calcium buffering and redox balance and, therefore, are considered common effectors of cell loss in MS and neurodegenerative diseases (Figure 1). During MS's earliest phases they are considered to be mainly triggered by autoimmunity, but whether their activation might progress independently from inflammation is currently under debate [46].

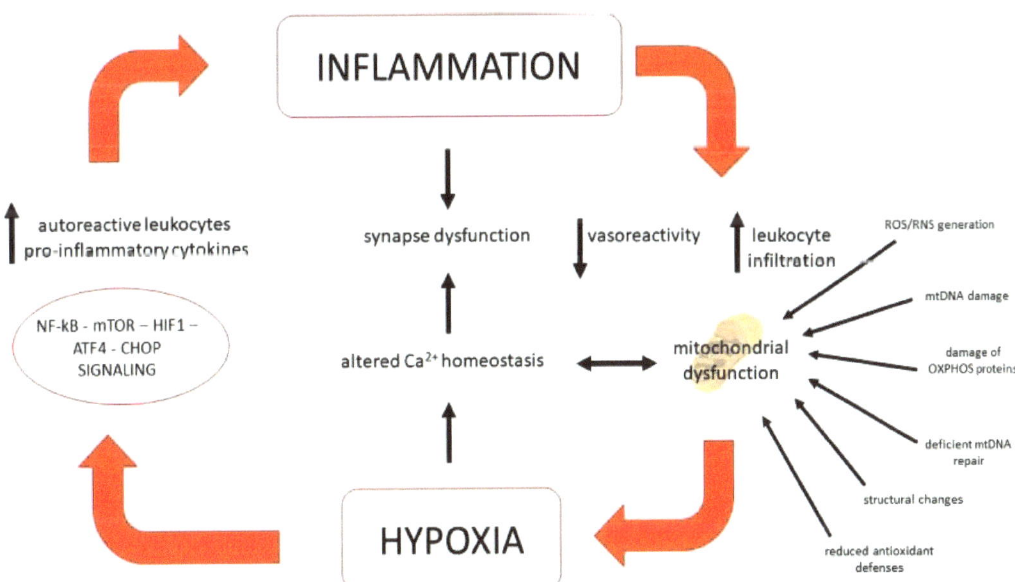

Figure 1. The positive feedback loop of hypoxia and inflammation. The low oxygen presence will lead to the activation of NF-κB, m-TOR, HIF1, ATF4, CHOP signaling, all regulators of inflammation. Increased levels of autoreactive leukocytes and pro-inflammatory cytokines can decrease vasoreactivity, and impair mitochondrial function, which could in turn exacerbate hypoxia.

5.2. Role of Mitochondria

Considering the pathophysiological analogies found in different experimental models of neurodegeneration, indicating a significant role of mitochondria in regulating cell fate, several lines of research have converged on mitochondrial impairment and related mechanisms in shaping MS pathology [45,48]. In fact, under a pathogenetic perspective, it has been observed in several disease models that the high energy consumption of nerve cells and their reliance on oxidative metabolism might render them particularly vulnerable to degenerative changes in contexts of impaired mitochondrial ATP production, potentially starting multiple interlinked deleterious processes.

It is well documented that mitochondria from MS patients are altered in morphology and distribution, carrying mutations in mtDNA while also showing diminished expression of elements of the respiratory chain and altered expression of heat shock proteins, resulting in ATP production impairment. Such changes are thought to be more relevant in progressive disease, albeit beginning from the earliest phases [46,47].

In accordance with the hypothesis of a pivotal role of mitochondria in MS, many cytotoxic agents, used to induce demyelination in animal models, such as cuprizone, lysolecithin or ethidium-bromide, may directly alter their number or disrupt respiratory chain complex expression [70,141,142].

Decreased energy production might alter ionic transmembrane gradients, sustaining calcium entry, heightening reactive oxygen species (ROS) generation, endoplasmic reticulum stress and stimulation of intracellular transducers, such as activating transcription factor 4 (ATF4), glucose regulated protein (GRP78) and C/EBP homologous protein (CHOP), which are closely tied to apoptosis and inflammation [143–145]. These interlinked processes might concur to decrease cell energy metabolism progressively, promoting a self-sustaining cycle of damage, which might lead to cell death, with consequent debris release and inflammation.

Such a sequence of events has been termed a "mitochondrial spiral" and is thought to occur in Alzheimer's dementia and stroke [146,147]. Despite striking differences in clinical course between stroke, primarily neurodegenerative diseases and MS, dysfunctional energetic homeostasis appears as a shared pathogenetic factor of critical importance [148].

5.3. Ion Homeostasis and Energy Metabolism Regulation

In MS, reduction in cerebral blood flow might impair ATP production, especially within demyelinated areas, whereas altered numbers and morphology of mitochondria might reflect a homeostatic response to increased metabolic demands or relative lack of oxygen and nutrients. Under a pathophysiological perspective, oxygen–glucose deprivation, leading to decreased ATP production, promotes sodium accumulation and calcium entry from the extracellular space, operated by the sodium calcium exchanger (NCX) reverse mode [149,150]. In an analogy to the biochemical changes triggered by hyperacute oxygen–glucose deprivation happening during ischemia, significant accumulation of sodium ions within active and inactive demyelinated areas has been detected through MRI in MS patients [151], supporting the hypothesis of lasting imbalances in calcium cycling.

Although NCX has been mostly perceived to promote excessive calcium influx after hypoxia, its reverse mode transport (sodium-dependent calcium influx) might be essential for the activation of ischemic conditioning [152] and might also play a pivotal role, due its close physical and functional coupling with neuronal and glial sodium-dependent glutamate transporters, in sustaining glutamate-induced ATP synthesis [152–154]. Further enquiry about the functional properties of distinct isoforms that display heterogeneous gating properties [155] and differential distribution within the CNS [156] is needed in order to clarify their pathophysiological significance.

In an analogy with data from acute damage models, a potential role for NCX in chronic neurodegenerative diseases, which is to be further characterized, has been suggested [157]. In parallel, sodium accumulation within demyelinated axons might modify the activity of other sodium-dependent transporters, including the sodium hydrogen exchanger (NHE) and sodium potassium chloride cotransporter (NKCC). These transporters have been implied in regulating cell death across several pathologic scenarios in the CNS, although the precise functional interactions between sodium-dependent transporters, energy metabolism, substrate uptake, inflammation and calcium cycling in MS need to be further elucidated.

Ultimately, deregulation of calcium homeostasis, among its widespread toxic effects, contributes to oxidative phosphorylation and ATP synthesis impairment, affecting at first detrimentally those functions mostly dependent on sustained energy synthesis, such as synaptic transmission and plasticity [158]. In addition, prolonged calcium accumulation, either by entrance through the plasma membrane or by excessive loading of internal stores, triggers mitochondrial-dependent pathways, such as MPTP opening, resulting in irreversible mitochondrial membrane depolarization and thus cell death [159].

In parallel to mechanisms inducing mitochondrial dysfunction during hypoxia, several signaling pathways related to cellular resistance to such challenges have been explored for a potential role in mitigating neuroaxonal loss in MS. In particular, signaling cascades related to ischemic conditioning, autophagy and metabolic reprogramming have stood out in preclinical models, also with potential implications for aberrant immunologic processing (Figure 1) [160].

At present, experimental models have highlighted a significant integration between the activation of cytoprotective pathways involved in preserving mitochondrial function during hypoxia, which affect oxidative stress and calcium overload, and the master signaling pathways modulating cell energy metabolism and inflammatory signaling [161].

The activity of potassium-dependent ATP channels, which are among the effectors of ischemic conditioning, has been associated with amelioration of the disease in preclinical models [162].

A common effector of cell responses to hypoxia and a key player in ischemic conditioning is hypoxia-inducible factor 1α (HIF1) [163]. Reduced energy production in MS might trigger HIF1 activation, adapting CNS cell energy metabolism, angiogenesis and ROS production to context-dependent cues, but also influencing iron accumulation and apoptosis [164]. On the other hand, sustained inflammation might heighten HIF1 activation and ROS production in continuously stimulated lymphocytes, leading to impaired responsiveness and senescence [165]. HIF1 induces expression of several genes, including vascular endothelial growth factor B (VEGF-B), whose levels have been found to be lower in MS patients during stable disease with respect to control subjects, suggesting that disease activity and metabolic stress might be associated [166].

A potential relationship between cascades involved in hypoxia and MS might be supported not only by evidence from experimental models, but also by the observation that remote ischemic preconditioning, a procedure thought to stimulate cell programs aimed at preserving the integrity of mitochondrial functions, might improve gait dysfunction in progressive MS patients [167–169].

Among regulators of metabolic programming, a critical cell pathway, implied in tuning the shift of metabolic resources in accordance to nutrient availability, is represented by mechanistic targeting of rapamycin (mTOR), a ubiquitous regulator of energy metabolism, proliferation and inflammation [170,171].

In addition to its well-known effects on lymphocyte proliferation and suppression, its role in diverting utilization of metabolic resources in glia and nerve cells by repurposing their phenotype towards anabolism or catabolism is being increasingly recognized, especially for potential implications for autophagy and remyelination [172].

Indeed, it has been observed that mTOR plays an important role in shifting metabolism towards aerobic glycolysis in activated microglia [96]. In addition, preliminary evidence coming from human studies has also suggested a potential efficacy in MS of therapies acting on the mTOR axis, either indirectly, such as metformin, or directly, such as rapamycin [173]. Among other cascades functionally related to the mTOR axis, recent studies have suggested involvement of DJ-1 and parkin, whose functional roles are tied to oxidative stress and mitophagy, in driving inflammation as well as cell death in MS [174–176].

5.4. Oxidative and Cell Stress Signaling Pathways

From a wider perspective, among other regulators of cellular resistance to metabolic stressors, klotho, an anti-aging protein involved in the FGF-23 signaling, oxidative stress and mitochondrial damage [177] has been recently associated with remyelination in experimental models and has also been suggested as a potential player in MS pathogenesis. In accordance with this hypothesis, it has been found in higher titers in serum from MS patients with respect to controls [178–180].

The involvement of cellular pathways related to aging is also suggested by the observation that sirtuins (SIRT), ubiquitary NAD-dependent enzymes which are also critical for lifespan regulation and epigenetic regulation, might influence disease phenotype in EAE. More specifically, it has been suggested that SIRT might contribute to MS pathogenesis by regulating oxidative stress, mitochondrial phosphorylative oxidation and autophagic networks [181]. In addition, they might poise activation of master regulators of inflammation such as NfKB, modulate antigen presentation by dendritic cells and activate either anti-inflammatory or pro-inflammatory responses. In particular, SIRT1 overexpression has been found to ameliorate EAE phenotype [88]. SIRT might also act in conjunction with nuclear erythroid factor 2 (Nrf2), a transcription factor involved in antioxidant production, mitochondrial biogenesis and oxidative phosphorylation, which is thought to play a role in neurodegeneration and MS pathogenesis [182].

Dimethylfumarate, a drug approved to treat RRMS, exerts a complex action on pathways regulating B and T cell survival, promoting emergence of regulatory cell subsets, while in neurons its effects are tied to Nrf2 activation, with a potential cytoprotective effect [183].

Another interesting area of research, which lies at the border between cell survival cascades, metabolism and stress signaling, is constituted by signaling lipids, such as sphingosine and ceramides. Ceramides in particular are considered a crucial switch for apoptosis due to their regulation of mitochondrial outer membrane potential and permeability [184]. Fingolimod and siponimod, oral therapies acting on sphingosine-1-phosphate receptors (S1PRs), have shown clinical efficacy by downregulating their expression on peripheral lymphocytes and thus inhibiting lymphocyte homing towards the CNS [185].

Follow-up of patients treated with S1P analogues has highlighted a potential protective effect on brain atrophy in addition to regulating immune cell trafficking [186], which might be related to fine-tuning in both neurons and astrocytes of lipid signaling cascades pertaining to endo/exocytotic vesicle cycling and neurotransmitter release. It has also been observed that these drugs possess the ability to dampen glial inflammatory phenotype changes induced by the disease [187–189].

5.5. Synaptic Aspects

In parallel with inflammation and the associated dysfunctional energy metabolism in the CNS, synapses exhibit a precocious dysfunction, which over time might become a bona fide "synaptopathy" [37]. Summarizing evidence from pathological studies, significant alterations in synaptic numbers and morphology have been described in lesions and within apparently normal gray and white matter underlying long-standing functional alterations [33]. In preclinical models, perturbation in pre- and post-synaptic protein expression, electrophysiology and synaptic demolition by the complement cascade, are well-recognized elements [37,190,191]. The main players involved in these processes are thought to be dysfunctional astrocytes and microglia primed by inflammatory changes, which might retain long-lasting pathologic phenotypes that outlive resolution of acute inflammation. Several efforts have been made to characterize, in more detail, these alterations, leading to a theory of the establishment of a long-lived imbalance between excitatory and inhibitory transmission, progressing to a complex dysfunction of synaptic potentiation and depression [192,193]. Despite morphological and functional abnormalities having been most extensively studied with regard to glutamatergic and GABAergic systems, other neurotransmitters such as neuropeptides and neurosteroids are being increasingly recognized as involved in synaptic dysfunction in MS [190,194].

Other less studied mechanisms, although increasingly recognized in MS pathogenesis, are constituted by BBB permeabilization and vascular and endothelial regulation, which are bidirectionally linked to synaptic activity, inflammation and non-physiological neurovascular coupling.

5.6. Vascular Aspects

Several studies have observed in MS elements of endothelial dysfunction, such as an increase in adhesion molecule (i.e., VCAM-1) expression, which might be related to inflammation-driven permeabilization of the BBB [195]. In addition, an epidemiological association between increased incidence of ischemic stroke and migraine, which are characterized by endothelial dysfunction [196], has been reported in MS patients [197,198]. Furthermore, global brain perfusion in MS patients is frequently decreased, suggesting the presence of a widespread disruption of autoregulation [199].

Cerebral vascular reactivity, measured as flow-mediated dilation (FMD) or response to hypercapnia, evaluated with neurosonologic methods, was found to be impaired in patients with SPMS or PPMS in comparison to RRMS [200,201]. Collaterally, a proinflammatory phenotype of platelets, characterized by increased endothelial adhesion, chronic activation, adhesion to astrocytes and neurons, has been described and is thought to promote lesion activity [202].

On the whole, MS appears to embrace and connect various aspects of neuronal and immune system physiology. Most pathogenetic mechanisms considered so far, either involving acute inflammation or dysfunction of neuronal and glial homeostatic processes, while mostly active within lesions, might affect apparently normal gray and white matter.

It is not well-known, however, which signals influence apparently normal areas at the beginning of the disease. These observations have suggested a potential pathogenetic role for mediators exerting their effects beyond the borders of the inflammatory milieu within lesions. From this perspective, in addition to cytokines, vasoactive peptides do stand out, given their role in the CNS as "volume transmitters", i.e., neuropeptides released by neurons from sites not restricted to synapses and therefore able to diffuse beyond synaptic borders [203].

5.7. Role of Neuropeptides

Neuropeptides are ubiquitous signaling molecules that in the PNS and CNS might be expressed by neurons and co-released with fast neurotransmitters, acting on local scales. Neuropeptides might also travel for longer distances, engaging more distant targets, in a manner akin to hormones [203]. Experimental models have shown that several neuropeptides, including endothelin-1 (ET-1), calcitonin gene-related peptide (CGRP) and vasoactive intestinal peptide (VIP) might be involved in regulation of synaptic potentiation/depression [204–206]. Additionally, pleiotropic effects including growth factor-like properties and potent regulatory effects on vascular tone, inflammation and immunity have been described [207,208].

Vasoactive peptides have been mostly studied for their relationship with BBB permeabilization, vascular tone and neurogenic inflammation. Recent research has highlighted in addition pleiotropic neuroprotective but also neurotoxic properties in cell and animal models. On the whole, despite the existence of different isoforms and receptors, vasodilatory peptides have been associated with neuroprotective properties, while vasoconstrictive peptides have been associated with a detrimental effect [209,210]; considering their action on multiple targets, they might be implied in MS pathogenesis at several levels, including innate and acquired immunity, vascular dysfunction but also neuron survival and glial dysfunction (Figure 2).

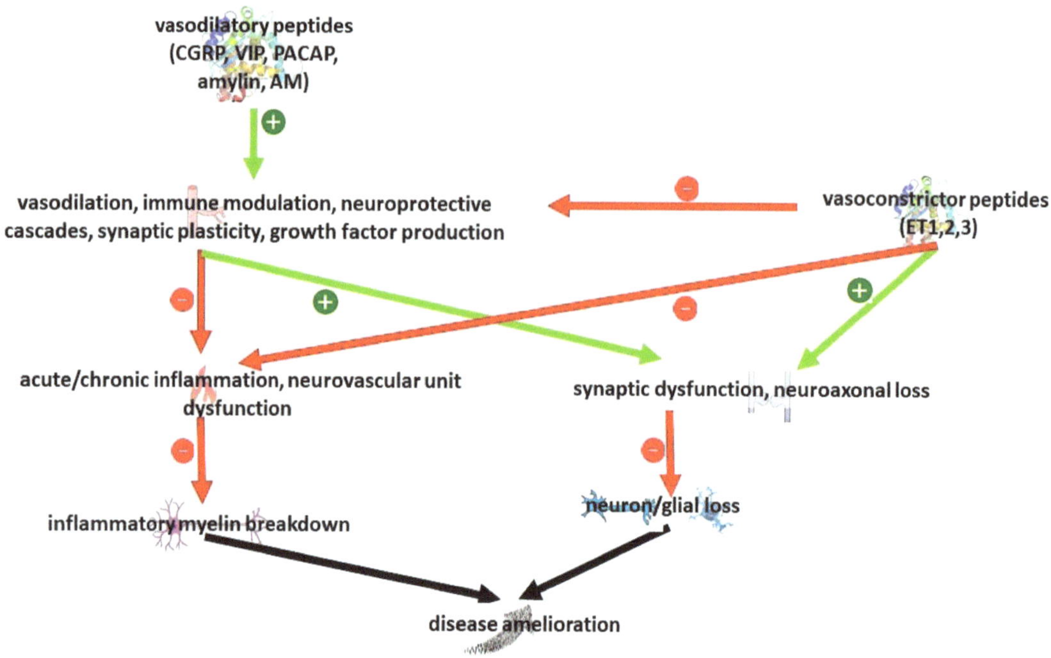

Figure 2. Overview of relevant pathways to MS pathology regulated by vasoactive peptides.

The vasoactive intestinal peptide (VIP) and pituitary adenylate cyclase-activating peptide (PACAP) have been extensively studied in EAE models, suggesting a complex bidirectional pathogenetic role in inflammation and demyelination. Activation of their shared receptors (VPAC 1-2) has been reported to ameliorate EAE severity, while selective VIP knockout or VPAC-1 receptor knockout or pharmacological blockade has been observed to confer resistance to EAE development [211,212].

Other neuropeptides, such as substance P and neuropeptide Y (NPY), have also been associated to a potential anti-inflammatory role in EAE models. Among vasoconstrictive peptides, the endothelin family (ETs), represented by endothelin 1 (ET-1), endothelin 2 (ET-2) and endothelin 3 (ET-3), stands out for a potential pathogenetic role. ETs are ubiquitous mediators considered potent vasoconstrictors that act on a local scale, with prominent actions on vascular tone, remodeling and endothelial dysfunction [213]. All the three peptides act in synergy on different receptor, resulting in highly regulated signals on vascular tone [214]. Among the three peptides, ET-1, of endothelial origin, is the most studied. On a cellular level ET-1, by activating endothelin A and endothelin B receptors, might modulate neuronal cascades implied in cell survival, such as CHOP and Jun [215], while it is produced by astrocytes following demyelination, with a consequent activation of the notch pathway, which has been associated with defective myelin repair [216,217]. Other investigations have also suggested that ET-1 might exert a pleiotropic role during acute neuronal injury. In fact, a recent study on a spinal cord hypoxia-reperfusion injury model has shown that endothelin receptor blockade might ameliorate tissue damage [218], while He and colleagues have observed that remote ischemic conditioning is abrogated by preemptive ET receptor blockade, thus requiring an increase in ET-1 signaling to stimulate neuroprotective cascades, such as Nrf2 [219]. In addition, ET-1 overexpression has been found to increase disease severity in transgenic mice, while receptor blockade has been associated with diminished EAE progression [220,221]. As for evidence coming from human studies, plasma levels of ET-1 and ET-3 are increased in MS patients with respect to control subjects, and increased CSF ET-1 concentrations have been associated with a poorer visual recovery in MS patients after an episode of optic neuritis [222,223].

VIP, PACAP and CGRP, which are vasodilatory, have been found to reduce the severity of neurologic dysfunction in EAE, via a modulatory action on inflammation and immune activation [224–226].

CGRP, as VIP and PACAP, possesses pleiotropic properties, with a contribution from its effects on various cell targets, including vascular smooth muscle, neurons, glia and immune cells [227]. In particular α-CGRP has been proposed as involved in the protective effects of ischemic postconditioning [228]. In murine stroke models, CGRP administration at reperfusion was found to reduce infarct size after middle cerebral artery occlusion [229], while CGRP knockout in a bilateral carotid stenosis model was found to reduce angiogenesis and to increase oxidative damage and demyelination [230].

As for inflammation and immune activation, CGRP has been shown to exert a context-dependent bidirectional effect. In particular, it has been found to dampen toll-like receptor (TLR) responses during lipopolysaccharide (LPS) stimulation, but also to poise excessive inflammation during sepsis, hypothetically through cAMP-dependent signaling; furthermore CGRP signaling might influence maturation of $CD4^{+}$- $Cd25^{+}$-$FOXP3^{+}$ lymphocytes [231,232].

In the CNS it is considered a primary effector of neurogenic inflammation in migraine [233], but has also been found to ameliorate EAE severity during disease induction through a complex regulation, in microglial elements, of the expression of proinflammatory immune activation markers, such as IL1-β and IL6, or anti-inflammatory markers, such as Ym1 and CD163 [226].

Furthermore α-CGRP is produced in the CNS by spinal motor neurons, which upregulate its synthesis after mechanical injury, such as after axotomy [234], or during inflammation, such as in the acute phase of EAE [235]. CGRP, beyond its role in acute inflammation and immunity, as a neurotransmitter, affects monoaminergic circuits and might be involved in pathophysiology of depression and cognitive impairment, which commonly occur during MS [236–238].

Due to its wealth of functions and the ubiquitous expression of CGRP receptors in the CNS [239], it might influence in a pleiotropic manner MS pathogenesis, not only regulating inflammatory cascades, but also through mechanisms involving regulation of growth factor production, survival cascades and synaptic plasticity [227,233,240]. In addition, its potent vasodilatory action might play a role in preserving the integrity of neurovascular unit functioning. Considering data from experimental models of CNS demyelination and the epidemiological association between migraine and MS, a pathogenetic relationship between CGRP and MS pathogenesis appears worthy of further study.

CGRP belongs to the amylin (AMY) family of neuropeptides and is structurally related to adrenomedullin (AM), which might act as a low-affinity agonist on CGRP receptors [241]. Similarly to CGRP, AM was found to reduce EAE severity in experimental models [242] while expression of its mRNA in choroid plexuses was found to be higher in progressive MS patients in comparison to controls in autoptic studies, paralleled by upregulation of other genes involved in neuroprotective cascades, including the HIF axis [243].

CGRP also bears a higher structural homology to amylin in comparison to AM [244]. Amylin, closely related to amyloid β (Aβ) and a major constituent of amyloid plaques, has been investigated in several preclinical models of neurodegeneration, which have shown significant effects on neuronal survival and proinflammatory signaling [245,246]. Amylin might, in the first place, exert its effects through binding to AMY receptors, which are involved in modulation cascades relevant to inflammation, energy metabolism and synaptic plasticity. CGRP, on the other hand, due to its structural homology to amylin, displays high affinity towards AMY1a receptors, potentially reinforcing amylin signaling at physiologic levels [231,244,247]. In addition to the effects mediated by signaling through their specific receptors, it has been observed that a hexameric peptide shared by amylin, tau protein, serum amyloid P and Aβ A4 might bind proinflammatory mediators in plasma and reduce polymerization of amyloid fibrils, eliciting a therapeutic effect in EAE [248,249]. Under a speculative perspective, such molecular motifs might also affect neurodegenerative changes, since recent studies have suggested a complex relationship between Aβ metabolism and remyelination [250]. Furthermore, in human biomarker studies, lower CSF Aβ concentration has been associated with a worse prognosis in MS [251].

Another potential implication for the amylin family of neuropeptides in MS pathogenesis is supported by the observation that AMY, AM, CGRP and Aβ share common catabolic pathways, represented by endopeptidases such as neprilysin (NEP) [252–255], endothelin converting enzyme [256] and insulin-degrading enzyme [257,258], which have been described as key players in regulating inflammation and degenerative changes within the CNS [259].

At present, NEP appears an interesting target in MS since data coming from experimental studies support a role in ameliorating EAE severity through catabolism of several vasoactive peptides, including those of the amylin family and endogenous opioids such as met-enkephalin [260]. In contrast, data coming from genomic studies point to an epidemiological association between a polymorphism in the MMEL1 gene, encoding NEP2 and MS susceptibility [261], although further studies are needed on this subject. Another enzyme involved in catabolism of vasoactive peptides, which could play a pathogenetic role in MS, is represented by CD26/dipeptidyl peptidase IV (DPP4), which primarily regulates systemic glucose metabolism by catabolizing glucagon-like peptide-1, glucagon inhibiting peptide and glucagon influencing insulin sensitivity and type II diabetes mellitus pathogenesis. More recently, it has also been implied in several brain disorders since its other substrates include neuropeptide Y, secretin, substance PACAP and amyloid peptides [262]. At present, lower soluble DPP4 expression in plasma samples from MS has been detected with respect to controls, while surface expression by $CD8^+$ circulating cells was increased [263]. Further studies are needed on the relationship between MS pathogenesis and CD26.

6. Conclusive Remarks

In MS, a wealth of mechanisms contemporarily concurs to pathogenesis, crosslinking innate and adaptive immunity, stress response and survival-related cascades in neural and glial cells. Acute and chronic inflammation appear the primary drivers of damage, although neurodegenerative changes, such as synaptic disruption and neuroaxonal loss, display early appearance and might progress independently from the resolution of acute inflammation. Significant clinical progress has been achieved through introduction of highly effective immunomodulating drugs in delaying the onset of disability and clinical conversion in RRMS. Unfortunately, therapeutic tools for progressive forms appear much less effective to date. It is increasingly recognized that disability might progress independently from inflammation, whereas irreversible decay of neurologic function might depend on the exhaustion of neuronal functional plasticity, which compensates for neuroaxonal loss through remyelination, synaptic remodeling and staminal precursor recruitment. In order to extend time to irreversible disability, approaches involving intensive immunosuppression in the earliest clinical phases have been advocated, although it is yet to be ascertained whether such therapies might influence in the long run degenerative processes pertaining to glial and neuronal cells.

Despite the identification of several potential neuroprotective agents in neurodegeneration and EAE models, none have to date shown similar, long-lasting effects in humans. Among current therapy regimens, only dimethylfumarate and S1P receptor agonists, in addition to their immunomodulatory properties acting on high-order regulatory pathways of inflammation, energy metabolism and cell survival, have shown a neuroprotective potential and might therefore speculatively represent a proof-of-concept for further drug development. A current etiology for the disease as well as its precise triggers are not known, although research has shed light in recent years on the existence of several physiological interlinked mechanisms, which might at the same time concur to aberrant immune activation but also to degenerative aspects and whose modulation could constitute an interesting therapeutic target. Among various putative targets, neuropeptides could speculatively play an important role, which is partly sustained by experimental and biomarker studies, in consideration of their ubiquitous distribution and their multifaceted actions on immunity and neuronal processes.

Therefore, in MS, it would be advisable for future studies to identify essential shared cell pathways underlying inflammation, cell proliferation and functional reprogramming of the neuroimmune axis. Such elements could constitute interesting targets for drug design, with potential implications towards other chronic neurologic diseases involving degeneration of nerve cells. In addition, the development of related biomarkers could play a significant role in focusing the field of study.

Author Contributions: Conceptualization, G.P., M.S., C.P. and S.L.; writing—original draft preparation, G.P.; writing—review and editing G.D., G.C. and S.A.; visualization, G.P.; supervision, S.L. and A.V. All authors have read and agreed to the published version of the manuscript.

Funding: This research received no external funding.

Institutional Review Board Statement: Not applicable.

Informed Consent Statement: Not applicable.

Data Availability Statement: Not applicable.

Conflicts of Interest: The authors declare no conflict of interest.

References

1. Lock, C.; Hermans, G.; Pedotti, R.; Brendolan, A.; Schadt, E.; Garren, H.; Langer-Gould, A.; Strober, S.; Cannella, B.; Allard, J.; et al. Gene-Microarray Analysis of Multiple Sclerosis Lesions Yields New Targets Validated in Autoimmune Encephalomyelitis. *Nat. Med.* **2002**, *8*, 500–508. [CrossRef] [PubMed]
2. Paul, A.; Comabella, M.; Gandhi, R. Biomarkers in Multiple Sclerosis. *Cold Spring Harb. Perspect. Med.* **2019**, *9*, a029058. [CrossRef] [PubMed]
3. Małecka, I.; Przybek-Skrzypecka, J.; Kurowska, K.; Mirowska-Guzel, D.; Członkowska, A. Clinical and Laboratory Parameters by Age for Patients Diagnosed with Multiple Sclerosis between 2000 and 2015. *Neurol. Neurochir. Pol.* **2021**, *55*, 387–393. [CrossRef] [PubMed]
4. Leray, E.; Moreau, T.; Fromont, A.; Edan, G. Epidemiology of Multiple Sclerosis. *Rev. Neurol.* **2016**, *172*, 3–13. [CrossRef] [PubMed]
5. Baecher-Allan, C.; Kaskow, B.J.; Weiner, H.L. Multiple Sclerosis: Mechanisms and Immunotherapy. *Neuron* **2018**, *97*, 742–768. [CrossRef]
6. Swank, R.L.; Lerstad, O.; Strøm, A.; Backer, J. Multiple Sclerosis in Rural Norway Its Geographic and Occupational Incidence in Relation to Nutrition. *N. Engl. J. Med.* **1952**, *246*, 722–728. [CrossRef]
7. van der Mei, I.A.; Ponsonby, A.L.; Blizzard, L.; Dwyer, T. Regional Variation in Multiple Sclerosis Prevalence in Australia and Its Association with Ambient Ultraviolet Radiation. *Neuroepidemiology* **2001**, *20*, 168–174. [CrossRef]
8. Hawkes, C.H.; Giovannoni, G.; Lechner-Scott, J.; Levy, M.; Waubant, E. Multiple Sclerosis and Migration Revisited. *Mult. Scler. Relat. Disord.* **2019**, *34*, A1–A2. [CrossRef]
9. Rosso, M.; Chitnis, T. Association Between Cigarette Smoking and Multiple Sclerosis. *JAMA Neurol.* **2020**, *77*, 245. [CrossRef]
10. Schreiner, T.-G.; Genes, T.-M. Obesity and Multiple Sclerosis-A Multifaceted Association. *J. Clin. Med.* **2021**, *10*, 2689. [CrossRef]
11. Bishir, M.; Bhat, A.; Essa, M.M.; Ekpo, O.; Ihunwo, A.O.; Veeraraghavan, V.P.; Mohan, S.K.; Mahalakshmi, A.M.; Ray, B.; Tuladhar, S.; et al. Sleep Deprivation and Neurological Disorders. *BioMed Res. Int.* **2020**, *2020*, 5764017. [CrossRef] [PubMed]
12. Bellesi, M.; de Vivo, L.; Chini, M.; Gilli, F.; Tononi, G.; Cirelli, C. Sleep Loss Promotes Astrocytic Phagocytosis and Microglial Activation in Mouse Cerebral Cortex. *J. Neurosci. Off. J. Soc. Neurosci.* **2017**, *37*, 5263–5273. [CrossRef]
13. Bellesi, M.; Pfister-Genskow, M.; Maret, S.; Keles, S.; Tononi, G.; Cirelli, C. Effects of Sleep and Wake on Oligodendrocytes and Their Precursors. *J. Neurosci.* **2013**, *33*, 14288–14300. [CrossRef] [PubMed]
14. Brändle, S.M.; Obermeier, B.; Senel, M.; Bruder, J.; Mentele, R.; Khademi, M.; Olsson, T.; Tumani, H.; Kristoferitsch, W.; Lottspeich, F.; et al. Distinct Oligoclonal Band Antibodies in Multiple Sclerosis Recognize Ubiquitous Self-Proteins. *Proc. Natl. Acad. Sci. USA* **2016**, *113*, 7864–7869. [CrossRef] [PubMed]
15. Chapenko, S.; Millers, A.; Nora, Z.; Logina, I.; Kukaine, R.; Murovska, M. Correlation between HHV-6 Reactivation and Multiple Sclerosis Disease Activity. *J. Med. Virol.* **2003**, *69*, 111–117. [CrossRef]

16. Voumvourakis, K.I.; Kitsos, D.K.; Tsiodras, S.; Petrikkos, G.; Stamboulis, E. Human Herpesvirus 6 Infection as a Trigger of Multiple Sclerosis. *Mayo Clin. Proc.* **2010**, *85*, 1023–1030. [CrossRef]
17. Castellazzi, M.; Contini, C.; Tamborino, C.; Fasolo, F.; Roversi, G.; Seraceni, S.; Rizzo, R.; Baldi, E.; Tola, M.R.; Bellini, T.; et al. Epstein-Barr Virus-Specific Intrathecal Oligoclonal IgG Production in Relapsing-Remitting Multiple Sclerosis Is Limited to a Subset of Patients and Is Composed of Low-Affinity Antibodies. *J. Neuroinflamm.* **2014**, *11*, 188. [CrossRef] [PubMed]
18. Guan, Y.; Jakimovski, D.; Ramanathan, M.; Weinstock-Guttman, B.; Zivadinov, R. The Role of Epstein-Barr Virus in Multiple Sclerosis: From Molecular Pathophysiology to in Vivo Imaging. *Neural Regen. Res.* **2019**, *14*, 373–386. [CrossRef]
19. Skorstad, G.; Vandvik, B.; Vartdal, F.; Holmøy, T. MS and Clinically Isolated Syndromes: Shared Specificity but Diverging Clonal Patterns of Virus-Specific IgG Antibodies Produced in Vivo and by CSF B Cells in Vitro. *Eur. J. Neurol.* **2009**, *16*, 1124–1129. [CrossRef]
20. Perron, H.; Garson, J.A.; Bedin, F.; Beseme, F.; Paranhos-Baccala, G.; Komurian-Pradel, F.; Mallet, F.; Tuke, P.W.; Voisset, C.; Blond, J.L.; et al. Molecular Identification of a Novel Retrovirus Repeatedly Isolated from Patients with Multiple Sclerosis. The Collaborative Research Group on Multiple Sclerosis. *Proc. Natl. Acad. Sci. USA* **1997**, *94*, 7583–7588. [CrossRef]
21. Saleh, A.; Macia, A.; Muotri, A.R. Transposable Elements, Inflammation, and Neurological Disease. *Front. Neurol.* **2019**, *10*, 894. [CrossRef] [PubMed]
22. Fainardi, E.; Castellazzi, M.; Tamborino, C.; Seraceni, S.; Tola, M.R.; Granieri, E.; Contini, C. Chlamydia Pneumoniae-Specific Intrathecal Oligoclonal Antibody Response Is Predominantly Detected in a Subset of Multiple Sclerosis Patients with Progressive Forms. *J. Neurovirol.* **2009**, *15*, 425–433. [CrossRef] [PubMed]
23. Libbey, J.E.; Cusick, M.F.; Fujinami, R.S. Role of Pathogens in Multiple Sclerosis. *Int. Rev. Immunol.* **2014**, *33*, 266–283. [CrossRef] [PubMed]
24. Lindsey, J.; Patel, S. PCR for Bacterial 16S Ribosomal DNA in Multiple Sclerosis Cerebrospinal Fluid. *Mult. Scler. Houndmills Basingstoke Engl.* **2008**, *14*, 147–152. [CrossRef] [PubMed]
25. Thompson, A.J.; Banwell, B.L.; Barkhof, F.; Carroll, W.M.; Coetzee, T.; Comi, G.; Correale, J.; Fazekas, F.; Filippi, M.; Freedman, M.S.; et al. Diagnosis of Multiple Sclerosis: 2017 Revisions of the McDonald Criteria. *Lancet Neurol.* **2018**, *17*, 162–173. [CrossRef] [PubMed]
26. Miller, D.H.; Chard, D.T.; Ciccarelli, O. Clinically Isolated Syndromes. *Lancet Neurol.* **2012**, *11*, 157–169. [CrossRef]
27. Lublin, F.D.; Reingold, S.C.; Cohen, J.A.; Cutter, G.R.; Sørensen, P.S.; Thompson, A.J.; Wolinsky, J.S.; Balcer, L.J.; Banwell, B.; Barkhof, F.; et al. Defining the Clinical Course of Multiple Sclerosis: The 2013 Revisions. *Neurology* **2014**, *83*, 278–286. [CrossRef] [PubMed]
28. Ontaneda, D.; Thompson, A.J.; Fox, R.J.; Cohen, J.A. Progressive Multiple Sclerosis: Prospects for Disease Therapy, Repair, and Restoration of Function. *Lancet* **2017**, *389*, 1357–1366. [CrossRef] [PubMed]
29. Trapp, B.D.; Bö, L.; Mörk, S.; Chang, A. Pathogenesis of Tissue Injury in MS Lesions. *J. Neuroimmunol.* **1999**, *98*, 49–56. [CrossRef] [PubMed]
30. Reynders, T.; D'haeseleer, M.; De Keyser, J.; Nagels, G.; D'hooghe, M.B. Definition, Prevalence and Predictive Factors of Benign Multiple Sclerosis. *eNeurologicalSci* **2017**, *7*, 37–43. [CrossRef] [PubMed]
31. Villarreal, J.V.; Abraham, M.J.; Acevedo, J.A.G.; Rai, P.K.; Thottempudi, N.; Fang, X.; Gogia, B. Tumefactive Multiple Sclerosis (TMS): A Case Series of This Challenging Variant of MS. *Mult. Scler. Relat. Disord.* **2021**, *48*, 102699. [CrossRef] [PubMed]
32. Rohani, M.; Ghourchian, S. Fulminant Multiple Sclerosis (MS). *Neurol. Sci. Off. J. Ital. Neurol. Soc. Ital. Soc. Clin. Neurophysiol.* **2011**, *32*, 953–957. [CrossRef] [PubMed]
33. Lassmann, H. Multiple Sclerosis Pathology. *Cold Spring Harb. Perspect. Med.* **2018**, *8*, a028936. [CrossRef] [PubMed]
34. Pirko, I.; Lucchinetti, C.F.; Sriram, S.; Bakshi, R. Gray Matter Involvement in Multiple Sclerosis. *Neurology* **2007**, *68*, 634–642. [CrossRef]
35. Jarius, S.; König, F.B.; Metz, I.; Ruprecht, K.; Paul, F.; Brück, W.; Wildemann, B. Pattern II and Pattern III MS Are Entities Distinct from Pattern I MS: Evidence from Cerebrospinal Fluid Analysis. *J. Neuroinflamm.* **2017**, *14*, 171. [CrossRef]
36. Lucchinetti, C.F.; Bruck, W.; Lassmann, H. Evidence for Pathogenic Heterogeneity in Multiple Sclerosis. *Ann. Neurol.* **2004**, *56*, 308. [CrossRef]
37. Bellingacci, L.; Mancini, A.; Gaetani, L.; Tozzi, A.; Parnetti, L.; Di Filippo, M. Synaptic Dysfunction in Multiple Sclerosis: A Red Thread from Inflammation to Network Disconnection. *Int. J. Mol. Sci.* **2021**, *22*, 9753. [CrossRef]
38. Lassmann, H. Mechanisms of White Matter Damage in Multiple Sclerosis. *Glia* **2014**, *62*, 1816–1830. [CrossRef]
39. Carotenuto, A.; Cacciaguerra, L.; Pagani, E.; Preziosa, P.; Filippi, M.; Rocca, M.A. Glymphatic System Impairment in Multiple Sclerosis: Relation with Brain Damage and Disability. *Brain J. Neurol.* **2022**, *145*, 2785–2795. [CrossRef]
40. Serafini, B.; Rosicarelli, B.; Magliozzi, R.; Stigliano, E.; Aloisi, F. Detection of Ectopic B-Cell Follicles with Germinal Centers in the Meninges of Patients with Secondary Progressive Multiple Sclerosis. *Brain Pathol. Zurich Switz.* **2004**, *14*, 164–174. [CrossRef]

41. Kutzelnigg, A.; Lucchinetti, C.F.; Stadelmann, C.; Brück, W.; Rauschka, H.; Bergmann, M.; Schmidbauer, M.; Parisi, J.E.; Lassmann, H. Cortical Demyelination and Diffuse White Matter Injury in Multiple Sclerosis. *Brain* **2005**, *128*, 2705–2712. [CrossRef] [PubMed]
42. Dusek, P.; Hofer, T.; Alexander, J.; Roos, P.M.; Aaseth, J.O. Cerebral Iron Deposition in Neurodegeneration. *Biomolecules* **2022**, *12*, 714. [CrossRef] [PubMed]
43. Stankiewicz, J.M.; Neema, M.; Ceccarelli, A. Iron and Multiple Sclerosis. *Neurobiol. Aging* **2014**, *35*, S51–S58. [CrossRef] [PubMed]
44. Hamdy, E.; Galeel, A.A.; Ramadan, I.; Gaber, D.; Mustafa, H.; Mekky, J. Iron Deposition in Multiple Sclerosis: Overall Load or Distribution Alteration? *Eur. Radiol. Exp.* **2022**, *6*, 49. [CrossRef] [PubMed]
45. O'Rourke, B.; Cortassa, S.; Aon, M.A. Mitochondrial Ion Channels: Gatekeepers of Life and Death. *Physiol. Bethesda Md* **2005**, *20*, 303–315. [CrossRef] [PubMed]
46. de Barcelos, I.P.; Troxell, R.M.; Graves, J.S. Mitochondrial Dysfunction and Multiple Sclerosis. *Biology* **2019**, *8*, 37. [CrossRef]
47. Campbell, G.; Mahad, D.J. Mitochondrial Dysfunction and Axon Degeneration in Progressive Multiple Sclerosis. *FEBS Lett.* **2018**, *592*, 1113–1121. [CrossRef]
48. Kennedy, P.G.E.; George, W.; Yu, X. The Possible Role of Neural Cell Apoptosis in Multiple Sclerosis. *Int. J. Mol. Sci.* **2022**, *23*, 7584. [CrossRef]
49. Li, X.; Chu, Y.; Ma, R.; Dou, M.; Li, S.; Song, Y.; Lv, Y.; Zhu, L. Ferroptosis as a Mechanism of Oligodendrocyte Loss and Demyelination in Experimental Autoimmune Encephalomyelitis. *J. Neuroimmunol.* **2022**, *373*, 577995. [CrossRef]
50. Ofengeim, D.; Ito, Y.; Najafov, A.; Zhang, Y.; Shan, B.; DeWitt, J.P.; Ye, J.; Zhang, X.; Chang, A.; Vakifahmetoglu-Norberg, H.; et al. Activation of Necroptosis in Multiple Sclerosis. *Cell Rep.* **2015**, *10*, 1836–1849. [CrossRef]
51. Prineas, J.W.; Barnard, R.O.; Kwon, E.E.; Sharer, L.R.; Cho, E.S. Multiple Sclerosis: Remyelination of Nascent Lesions. *Ann. Neurol.* **1993**, *33*, 137–151. [CrossRef] [PubMed]
52. Patrikios, P.; Stadelmann, C.; Kutzelnigg, A.; Rauschka, H.; Schmidbauer, M.; Laursen, H.; Sorensen, P.S.; Brück, W.; Lucchinetti, C.; Lassmann, H. Remyelination Is Extensive in a Subset of Multiple Sclerosis Patients. *Brain J. Neurol.* **2006**, *129*, 3165–3172. [CrossRef]
53. Franklin, R.J.M.; Frisén, J.; Lyons, D.A. Revisiting Remyelination: Towards a Consensus on the Regeneration of CNS Myelin. *Semin. Cell Dev. Biol.* **2021**, *116*, 3–9. [CrossRef] [PubMed]
54. Sim, F.J.; Zhao, C.; Penderis, J.; Franklin, R.J.M. The Age-Related Decrease in CNS Remyelination Efficiency Is Attributable to an Impairment of Both Oligodendrocyte Progenitor Recruitment and Differentiation. *J. Neurosci.* **2002**, *22*, 2451–2459. [CrossRef] [PubMed]
55. Yuen, T.J.; Silbereis, J.C.; Griveau, A.; Chang, S.M.; Daneman, R.; Fancy, S.P.J.; Zahed, H.; Maltepe, E.; Rowitch, D.H. Oligodendrocyte-Encoded HIF Function Couples Postnatal Myelination and White Matter Angiogenesis. *Cell* **2014**, *158*, 383–396. [CrossRef]
56. Akay, L.A.; Effenberger, A.H.; Tsai, L.-H. Cell of All Trades: Oligodendrocyte Precursor Cells in Synaptic, Vascular, and Immune Function. *Genes Dev.* **2021**, *35*, 180–198. [CrossRef]
57. Albert, M.; Antel, J.; Brück, W.; Stadelmann, C. Extensive Cortical Remyelination in Patients with Chronic Multiple Sclerosis. *Brain Pathol. Zurich Switz.* **2007**, *17*, 129–138. [CrossRef]
58. Yeung, M.S.Y.; Djelloul, M.; Steiner, E.; Bernard, S.; Salehpour, M.; Possnert, G.; Brundin, L.; Frisén, J. Dynamics of Oligodendrocyte Generation in Multiple Sclerosis. *Nature* **2019**, *566*, 538–542. [CrossRef]
59. Yeung, M.S.Y.; Zdunek, S.; Bergmann, O.; Bernard, S.; Salehpour, M.; Alkass, K.; Perl, S.; Tisdale, J.; Possnert, G.; Brundin, L.; et al. Dynamics of Oligodendrocyte Generation and Myelination in the Human Brain. *Cell* **2014**, *159*, 766–774. [CrossRef]
60. Baaklini, C.S.; Rawji, K.S.; Duncan, G.J.; Ho, M.F.S.; Plemel, J.R. Central Nervous System Remyelination: Roles of Glia and Innate Immune Cells. *Front. Mol. Neurosci.* **2019**, *12*, 225. [CrossRef]
61. Clemente, D.; Ortega, M.C.; Melero-Jerez, C.; de Castro, F. The Effect of Glia-Glia Interactions on Oligodendrocyte Precursor Cell Biology during Development and in Demyelinating Diseases. *Front. Cell. Neurosci.* **2013**, *7*, 268. [CrossRef] [PubMed]
62. Bramow, S.; Frischer, J.M.; Lassmann, H.; Koch-Henriksen, N.; Lucchinetti, C.F.; Sørensen, P.S.; Laursen, H. Demyelination versus Remyelination in Progressive Multiple Sclerosis. *Brain* **2010**, *133*, 2983–2998. [CrossRef] [PubMed]
63. Zambonin, J.L.; Zhao, C.; Ohno, N.; Campbell, G.R.; Engeham, S.; Ziabreva, I.; Schwarz, N.; Lee, S.E.; Frischer, J.M.; Turnbull, D.M.; et al. Increased Mitochondrial Content in Remyelinated Axons: Implications for Multiple Sclerosis. *Brain J. Neurol.* **2011**, *134*, 1901–1913. [CrossRef] [PubMed]
64. Lampron, A.; Larochelle, A.; Laflamme, N.; Préfontaine, P.; Plante, M.-M.; Sánchez, M.G.; Yong, V.W.; Stys, P.K.; Tremblay, M.-È.; Rivest, S. Inefficient Clearance of Myelin Debris by Microglia Impairs Remyelinating Processes. *J. Exp. Med.* **2015**, *212*, 481–495. [CrossRef]
65. Liu, A.; Li, J.; Marin-Husstege, M.; Kageyama, R.; Fan, Y.; Gelinas, C.; Casaccia-Bonnefil, P. A Molecular Insight of Hes5-Dependent Inhibition of Myelin Gene Expression: Old Partners and New Players. *EMBO J.* **2006**, *25*, 4833–4842. [CrossRef]

66. Natrajan, M.S.; de la Fuente, A.G.; Crawford, A.H.; Linehan, E.; Nuñez, V.; Johnson, K.R.; Wu, T.; Fitzgerald, D.C.; Ricote, M.; Bielekova, B.; et al. Retinoid X Receptor Activation Reverses Age-Related Deficiencies in Myelin Debris Phagocytosis and Remyelination. *Brain* **2015**, *138*, 3581–3597. [CrossRef]
67. Reichert, F.; Rotshenker, S. Galectin-3 (MAC-2) Controls Microglia Phenotype Whether Amoeboid and Phagocytic or Branched and Non-Phagocytic by Regulating the Cytoskeleton. *Front. Cell. Neurosci.* **2019**, *13*, 90. [CrossRef]
68. Mi, S.; Hu, B.; Hahm, K.; Luo, Y.; Kam Hui, E.S.; Yuan, Q.; Wong, W.M.; Wang, L.; Su, H.; Chu, T.-H.; et al. LINGO-1 Antagonist Promotes Spinal Cord Remyelination and Axonal Integrity in MOG-Induced Experimental Autoimmune Encephalomyelitis. *Nat. Med.* **2007**, *13*, 1228–1233. [CrossRef]
69. Ahmed, Z.; Fulton, D.; Douglas, M.R. Opicinumab: Is It a Potential Treatment for Multiple Sclerosis? *Ann. Transl. Med.* **2020**, *8*, 892. [CrossRef]
70. Varhaug, K.N.; Kråkenes, T.; Alme, M.N.; Vedeler, C.A.; Bindoff, L.A. Mitochondrial Complex IV Is Lost in Neurons in the Cuprizone Mouse Model. *Mitochondrion* **2020**, *50*, 58–62. [CrossRef]
71. Constantinescu, C.S.; Farooqi, N.; O'Brien, K.; Gran, B. Experimental Autoimmune Encephalomyelitis (EAE) as a Model for Multiple Sclerosis (MS). *Br. J. Pharmacol.* **2011**, *164*, 1079–1106. [CrossRef] [PubMed]
72. Omura, S.; Kawai, E.; Sato, F.; Martinez, N.E.; Minagar, A.; Al-Kofahi, M.; Yun, J.W.; Cvek, U.; Trutschl, M.; Alexander, J.S.; et al. Theiler's Virus-Mediated Immunopathology in the CNS and Heart: Roles of Organ-Specific Cytokine and Lymphatic Responses. *Front. Immunol.* **2018**, *9*, 2870. [CrossRef] [PubMed]
73. Medhasi, S.; Chantratita, N. Human Leukocyte Antigen (HLA) System: Genetics and Association with Bacterial and Viral Infections. *J. Immunol. Res.* **2022**, *2022*, 9710376. [CrossRef] [PubMed]
74. Choo, S.Y. The HLA System: Genetics, Immunology, Clinical Testing, and Clinical Implications. *Yonsei Med. J.* **2007**, *48*, 11. [CrossRef] [PubMed]
75. Wyatt, R.C.; Lanzoni, G.; Russell, M.A.; Gerling, I.; Richardson, S.J. What the HLA-I!—Classical and Non-Classical HLA Class I and Their Potential Roles in Type 1 Diabetes. *Curr. Diab. Rep.* **2019**, *19*, 159. [CrossRef] [PubMed]
76. Chen, B.; Khodadoust, M.S.; Olsson, N.; Wagar, L.E.; Fast, E.; Liu, C.L.; Muftuoglu, Y.; Sworder, B.J.; Diehn, M.; Levy, R.; et al. Predicting HLA Class II Antigen Presentation through Integrated Deep Learning. *Nat. Biotechnol.* **2019**, *37*, 1332–1343. [CrossRef] [PubMed]
77. Patsopoulos, N.A. Genetics of Multiple Sclerosis: An Overview and New Directions. *Cold Spring Harb. Perspect. Med.* **2018**, *8*, a028951. [CrossRef]
78. Perez-Miralles, F.C. Daclizumab in Multiple Sclerosis. *Rev. Neurol.* **2018**, *66*, 271–282.
79. Lee, S.Y.; Goverman, J.M. The Influence of T Cell Ig Mucin-3 Signaling on Central Nervous System Autoimmune Disease Is Determined by the Effector Function of the Pathogenic T Cells. *J. Immunol. Baltim. Md 1950* **2013**, *190*, 4991–4999. [CrossRef]
80. Huber, M.; Heink, S.; Pagenstecher, A.; Reinhard, K.; Ritter, J.; Visekruna, A.; Guralnik, A.; Bollig, N.; Jeltsch, K.; Heinemann, C.; et al. IL-17A Secretion by CD8+ T Cells Supports Th17-Mediated Autoimmune Encephalomyelitis. *J. Clin. Investig.* **2013**, *123*, 247–260. [CrossRef]
81. Reich, D.S.; Lucchinetti, C.F.; Calabresi, P.A. Multiple Sclerosis. *N. Engl. J. Med.* **2018**, *378*, 169–180. [CrossRef] [PubMed]
82. Hauser, S.L.; Bhan, A.K.; Gilles, F.; Kemp, M.; Kerr, C.; Weiner, H.L. Immunohistochemical Analysis of the Cellular Infiltrate in Multiple Sclerosis Lesions. *Ann. Neurol.* **1986**, *19*, 578–587. [CrossRef] [PubMed]
83. Martin, R.; Sospedra, M.; Rosito, M.; Engelhardt, B. Current Multiple Sclerosis Treatments Have Improved Our Understanding of MS Autoimmune Pathogenesis. *Eur. J. Immunol.* **2016**, *46*, 2078–2090. [CrossRef]
84. Schrempf, W.; Ziemssen, T. Glatiramer Acetate: Mechanisms of Action in Multiple Sclerosis. *Autoimmun. Rev.* **2007**, *6*, 469–475. [CrossRef] [PubMed]
85. Bielekova, B.; Catalfamo, M.; Reichert-Scrivner, S.; Packer, A.; Cerna, M.; Waldmann, T.A.; McFarland, H.; Henkart, P.A.; Martin, R. Regulatory CD56 Bright Natural Killer Cells Mediate Immunomodulatory Effects of IL-2Rα-Targeted Therapy (Daclizumab) in Multiple Sclerosis. *Proc. Natl. Acad. Sci. USA* **2006**, *103*, 5941–5946. [CrossRef]
86. Sinha, S.; Boyden, A.W.; Itani, F.R.; Crawford, M.P.; Karandikar, N.J. CD8(+) T-Cells as Immune Regulators of Multiple Sclerosis. *Front. Immunol.* **2015**, *6*, 619. [CrossRef]
87. Laroni, A.; Armentani, E.; Kerlero de Rosbo, N.; Ivaldi, F.; Marcenaro, E.; Sivori, S.; Gandhi, R.; Weiner, H.L.; Moretta, A.; Mancardi, G.L.; et al. Dysregulation of Regulatory CD56(Bright) NK Cells/T Cells Interactions in Multiple Sclerosis. *J. Autoimmun.* **2016**, *72*, 8–18. [CrossRef]
88. Piacente, F.; Bottero, M.; Benzi, A.; Vigo, T.; Uccelli, A.; Bruzzone, S.; Ferrara, G. Neuroprotective Potential of Dendritic Cells and Sirtuins in Multiple Sclerosis. *Int. J. Mol. Sci.* **2022**, *23*, 4352. [CrossRef]
89. Matsushita, T. Regulatory and Effector B Cells: Friends or Foes? *J. Dermatol. Sci.* **2019**, *93*, 2–7. [CrossRef]
90. Montalban, X.; Hauser, S.L.; Kappos, L.; Arnold, D.L.; Bar-Or, A.; Comi, G.; de Seze, J.; Giovannoni, G.; Hartung, H.-P.; Hemmer, B.; et al. Ocrelizumab versus Placebo in Primary Progressive Multiple Sclerosis. *N. Engl. J. Med.* **2017**, *376*, 209–220. [CrossRef]

91. Xiang, W.; Xie, C.; Guan, Y. The Identification, Development and Therapeutic Potential of IL-10-Producing Regulatory B Cells in Multiple Sclerosis. *J. Neuroimmunol.* **2021**, *354*, 577520. [CrossRef] [PubMed]
92. Xia, S.; Liu, X.; Cao, X.; Xu, S. T-Cell Expression of Bruton's Tyrosine Kinase Promotes Autoreactive T-Cell Activation and Exacerbates Aplastic Anemia. *Cell. Mol. Immunol.* **2020**, *17*, 1042–1052. [CrossRef] [PubMed]
93. Martin, E.; Aigrot, M.-S.; Grenningloh, R.; Stankoff, B.; Lubetzki, C.; Boschert, U.; Zalc, B. Bruton's Tyrosine Kinase Inhibition Promotes Myelin Repair. *Brain Plast.* **2020**, *5*, 123–133. [CrossRef]
94. Steinmaurer, A.; Wimmer, I.; Berger, T.; Rommer, P.S.; Sellner, J. Bruton's Tyrosine Kinase Inhibition in the Treatment of Preclinical Models and Multiple Sclerosis. *Curr. Pharm. Des.* **2022**, *28*, 437–444. [CrossRef] [PubMed]
95. Neys, S.F.H.; Rip, J.; Hendriks, R.W.; Corneth, O.B.J. Bruton's Tyrosine Kinase Inhibition as an Emerging Therapy in Systemic Autoimmune Disease. *Drugs* **2021**, *81*, 1605–1626. [CrossRef] [PubMed]
96. Kaushik, D.K.; Yong, V.W. Metabolic Needs of Brain-Infiltrating Leukocytes and Microglia in Multiple Sclerosis. *J. Neurochem.* **2021**, *158*, 14–24. [CrossRef] [PubMed]
97. De Riccardis, L.; Rizzello, A.; Ferramosca, A.; Urso, E.; De Robertis, F.; Danieli, A.; Giudetti, A.M.; Trianni, G.; Zara, V.; Maffia, M. Bioenergetics Profile of CD4 + T Cells in Relapsing Remitting Multiple Sclerosis Subjects. *J. Biotechnol.* **2015**, *202*, 31–39. [CrossRef]
98. Chen, K.; Lai, C.; Su, Y.; Bao, W.D.; Yang, L.N.; Xu, P.-P.; Zhu, L.-Q. CGAS-STING-Mediated IFN-I Response in Host Defense and Neuroinflammatory Diseases. *Curr. Neuropharmacol.* **2022**, *20*, 362–371. [CrossRef]
99. Zahid, M.; Busmail, A.; Penumetcha, S.S.; Ahluwalia, S.; Irfan, R.; Khan, S.A.; Rohit Reddy, S.; Vasquez Lopez, M.E.; Mohammed, L. Tumor Necrosis Factor Alpha Blockade and Multiple Sclerosis: Exploring New Avenues. *Cureus* **2021**, *13*, e18847. [CrossRef]
100. Kemanetzoglou, E.; Andreadou, E. CNS Demyelination with TNF-α Blockers. *Curr. Neurol. Neurosci. Rep.* **2017**, *17*, 36. [CrossRef]
101. Piehl, F. Current and Emerging Disease-modulatory Therapies and Treatment Targets for Multiple Sclerosis. *J. Intern. Med.* **2021**, *289*, 771–791. [CrossRef] [PubMed]
102. Johnson, B.M.; Uchimura, T.; Gallovic, M.D.; Thamilarasan, M.; Chou, W.-C.; Gibson, S.A.; Deng, M.; Tam, J.W.; Batty, C.J.; Williams, J.; et al. STING Agonist Mitigates Experimental Autoimmune Encephalomyelitis by Stimulating Type I IFN-Dependent and -Independent Immune-Regulatory Pathways. *J. Immunol. Baltim. Md 1950* **2021**, *206*, 2015–2028. [CrossRef] [PubMed]
103. Masanneck, L.; Eichler, S.; Vogelsang, A.; Korsen, M.; Wiendl, H.; Budde, T.; Meuth, S.G. The STING-IFN-β-Dependent Axis Is Markedly Low in Patients with Relapsing-Remitting Multiple Sclerosis. *Int. J. Mol. Sci.* **2020**, *21*, 9249. [CrossRef]
104. Zhang, X.; Shi, H.; Wu, J.; Zhang, X.; Sun, L.; Chen, C.; Chen, Z.J. Cyclic GMP-AMP Containing Mixed Phosphodiester Linkages Is An Endogenous High-Affinity Ligand for STING. *Mol. Cell* **2013**, *51*, 226–235. [CrossRef] [PubMed]
105. Fryer, A.L.; Abdullah, A.; Taylor, J.M.; Crack, P.J. The Complexity of the CGAS-STING Pathway in CNS Pathologies. *Front. Neurosci.* **2021**, *15*, 621501. [CrossRef]
106. Ma, F.; Li, B.; Yu, Y.; Iyer, S.S.; Sun, M.; Cheng, G. Positive Feedback Regulation of Type I Interferon by the Interferon-Stimulated Gene STING. *EMBO Rep.* **2015**, *16*, 202–212. [CrossRef]
107. Watson, R.O.; Bell, S.L.; MacDuff, D.A.; Kimmey, J.M.; Diner, E.J.; Olivas, J.; Vance, R.E.; Stallings, C.L.; Virgin, H.W.; Cox, J.S. The Cytosolic Sensor CGAS Detects Mycobacterium Tuberculosis DNA to Induce Type I Interferons and Activate Autophagy. *Cell Host Microbe* **2015**, *17*, 811–819. [CrossRef]
108. Dos Santos, A.C.; Roffê, E.; Arantes, R.M.E.; Juliano, L.; Pesquero, J.L.; Pesquero, J.B.; Bader, M.; Teixeira, M.M.; Carvalho-Tavares, J. Kinin B2 Receptor Regulates Chemokines CCL2 and CCL5 Expression and Modulates Leukocyte Recruitment and Pathology in Experimental Autoimmune Encephalomyelitis (EAE) in Mice. *J. Neuroinflamm.* **2008**, *5*, 49. [CrossRef]
109. Huang, L.; Liu, M.; Jiang, W.; Ding, H.; Han, Y.; Wen, M.; Li, Y.; Liu, X.; Zeng, H. Bradykinin/Bradykinin 1 Receptor Promotes Brain Microvascular Endothelial Cell Permeability and Proinflammatory Cytokine Release by Downregulating Wnt3a. *J. Biochem. Mol. Toxicol.* **2022**, *36*, e23213. [CrossRef]
110. Uzawa, A.; Mori, M.; Taniguchi, J.; Kuwabara, S. Modulation of the Kallikrein/Kinin System by the Angiotensin-Converting Enzyme Inhibitor Alleviates Experimental Autoimmune Encephalomyelitis. *Clin. Exp. Immunol.* **2014**, *178*, 245–252. [CrossRef]
111. Prat, A.; Weinrib, L.; Becher, B.; Poirier, J.; Duquette, P.; Couture, R.; Antel, J.P. Bradykinin B1 Receptor Expression and Function on T Lymphocytes in Active Multiple Sclerosis. *Neurology* **1999**, *53*, 2087–2092. [CrossRef]
112. Tatomir, A.; Talpos-Caia, A.; Anselmo, F.; Kruszewski, A.M.; Boodhoo, D.; Rus, V.; Rus, H. The Complement System as a Biomarker of Disease Activity and Response to Treatment in Multiple Sclerosis. *Immunol. Res.* **2017**, *65*, 1103–1109. [CrossRef] [PubMed]
113. Rus, H.G.; Kim, L.M.; Niculescu, F.I.; Shin, M.L. Induction of C3 Expression in Astrocytes Is Regulated by Cytokines and Newcastle Disease Virus. *J. Immunol. Baltim. Md 1950* **1992**, *148*, 928–933. [CrossRef]
114. Soane, L.; Cho, H.J.; Niculescu, F.; Rus, H.; Shin, M.L. C5b-9 Terminal Complement Complex Protects Oligodendrocytes from Death by Regulating Bad through Phosphatidylinositol 3-Kinase/Akt Pathway. *J. Immunol. Baltim. Md 1950* **2001**, *167*, 2305–2311. [CrossRef] [PubMed]

115. Presumey, J.; Bialas, A.R.; Carroll, M.C. Complement System in Neural Synapse Elimination in Development and Disease. *Adv. Immunol.* **2017**, *135*, 53–79. [CrossRef] [PubMed]
116. Vasek, M.J.; Garber, C.; Dorsey, D.; Durrant, D.M.; Bollman, B.; Soung, A.; Yu, J.; Perez-Torres, C.; Frouin, A.; Wilton, D.K.; et al. A Complement-Microglial Axis Drives Synapse Loss during Virus-Induced Memory Impairment. *Nature* **2016**, *534*, 538–543. [CrossRef] [PubMed]
117. Aeinehband, S.; Lindblom, R.P.F.; Al Nimer, F.; Vijayaraghavan, S.; Sandholm, K.; Khademi, M.; Olsson, T.; Nilsson, B.; Ekdahl, K.N.; Darreh-Shori, T.; et al. Complement Component C3 and Butyrylcholinesterase Activity Are Associated with Neurodegeneration and Clinical Disability in Multiple Sclerosis. *PLoS ONE* **2015**, *10*, e0122048. [CrossRef]
118. Ingram, G.; Hakobyan, S.; Robertson, N.P.; Morgan, B.P. Elevated Plasma C4a Levels in Multiple Sclerosis Correlate with Disease Activity. *J. Neuroimmunol.* **2010**, *223*, 124–127. [CrossRef]
119. Allinovi, M.; Bellinvia, A.; Pesce, F.; Milan Manani, S.; Razzolini, L.; Brezzi, B.; Protopapa, P.; Mantero, V.; Caroti, L.; Cirami, C.L.; et al. Safety and Efficacy of Eculizumab Therapy in Multiple Sclerosis: A Case Series. *Brain Sci.* **2021**, *11*, 1341. [CrossRef]
120. Huynh, J.L.; Casaccia, P. Epigenetic Mechanisms in Multiple Sclerosis: Implications for Pathogenesis and Treatment. *Lancet Neurol.* **2013**, *12*, 195–206. [CrossRef]
121. Ma, N.; He, T.; Johnston, L.J.; Ma, X. Host-Microbiome Interactions: The Aryl Hydrocarbon Receptor as a Critical Node in Tryptophan Metabolites to Brain Signaling. *Gut Microbes* **2020**, *11*, 1203–1219. [CrossRef]
122. Rothhammer, V.; Mascanfroni, I.D.; Bunse, L.; Takenaka, M.C.; Kenison, J.E.; Mayo, L.; Chao, C.-C.; Patel, B.; Yan, R.; Blain, M.; et al. Type I Interferons and Microbial Metabolites of Tryptophan Modulate Astrocyte Activity and Central Nervous System Inflammation via the Aryl Hydrocarbon Receptor. *Nat. Med.* **2016**, *22*, 586–597. [CrossRef]
123. Giovannoni, G.; Knappertz, V.; Steinerman, J.R.; Tansy, A.P.; Li, T.; Krieger, S.; Uccelli, A.; Uitdehaag, B.M.J.; Montalban, X.; Hartung, H.-P.; et al. A Randomized, Placebo-Controlled, Phase 2 Trial of Laquinimod in Primary Progressive Multiple Sclerosis. *Neurology* **2020**, *95*, e1027–e1040. [CrossRef]
124. Rothhammer, V.; Kenison, J.E.; Li, Z.; Tjon, E.; Takenaka, M.C.; Chao, C.-C.; Alves de Lima, K.; Borucki, D.M.; Kaye, J.; Quintana, F.J. Aryl Hydrocarbon Receptor Activation in Astrocytes by Laquinimod Ameliorates Autoimmune Inflammation in the CNS. *Neurol. Neuroimmunol. Neuroinflamm.* **2021**, *8*, 946. [CrossRef]
125. Ntranos, A.; Park, H.-J.; Wentling, M.; Tolstikov, V.; Amatruda, M.; Inbar, B.; Kim-Schulze, S.; Frazier, C.; Button, J.; Kiebish, M.A.; et al. Bacterial Neurotoxic Metabolites in Multiple Sclerosis Cerebrospinal Fluid and Plasma. *Brain J. Neurol.* **2022**, *145*, 569–583. [CrossRef]
126. Lünemann, J.D.; Ruck, T.; Muraro, P.A.; Bar-Or, A.; Wiendl, H. Immune Reconstitution Therapies: Concepts for Durable Remission in Multiple Sclerosis. *Nat. Rev. Neurol.* **2020**, *16*, 56–62. [CrossRef]
127. Sorensen, P.S.; Sellebjerg, F. Pulsed Immune Reconstitution Therapy in Multiple Sclerosis. *Ther. Adv. Neurol. Disord.* **2019**, *12*, 1756286419836913. [CrossRef]
128. AlSharoqi, I.A.; Aljumah, M.; Bohlega, S.; Boz, C.; Daif, A.; El-Koussa, S.; Inshasi, J.; Kurtuncu, M.; Müller, T.; Retief, C.; et al. Immune Reconstitution Therapy or Continuous Immunosuppression for the Management of Active Relapsing-Remitting Multiple Sclerosis Patients? A Narrative Review. *Neurol. Ther.* **2020**, *9*, 55–66. [CrossRef]
129. Amor, S.; Monson, N.; Sellner, J.; Van Luijn, M.M.; Van Langelaar, J.; Rijvers, L.; Smolders, J. B and T Cells Driving Multiple Sclerosis: Identity, Mechanisms and Potential Triggers. *Front. Immunol.* **2020**, *11*, 760. [CrossRef]
130. Pucci, E.; Giuliani, G.; Solari, A.; Simi, S.; Minozzi, S.; Di Pietrantonj, C.; Galea, I. Natalizumab for Relapsing Remitting Multiple Sclerosis. *Cochrane Database Syst. Rev.* **2011**, *10*, CD007621. [CrossRef]
131. Kapoor, R.; Ho, P.-R.; Campbell, N.; Chang, I.; Deykin, A.; Forrestal, F.; Lucas, N.; Yu, B.; Arnold, D.L.; Freedman, M.S.; et al. Effect of Natalizumab on Disease Progression in Secondary Progressive Multiple Sclerosis (ASCEND): A Phase 3, Randomised, Double-Blind, Placebo-Controlled Trial with an Open-Label Extension. *Lancet Neurol.* **2018**, *17*, 405–415. [CrossRef]
132. Sorensen, P.S.; Koch-Henriksen, N.; Petersen, T.; Ravnborg, M.; Oturai, A.; Sellebjerg, F. Recurrence or Rebound of Clinical Relapses after Discontinuation of Natalizumab Therapy in Highly Active MS Patients. *J. Neurol.* **2014**, *261*, 1170–1177. [CrossRef]
133. Hartung, H.-P.; Derfuss, T.; Cree, B.A.; Sormani, M.P.; Selmaj, K.; Stutters, J.; Prados, F.; MacManus, D.; Schneble, H.-M.; Lambert, E.; et al. Efficacy and Safety of Temelimab in Multiple Sclerosis: Results of a Randomized Phase 2b and Extension Study. *Mult. Scler. Houndmills Basingstoke Engl.* **2022**, *28*, 429–440. [CrossRef]
134. DiSabato, D.J.; Quan, N.; Godbout, J.P. Neuroinflammation: The Devil Is in the Details. *J. Neurochem.* **2016**, *139*, 136–153. [CrossRef]
135. Blutstein, T.; Haydon, P.G. The Tripartite Synapse. In *The Synapse*; Elsevier: Amsterdam, The Netherlands, 2014; pp. 155–172.
136. Bachiller, S.; Jiménez-Ferrer, I.; Paulus, A.; Yang, Y.; Swanberg, M.; Deierborg, T.; Boza-Serrano, A. Microglia in Neurological Diseases: A Road Map to Brain-Disease Dependent-Inflammatory Response. *Front. Cell. Neurosci.* **2018**, *12*, 488. [CrossRef] [PubMed]
137. Bradl, M.; Lassmann, H. Oligodendrocytes: Biology and Pathology. *Acta Neuropathol.* **2010**, *119*, 37–53. [CrossRef] [PubMed]

138. Perea, G.; Navarrete, M.; Araque, A. Tripartite Synapses: Astrocytes Process and Control Synaptic Information. *Trends Neurosci.* **2009**, *32*, 421–431. [CrossRef] [PubMed]
139. Escartin, C.; Galea, E.; Lakatos, A.; O'Callaghan, J.P.; Petzold, G.C.; Serrano-Pozo, A.; Steinhäuser, C.; Volterra, A.; Carmignoto, G.; Agarwal, A.; et al. Reactive Astrocyte Nomenclature, Definitions, and Future Directions. *Nat. Neurosci.* **2021**, *24*, 312–325. [CrossRef] [PubMed]
140. Mao, P.; Reddy, P.H. Is Multiple Sclerosis a Mitochondrial Disease? *Biochim. Biophys. Acta* **2010**, *1802*, 66–79. [CrossRef] [PubMed]
141. Bondan, E.F.; Custódio, P.R.; Lallo, M.A.; Bentubo, H.D.L.; Graça, D.L. Ethidium Bromide-Induced Demyelination in the Sciatic Nerve of Diabetic Rats. *Arq. Neuropsiquiatr.* **2009**, *67*, 1066–1070. [CrossRef]
142. Licht-Mayer, S.; Campbell, G.R.; Mehta, A.R.; McGill, K.; Symonds, A.; Al-Azki, S.; Pryce, G.; Zandee, S.; Zhao, C.; Kipp, M.; et al. Axonal Response of Mitochondria to Demyelination and Complex IV Activity within Demyelinated Axons in Experimental Models of Multiple Sclerosis. *Neuropathol. Appl. Neurobiol.* **2022**, *49*, e12851. [CrossRef]
143. Sprenkle, N.T.; Sims, S.G.; Sánchez, C.L.; Meares, G.P. Endoplasmic Reticulum Stress and Inflammation in the Central Nervous System. *Mol. Neurodegener.* **2017**, *12*, 42. [CrossRef]
144. Cunnea, P.; Mháille, A.N.; McQuaid, S.; Farrell, M.; McMahon, J.; FitzGerald, U. Expression Profiles of Endoplasmic Reticulum Stress-Related Molecules in Demyelinating Lesions and Multiple Sclerosis. *Mult. Scler. Houndmills Basingstoke Engl.* **2011**, *17*, 808–818. [CrossRef]
145. Yu, Z.; Luo, H.; Fu, W.; Mattson, M.P. The Endoplasmic Reticulum Stress-Responsive Protein GRP78 Protects Neurons against Excitotoxicity and Apoptosis: Suppression of Oxidative Stress and Stabilization of Calcium Homeostasis. *Exp. Neurol.* **1999**, *155*, 302–314. [CrossRef]
146. Blass, J.P. The Mitochondrial Spiral. An Adequate Cause of Dementia in the Alzheimer's Syndrome. *Ann. N. Y. Acad. Sci.* **2000**, *924*, 170–183. [CrossRef]
147. Blass, J.P. Brain Metabolism and Brain Disease: Is Metabolic Deficiency the Proximate Cause of Alzheimer Dementia? *J. Neurosci. Res.* **2001**, *66*, 851–856. [CrossRef]
148. Camara-Lemarroy, C.R.; Metz, L.; Smith, E.E.; Dunn, J.F.; Yong, V.W. Expanding the Potential Therapeutic Options for Remote Ischemic Preconditioning: Use in Multiple Sclerosis. *Front. Neurol.* **2018**, *9*, 475. [CrossRef]
149. Kang, T.M.; Hilgemann, D.W. Multiple Transport Modes of the Cardiac Na+/Ca2+ Exchanger. *Nature* **2004**, *427*, 544–548. [CrossRef]
150. Hilgemann, D.W. Steady-State and Dynamic Properties of Cardiac Sodium-Calcium Exchange. Sodium-Dependent Inactivation. *J. Gen. Physiol.* **1992**, *100*, 905–932. [CrossRef]
151. Inglese, M.; Madelin, G.; Oesingmann, N.; Babb, J.S.; Wu, W.; Stoeckel, B.; Herbert, J.; Johnson, G. Brain Tissue Sodium Concentration in Multiple Sclerosis: A Sodium Imaging Study at 3 Tesla. *Brain J. Neurol.* **2010**, *133*, 847–857. [CrossRef]
152. Maiolino, M.; Castaldo, P.; Lariccia, V.; Piccirillo, S.; Amoroso, S.; Magi, S. Essential Role of the Na+-Ca2+ Exchanger (NCX) in Glutamate-Enhanced Cell Survival in Cardiac Cells Exposed to Hypoxia/Reoxygenation. *Sci. Rep.* **2017**, *7*, 13073. [CrossRef] [PubMed]
153. Magi, S.; Lariccia, V.; Castaldo, P.; Arcangeli, S.; Nasti, A.A.; Giordano, A.; Amoroso, S. Physical and Functional Interaction of NCX1 and EAAC1 Transporters Leading to Glutamate-Enhanced ATP Production in Brain Mitochondria. *PLoS ONE* **2012**, *7*, e34015. [CrossRef] [PubMed]
154. Magi, S.; Arcangeli, S.; Castaldo, P.; Nasti, A.A.; Berrino, L.; Piegari, E.; Bernardini, R.; Amoroso, S.; Lariccia, V. Glutamate-Induced ATP Synthesis: Relationship between Plasma Membrane Na+/Ca2+ Exchanger and Excitatory Amino Acid Transporters in Brain and Heart Cell Models. *Mol. Pharmacol.* **2013**, *84*, 603–614. [CrossRef] [PubMed]
155. Lariccia, V.; Amoroso, S. Calcium- and ATP-Dependent Regulation of Na/Ca Exchange Function in BHK Cells: Comparison of NCX1 and NCX3 Exchangers. *Cell Calcium* **2018**, *73*, 95–103. [CrossRef]
156. Minelli, A.; Castaldo, P.; Gobbi, P.; Salucci, S.; Magi, S.; Amoroso, S. Cellular and Subcellular Localization of Na+-Ca2+ Exchanger Protein Isoforms, NCX1, NCX2, and NCX3 in Cerebral Cortex and Hippocampus of Adult Rat. *Cell Calcium* **2007**, *41*, 221–234. [CrossRef]
157. Magi, S.; Castaldo, P.; Macrì, M.L.; Maiolino, M.; Matteucci, A.; Bastioli, G.; Gratteri, S.; Amoroso, S.; Lariccia, V. Intracellular Calcium Dysregulation: Implications for Alzheimer's Disease. *BioMed Res. Int.* **2016**, *2016*, 6701324. [CrossRef]
158. Stirling, D.P.; Stys, P.K. Mechanisms of Axonal Injury: Internodal Nanocomplexes and Calcium Deregulation. *Trends Mol. Med.* **2010**, *16*, 160–170. [CrossRef]
159. Kinnally, K.W.; Peixoto, P.M.; Ryu, S.-Y.; Dejean, L.M. Is MPTP the Gatekeeper for Necrosis, Apoptosis, or Both? *Biochim. Biophys. Acta* **2011**, *1813*, 616–622. [CrossRef]
160. Correia, S.C.; Santos, R.X.; Perry, G.; Zhu, X.; Moreira, P.I.; Smith, M.A. Mitochondria: The Missing Link between Preconditioning and Neuroprotection. *J. Alzheimers Dis. JAD* **2010**, *20* (Suppl 2), S475–S485. [CrossRef]
161. Yang, R.; Dunn, J.F. Multiple Sclerosis Disease Progression: Contributions from a Hypoxia-Inflammation Cycle. *Mult. Scler. Houndmills Basingstoke Engl.* **2019**, *25*, 1715–1718. [CrossRef]
162. Virgili, N.; Espinosa-Parrilla, J.F.; Mancera, P.; Pastén-Zamorano, A.; Gimeno-Bayon, J.; Rodríguez, M.J.; Mahy, N.; Pugliese, M. Oral Administration of the KATP Channel Opener Diazoxide Ameliorates Disease Progression in a Murine Model of Multiple Sclerosis. *J. Neuroinflamm.* **2011**, *8*, 149. [CrossRef] [PubMed]

163. Du, X.; Yang, J.; Liu, C.; Wang, S.; Zhang, C.; Zhao, H.; Du, H.; Geng, X. Hypoxia-Inducible Factor 1α and 2α Have Beneficial Effects in Remote Ischemic Preconditioning Against Stroke by Modulating Inflammatory Responses in Aged Rats. *Front. Aging Neurosci.* **2020**, *12*, 54. [CrossRef] [PubMed]
164. Merelli, A.; Rodríguez, J.C.G.; Folch, J.; Regueiro, M.R.; Camins, A.; Lazarowski, A. Understanding the Role of Hypoxia Inducible Factor During Neurodegeneration for New Therapeutics Opportunities. *Curr. Neuropharmacol.* **2018**, *16*, 1484–1498. [CrossRef] [PubMed]
165. Scharping, N.E.; Rivadeneira, D.B.; Menk, A.V.; Vignali, P.D.A.; Ford, B.R.; Rittenhouse, N.L.; Peralta, R.; Wang, Y.; Wang, Y.; DePeaux, K.; et al. Mitochondrial Stress Induced by Continuous Stimulation under Hypoxia Rapidly Drives T Cell Exhaustion. *Nat. Immunol.* **2021**, *22*, 205–215. [CrossRef] [PubMed]
166. Cirac, A.; Tsaktanis, T.; Beyer, T.; Linnerbauer, M.; Andlauer, T.; Grummel, V.; Nirschl, L.; Loesslein, L.; Quintana, F.J.; Hemmer, B.; et al. The Aryl Hydrocarbon Receptor-Dependent TGF-α/VEGF-B Ratio Correlates With Disease Subtype and Prognosis in Multiple Sclerosis. *Neurol. Neuroimmunol. Neuroinflamm.* **2021**, *8*, e1043. [CrossRef] [PubMed]
167. Javadov, S.; Karmazyn, M.; Escobales, N. Mitochondrial Permeability Transition Pore Opening as a Promising Therapeutic Target in Cardiac Diseases. *J. Pharmacol. Exp. Ther.* **2009**, *330*, 670–678. [CrossRef] [PubMed]
168. Hausenloy, D.J. Signalling Pathways in Ischaemic Postconditioning. *Thromb. Haemost.* **2009**, *101*, 626–634. [CrossRef]
169. Chotiyarnwong, C.; Nair, K.; Angelini, L.; Buckley, E.; Mazza, C.; Heyes, D.; Ramiz, R.; Baster, K.; Ismail, A.; Das, J.; et al. Effect of Remote Ischaemic Preconditioning on Walking in People with Multiple Sclerosis: Double-Blind Randomised Controlled Trial. *BMJ Neurol. Open* **2020**, *2*, e000022. [CrossRef]
170. Misrielal, C.; Mauthe, M.; Reggiori, F.; Eggen, B.J.L. Autophagy in Multiple Sclerosis: Two Sides of the Same Coin. *Front. Cell. Neurosci.* **2020**, *14*, 603710. [CrossRef]
171. Crino, P.B. The MTOR Signalling Cascade: Paving New Roads to Cure Neurological Disease. *Nat. Rev. Neurol.* **2016**, *12*, 379–392. [CrossRef]
172. Dello Russo, C.; Lisi, L.; Feinstein, D.L.; Navarra, P. MTOR Kinase, a Key Player in the Regulation of Glial Functions: Relevance for the Therapy of Multiple Sclerosis. *Glia* **2013**, *61*, 301–311. [CrossRef]
173. Sanadgol, N.; Barati, M.; Houshmand, F.; Hassani, S.; Clarner, T.; Shahlaei, M.; Golab, F. Metformin Accelerates Myelin Recovery and Ameliorates Behavioral Deficits in the Animal Model of Multiple Sclerosis via Adjustment of AMPK/Nrf2/MTOR Signaling and Maintenance of Endogenous Oligodendrogenesis during Brain Self-Repairing Period. *Pharmacol. Rep. PR* **2020**, *72*, 641–658. [CrossRef] [PubMed]
174. Zhang, L.; Wang, J.; Wang, J.; Yang, B.; He, Q.; Weng, Q. Role of DJ-1 in Immune and Inflammatory Diseases. *Front. Immunol.* **2020**, *11*, 994. [CrossRef] [PubMed]
175. Hirotani, M.; Maita, C.; Niino, M.; Iguchi-Ariga, S.; Hamada, S.; Ariga, H.; Sasaki, H. Correlation between DJ-1 Levels in the Cerebrospinal Fluid and the Progression of Disabilities in Multiple Sclerosis Patients. *Mult. Scler. Houndmills Basingstoke Engl.* **2008**, *14*, 1056–1060. [CrossRef] [PubMed]
176. McCoy, M.K.; Cookson, M.R. DJ-1 Regulation of Mitochondrial Function and Autophagy through Oxidative Stress. *Autophagy* **2011**, *7*, 531–532. [CrossRef]
177. Zeldich, E.; Chen, C.-D.; Avila, R.; Medicetty, S.; Abraham, C.R. The Anti-Aging Protein Klotho Enhances Remyelination Following Cuprizone-Induced Demyelination. *J. Mol. Neurosci. MN* **2015**, *57*, 185–196. [CrossRef]
178. Ellidag, H.Y.; Yilmaz, N.; Kurtulus, F.; Aydin, O.; Eren, E.; Inci, A.; Dolu, S.; Ince, F.D.A.; Giray, Ö.; Yaman, A. The Three Sisters of Fate in Multiple Sclerosis: Klotho (Clotho), Fibroblast Growth Factor-23 (Lachesis), and Vitamin D (Atropos). *Ann. Neurosci.* **2016**, *23*, 155–161. [CrossRef]
179. Moos, W.H.; Faller, D.V.; Glavas, I.P.; Harpp, D.N.; Kanara, I.; Mavrakis, A.N.; Pernokas, J.; Pernokas, M.; Pinkert, C.A.; Powers, W.R.; et al. Klotho Pathways, Myelination Disorders, Neurodegenerative Diseases, and Epigenetic Drugs. *BioResearch Open Access* **2020**, *9*, 94–105. [CrossRef]
180. Torbus-Paluszczak, M.; Bartman, W.; Adamczyk-Sowa, M. Klotho Protein in Neurodegenerative Disorders. *Neurol. Sci. Off. J. Ital. Neurol. Soc. Ital. Soc. Clin. Neurophysiol.* **2018**, *39*, 1677–1682. [CrossRef]
181. Foolad, F.; Khodagholi, F.; Javan, M. Sirtuins in Multiple Sclerosis: The Crossroad of Neurodegeneration, Autoimmunity and Metabolism. *Mult. Scler. Relat. Disord.* **2019**, *34*, 47–58. [CrossRef]
182. Dinkova-Kostova, A.T.; Abramov, A.Y. The Emerging Role of Nrf2 in Mitochondrial Function. *Free Radic. Biol. Med.* **2015**, *88*, 179–188. [CrossRef] [PubMed]
183. Mills, E.A.; Ogrodnik, M.A.; Plave, A.; Mao-Draayer, Y. Emerging Understanding of the Mechanism of Action for Dimethyl Fumarate in the Treatment of Multiple Sclerosis. *Front. Neurol.* **2018**, *9*, 5. [CrossRef] [PubMed]
184. Fisher-Wellman, K.H.; Hagen, J.T.; Neufer, P.D.; Kassai, M.; Cabot, M.C. On the Nature of Ceramide-Mitochondria Interactions—Dissection Using Comprehensive Mitochondrial Phenotyping. *Cell. Signal.* **2021**, *78*, 109838. [CrossRef] [PubMed]
185. McGinley, M.P.; Cohen, J.A. Sphingosine 1-Phosphate Receptor Modulators in Multiple Sclerosis and Other Conditions. *Lancet Lond. Engl.* **2021**, *398*, 1184–1194. [CrossRef]
186. De Stefano, N.; Silva, D.G.; Barnett, M.H. Effect of Fingolimod on Brain Volume Loss in Patients with Multiple Sclerosis. *CNS Drugs* **2017**, *31*, 289–305. [CrossRef]

187. Darios, F.; Wasser, C.; Shakirzyanova, A.; Giniatullin, A.; Goodman, K.; Munoz-Bravo, J.L.; Raingo, J.; Jorgacevski, J.; Kreft, M.; Zorec, R.; et al. Sphingosine Facilitates SNARE Complex Assembly and Activates Synaptic Vesicle Exocytosis. *Neuron* **2009**, *62*, 683–694. [CrossRef]
188. Stenovec, M.; Trkov, S.; Kreft, M.; Zorec, R. Alterations of Calcium Homoeostasis in Cultured Rat Astrocytes Evoked by Bioactive Sphingolipids. *Acta Physiol. Oxf. Engl.* **2014**, *212*, 49–61. [CrossRef]
189. Trkov Bobnar, S.; Stenovec, M.; Miš, K.; Pirkmajer, S.; Zorec, R. Fingolimod Suppresses the Proinflammatory Status of Interferon-γ-Activated Cultured Rat Astrocytes. *Mol. Neurobiol.* **2019**, *56*, 5971–5986. [CrossRef]
190. Mandolesi, G.; Gentile, A.; Musella, A.; Fresegna, D.; De Vito, F.; Bullitta, S.; Sepman, H.; Marfia, G.A.; Centonze, D. Synaptopathy Connects Inflammation and Neurodegeneration in Multiple Sclerosis. *Nat. Rev. Neurol.* **2015**, *11*, 711–724. [CrossRef]
191. Mandolesi, G.; De Vito, F.; Musella, A.; Gentile, A.; Bullitta, S.; Fresegna, D.; Sepman, H.; Di Sanza, C.; Haji, N.; Mori, F.; et al. MiR-142-3p Is a Key Regulator of IL-1β-Dependent Synaptopathy in Neuroinflammation. *J. Neurosci. Off. J. Soc. Neurosci.* **2017**, *37*, 546–561. [CrossRef]
192. Weiss, S.; Mori, F.; Rossi, S.; Centonze, D. Disability in Multiple Sclerosis: When Synaptic Long-Term Potentiation Fails. *Neurosci. Biobehav. Rev.* **2014**, *43*, 88–99. [CrossRef] [PubMed]
193. Mori, F.; Nisticò, R.; Mandolesi, G.; Piccinin, S.; Mango, D.; Kusayanagi, H.; Berretta, N.; Bergami, A.; Gentile, A.; Musella, A.; et al. Interleukin-1β Promotes Long-Term Potentiation in Patients with Multiple Sclerosis. *Neuromolecular Med.* **2014**, *16*, 38–51. [CrossRef] [PubMed]
194. Luchetti, S.; Huitinga, I.; Swaab, D.F. Neurosteroid and GABA-A Receptor Alterations in Alzheimer's Disease, Parkinson's Disease and Multiple Sclerosis. *Neuroscience* **2011**, *191*, 6–21. [CrossRef] [PubMed]
195. Dubchenko, E.; Ivanov, A.; Spirina, N.; Smirnova, N.; Melnikov, M.; Boyko, A.; Gusev, E.; Kubatiev, A. Hyperhomocysteinemia and Endothelial Dysfunction in Multiple Sclerosis. *Brain Sci.* **2020**, *10*, 637. [CrossRef]
196. Paolucci, M.; Altamura, C.; Vernieri, F. The Role of Endothelial Dysfunction in the Pathophysiology and Cerebrovascular Effects of Migraine: A Narrative Review. *J. Clin. Neurol. Seoul Korea* **2021**, *17*, 164–175. [CrossRef]
197. D'haeseleer, M.; Cambron, M.; Vanopdenbosch, L.; De Keyser, J. Vascular Aspects of Multiple Sclerosis. *Lancet Neurol.* **2011**, *10*, 657–666. [CrossRef]
198. Mirmosayyeb, O.; Barzegar, M.; Nehzat, N.; Shaygannejad, V.; Sahraian, M.A.; Ghajarzadeh, M. The Prevalence of Migraine in Multiple Sclerosis (MS): A Systematic Review and Meta-Analysis. *J. Clin. Neurosci. Off. J. Neurosurg. Soc. Australas.* **2020**, *79*, 33–38. [CrossRef]
199. D'haeseleer, M.; Hostenbach, S.; Peeters, I.; Sankari, S.E.; Nagels, G.; De Keyser, J.; D'hooghe, M.B. Cerebral Hypoperfusion: A New Pathophysiologic Concept in Multiple Sclerosis? *J. Cereb. Blood Flow Metab. Off. J. Int. Soc. Cereb. Blood Flow Metab.* **2015**, *35*, 1406–1410. [CrossRef]
200. Senzaki, K.; Okada, Y.; Ochi, H.; Ochi, M.; Takei, S.I.; Miura, S.; Igase, M.; Ohyagi, Y. Vascular Endothelial Dysfunction Associated with Severity in Multiple Sclerosis. *Mult. Scler. Relat. Disord.* **2021**, *54*, 103135. [CrossRef]
201. Lattanzi, S.; Acciarri, M.C.; Danni, M.; Taffi, R.; Cerqua, R.; Rocchi, C.; Silvestrini, M. Cerebral Hemodynamics in Patients with Multiple Sclerosis. *Mult. Scler. Relat. Disord.* **2020**, *44*, 102309. [CrossRef]
202. Orian, J.M.; D'Souza, C.S.; Kocovski, P.; Krippner, G.; Hale, M.W.; Wang, X.; Peter, K. Platelets in Multiple Sclerosis: Early and Central Mediators of Inflammation and Neurodegeneration and Attractive Targets for Molecular Imaging and Site-Directed Therapy. *Front. Immunol.* **2021**, *12*, 620963. [CrossRef] [PubMed]
203. van den Pol, A.N. Neuropeptide Transmission in Brain Circuits. *Neuron* **2012**, *76*, 98–115. [CrossRef] [PubMed]
204. Drew, G.M.; Coussens, C.M.; Abraham, W.C. Effects of Endothelin-1 on Hippocampal Synaptic Plasticity. *Neuroreport* **1998**, *9*, 1827–1830. [CrossRef] [PubMed]
205. Yang, K.; Trepanier, C.H.; Li, H.; Beazely, M.A.; Lerner, E.A.; Jackson, M.F.; MacDonald, J.F. Vasoactive Intestinal Peptide Acts via Multiple Signal Pathways to Regulate Hippocampal NMDA Receptors and Synaptic Transmission. *Hippocampus* **2009**, *19*, 779–789. [CrossRef] [PubMed]
206. Liu, Y.; Chen, Q.-Y.; Lee, J.H.; Li, X.-H.; Yu, S.; Zhuo, M. Cortical Potentiation Induced by Calcitonin Gene-Related Peptide (CGRP) in the Insular Cortex of Adult Mice. *Mol. Brain* **2020**, *13*, 36. [CrossRef]
207. Gressens, P.; Hill, J.M.; Gozes, I.; Fridkin, M.; Brenneman, D.E. Growth Factor Function of Vasoactive Intestinal Peptide in Whole Cultured Mouse Embryos. *Nature* **1993**, *362*, 155–158. [CrossRef]
208. Gressens, P.; Paindaveine, B.; Hill, J.M.; Brenneman, D.E.; Evrard, P. Growth Factor Properties of VIP during Early Brain Development.: Whole Embryo Culture and in Vivo Studies. *Ann. N. Y. Acad. Sci.* **1997**, *814*, 152–160. [CrossRef]
209. Deng, G.; Jin, L. The Effects of Vasoactive Intestinal Peptide in Neurodegenerative Disorders. *Neurol. Res.* **2017**, *39*, 65–72. [CrossRef]
210. Solés-Tarrés, I.; Cabezas-Llobet, N.; Vaudry, D.; Xifró, X. Protective Effects of Pituitary Adenylate Cyclase-Activating Polypeptide and Vasoactive Intestinal Peptide Against Cognitive Decline in Neurodegenerative Diseases. *Front. Cell. Neurosci.* **2020**, *14*, 221. [CrossRef]
211. Van, C.; Condro, M.C.; Ko, H.H.; Hoang, A.Q.; Zhu, R.; Lov, K.; Ricaflanca, P.T.; Diep, A.L.; Nguyen, N.N.M.; Lipshutz, G.S.; et al. Targeted Deletion of PAC1 Receptors in Retinal Neurons Enhances Neuron Loss and Axonopathy in a Model of Multiple Sclerosis and Optic Neuritis. *Neurobiol. Dis.* **2021**, *160*, 105524. [CrossRef]

212. Abad, C.; Jayaram, B.; Becquet, L.; Wang, Y.; O'Dorisio, M.S.; Waschek, J.A.; Tan, Y.-V. VPAC1 Receptor (Vipr1)-Deficient Mice Exhibit Ameliorated Experimental Autoimmune Encephalomyelitis, with Specific Deficits in the Effector Stage. *J. Neuroinflamm.* **2016**, *13*, 169. [CrossRef]
213. Masaki, T.; Sawamura, T. Endothelin and Endothelial Dysfunction. *Proc. Jpn. Acad. Ser. B Phys. Biol. Sci.* **2006**, *82*, 17–24. [CrossRef]
214. Masaki, T. Historical Review: Endothelin. *Trends Pharmacol. Sci.* **2004**, *25*, 219–224. [CrossRef]
215. Marola, O.J.; Syc-Mazurek, S.B.; Howell, G.R.; Libby, R.T. Endothelin 1-Induced Retinal Ganglion Cell Death Is Largely Mediated by JUN Activation. *Cell Death Dis.* **2020**, *11*, 811. [CrossRef]
216. Hammond, T.R.; Gadea, A.; Dupree, J.; Kerninon, C.; Nait-Oumesmar, B.; Aguirre, A.; Gallo, V. Astrocyte-Derived Endothelin-1 Inhibits Remyelination through Notch Activation. *Neuron* **2014**, *81*, 588–602. [CrossRef] [PubMed]
217. Hammond, T.R.; McEllin, B.; Morton, P.D.; Raymond, M.; Dupree, J.; Gallo, V. Endothelin-B Receptor Activation in Astrocytes Regulates the Rate of Oligodendrocyte Regeneration during Remyelination. *Cell Rep.* **2015**, *13*, 2090–2097. [CrossRef] [PubMed]
218. Gong, S.; Peng, L.; Yan, B.; Dong, Q.; Seng, Z.; Wang, W.; Lv, J.; He, X. Bosentan Reduces Neuronal Apoptosis Following Spinal Cord Ischemic Reperfusion Injury. *Spinal Cord* **2014**, *52*, 181–185. [CrossRef] [PubMed]
219. He, J.-T.; Li, H.; Yang, L.; Cheng, K.-L. Involvement of Endothelin-1, H2S and Nrf2 in Beneficial Effects of Remote Ischemic Preconditioning in Global Cerebral Ischemia-Induced Vascular Dementia in Mice. *Cell. Mol. Neurobiol.* **2019**, *39*, 671–686. [CrossRef]
220. Jin, Y.-H.; Kang, B.; Kang, H.S.; Koh, C.-S.; Kim, B.S. Endothelin-1 Contributes to the Development of Virus-Induced Demyelinating Disease. *J. Neuroinflamm.* **2020**, *17*, 307. [CrossRef]
221. Guo, Y.; Chung, S.K.; Siu, C.-W.; Kwan, S.-C.; Ho, P.W.-L.; Yeung, P.K.-K.; Chan, K.-H. Endothelin-1 Overexpression Exacerbate Experimental Allergic Encephalomyelitis. *J. Neuroimmunol.* **2014**, *276*, 64–70. [CrossRef]
222. Castellazzi, M.; Lamberti, G.; Resi, M.V.; Baldi, E.; Caniatti, L.M.; Galante, G.; Perri, P.; Pugliatti, M. Increased Levels of Endothelin-1 in Cerebrospinal Fluid Are a Marker of Poor Visual Recovery after Optic Neuritis in Multiple Sclerosis Patients. *Dis. Markers* **2019**, *2019*, 9320791. [CrossRef] [PubMed]
223. Monti, L.; Arrigucci, U.; Rossi, A. Insights into Endothelin-3 and Multiple Sclerosis. *Biomol. Concepts* **2020**, *11*, 137–141. [CrossRef] [PubMed]
224. Gonzalez-Rey, E.; Fernandez-Martin, A.; Chorny, A.; Martin, J.; Pozo, D.; Ganea, D.; Delgado, M. Therapeutic Effect of Vasoactive Intestinal Peptide on Experimental Autoimmune Encephalomyelitis. *Am. J. Pathol.* **2006**, *168*, 1179–1188. [CrossRef] [PubMed]
225. Kato, H.; Ito, A.; Kawanokuchi, J.; Jin, S.; Mizuno, T.; Ojika, K.; Ueda, R.; Suzumura, A. Pituitary Adenylate Cyclase-Activating Polypeptide (PACAP) Ameliorates Experimental Autoimmune Encephalomyelitis by Suppressing the Functions of Antigen Presenting Cells. *Mult. Scler. Houndmills Basingstoke Engl.* **2004**, *10*, 651–659. [CrossRef]
226. Rossetti, I.; Zambusi, L.; Finardi, A.; Bodini, A.; Provini, L.; Furlan, R.; Morara, S. Calcitonin Gene-Related Peptide Decreases IL-1beta, IL-6 as Well as Ym1, Arg1, CD163 Expression in a Brain Tissue Context-Dependent Manner While Ameliorating Experimental Autoimmune Encephalomyelitis. *J. Neuroimmunol.* **2018**, *323*, 94–104. [CrossRef]
227. Russell, F.A.; King, R.; Smillie, S.J.; Kodji, X.; Brain, S.D. Calcitonin Gene-Related Peptide: Physiology and Pathophysiology. *Physiol. Rev.* **2014**, *94*, 1099–1142. [CrossRef]
228. Guo, Z.; Liu, N.; Chen, L.; Zhao, X.; Li, M.-R. Independent Roles of CGRP in Cardioprotection and Hemodynamic Regulation in Ischemic Postconditioning. *Eur. J. Pharmacol.* **2018**, *828*, 18–25. [CrossRef]
229. Liu, Z.; Liu, Q.; Cai, H.; Xu, C.; Liu, G.; Li, Z. Calcitonin Gene-Related Peptide Prevents Blood–Brain Barrier Injury and Brain Edema Induced by Focal Cerebral Ischemia Reperfusion. *Regul. Pept.* **2011**, *171*, 19–25. [CrossRef]
230. Zhai, L.; Sakurai, T.; Kamiyoshi, A.; Ichikawa-Shindo, Y.; Kawate, H.; Tanaka, M.; Xian, X.; Hirabayashi, K.; Dai, K.; Cui, N.; et al. Endogenous Calcitonin Gene-Related Peptide Suppresses Ischemic Brain Injuries and Progression of Cognitive Decline. *J. Hypertens.* **2018**, *36*, 876–891. [CrossRef]
231. Hay, D.L.; Garelja, M.L.; Poyner, D.R.; Walker, C.S. Update on the Pharmacology of Calcitonin/CGRP Family of Peptides: IUPHAR Review 25. *Br. J. Pharmacol.* **2018**, *175*, 3–17. [CrossRef]
232. Gingell, J.J.; Hendrikse, E.R.; Hay, D.L. New Insights into the Regulation of CGRP-Family Receptors. *Trends Pharmacol. Sci.* **2019**, *40*, 71–83. [CrossRef]
233. Borkum, J.M. CGRP and Brain Functioning: Cautions for Migraine Treatment. *Headache* **2019**, *59*, 1339–1357. [CrossRef]
234. Piehl, F.; Arvidsson, U.; Johnson, H.; Cullheim, S.; Dagerlind, A.; Ulfhake, B.; Cao, Y.; Elde, R.; Pettersson, R.F.; Terenius, L. GAP-43, AFGF, CCK and Alpha- and Beta-CGRP in Rat Spinal Motoneurons Subjected to Axotomy and/or Dorsal Root Severance. *Eur. J. Neurosci.* **1993**, *5*, 1321–1333. [CrossRef] [PubMed]
235. Giardino, L.; Giuliani, A.; Fernandez, M.; Calzà, L. Spinal Motoneurone Distress during Experimental Allergic Encephalomyelitis. *Neuropathol. Appl. Neurobiol.* **2004**, *30*, 522–531. [CrossRef]
236. Mathé, A.A.; Ågren, H.; Lindström, L.; Theodorsson, E. Increased Concentration of Calcitonin Gene-Related Peptide in Cerebrospinal Fluid of Depressed Patients. A Possible Trait Marker of Major Depressive Disorder. *Neurosci. Lett.* **1994**, *182*, 138–142. [CrossRef] [PubMed]
237. Mathé, A.A.; Hertel, P.; Nomikos, G.G.; Gruber, S.; Mathé, J.M.; Svensson, T.H. The Psychotomimetic Drugs D-Amphetamine and Phencyclidine Release Calcitonin Gene-Related Peptide in the Limbic Forebrain of the Rat. *J. Neurosci. Res.* **1996**, *46*, 316–323. [CrossRef]

238. Siegert, R.J.; Abernethy, D.A. Depression in Multiple Sclerosis: A Review. *J. Neurol. Neurosurg. Psychiatry* **2005**, *76*, 469–475. [CrossRef]
239. Warfvinge, K.; Edvinsson, L.; Pickering, D.S.; Sheykhzade, M. The Presence of Calcitonin Gene-Related Peptide and Its Receptors in Rat, Pig and Human Brain: Species Differences in Calcitonin Gene-Related Peptide Pharmacology. *Pharmacology* **2019**, *104*, 332–341. [CrossRef]
240. Kaiser, E.A.; Rea, B.J.; Kuburas, A.; Kovacevich, B.R.; Garcia-, L.F.; Recober, A.; Russo, A.F.; City, I.; States, U.; City, I.; et al. Negative Regulation of TLR Responses by the Neuropeptide CGRP Is Mediated by the Transcriptional Repressor ICER. *Sci. Rep.* **2017**, *323*, 607–615. [CrossRef]
241. Kee, Z.; Kodji, X.; Brain, S.D. The Role of Calcitonin Gene Related Peptide (CGRP) in Neurogenic Vasodilation and Its Cardioprotective Effects. *Front. Physiol.* **2018**, *9*, 1249. [CrossRef]
242. Pedreño, M.; Morell, M.; Robledo, G.; Souza-Moreira, L.; Forte-Lago, I.; Caro, M.; O'Valle, F.; Ganea, D.; Gonzalez-Rey, E. Adrenomedullin Protects from Experimental Autoimmune Encephalomyelitis at Multiple Levels. *Brain. Behav. Immun.* **2014**, *37*, 152–163. [CrossRef]
243. Rodríguez-Lorenzo, S.; Ferreira Francisco, D.M.; Vos, R.; van Het Hof, B.; Rijnsburger, M.; Schroten, H.; Ishikawa, H.; Beaino, W.; Bruggmann, R.; Kooij, G.; et al. Altered Secretory and Neuroprotective Function of the Choroid Plexus in Progressive Multiple Sclerosis. *Acta Neuropathol. Commun.* **2020**, *8*, 35. [CrossRef] [PubMed]
244. Hay, D.L.; Chen, S.; Lutz, T.A.; Parkes, D.G.; Roth, J.D. Amylin: Pharmacology, Physiology, and Clinical Potential. *Pharmacol. Rev.* **2015**, *67*, 564–600. [CrossRef] [PubMed]
245. Wang, E.; Zhu, H.; Wang, X.; Gower, A.C.; Wallack, M.; Blusztajn, J.K.; Kowall, N.; Qiu, W.Q. Amylin Treatment Reduces Neuroinflammation and Ameliorates Abnormal Patterns of Gene Expression in the Cerebral Cortex of an Alzheimer's Disease Mouse Model. *J. Alzheimers Dis.* **2017**, *56*, 47–61. [CrossRef] [PubMed]
246. Grizzanti, J.; Corrigan, R.; Casadesus, G. Neuroprotective Effects of Amylin Analogues on Alzheimer's Disease Pathogenesis and Cognition. *J. Alzheimers Dis. JAD* **2018**, *66*, 11–23. [CrossRef]
247. Walker, C.S.; Conner, A.C.; Poyner, D.R.; Hay, D.L. Regulation of Signal Transduction by Calcitonin Gene-Related Peptide Receptors. *Trends Pharmacol. Sci.* **2010**, *31*, 476–483. [CrossRef] [PubMed]
248. Kurnellas, M.P.; Adams, C.M.; Sobel, R.A.; Steinman, L.; Rothbard, J.B. Amyloid Fibrils Composed of Hexameric Peptides Attenuate Neuroinflammation. *Sci. Transl. Med.* **2013**, *5*, 179ra42. [CrossRef]
249. Steinman, L.; Rothbard, J.B.; Kurnellas, M.P. Janus Faces of Amyloid Proteins in Neuroinflammation. *J. Clin. Immunol.* **2014**, *34* (Suppl 1), S61–S63. [CrossRef]
250. Pietroboni, A.M.; Colombi, A.; Carandini, T.; Scarpini, E.; Galimberti, D.; Bozzali, M. The Role of Amyloid-ß in White Matter Damage: Possible Common Pathogenetic Mechanisms in Neurodegenerative and Demyelinating Diseases. *J. Alzheimers Dis.* **2020**, *78*, 13–22. [CrossRef]
251. Pietroboni, A.M.; Caprioli, M.; Carandini, T.; Scarioni, M.; Ghezzi, L.; Arighi, A.; Cioffi, S.; Cinnante, C.; Fenoglio, C.; Oldoni, E.; et al. CSF β-Amyloid Predicts Prognosis in Patients with Multiple Sclerosis. *Mult. Scler. Houndmills Basingstoke Engl.* **2019**, *25*, 1223–1231. [CrossRef]
252. Bozkurt, B.; Nair, A.P.; Misra, A.; Scott, C.Z.; Mahar, J.H.; Fedson, S. Neprilysin Inhibitors in Heart Failure. *JACC Basic Transl. Sci.* **2022**, *8*, 88–105. [CrossRef] [PubMed]
253. Scuteri, D.; Adornetto, A.; Rombolà, L.; Naturale, M.D.; Morrone, L.A.; Bagetta, G.; Tonin, P.; Corasaniti, M.T. New Trends in Migraine Pharmacology: Targeting Calcitonin Gene–Related Peptide (CGRP) With Monoclonal Antibodies. *Front. Pharmacol.* **2019**, *10*, 363. [CrossRef] [PubMed]
254. Hersh, L.B.; Rodgers, D.W. Neprilysin and Amyloid Beta Peptide Degradation. *Curr. Alzheimer Res.* **2008**, *5*, 225–231. [CrossRef] [PubMed]
255. Guan, H.; Chow, K.M.; Shah, R.; Rhodes, C.J.; Hersh, L.B. Degradation of Islet Amyloid Polypeptide by Neprilysin. *Diabetologia* **2012**, *55*, 2989–2998. [CrossRef]
256. Eckman, E.A.; Reed, D.K.; Eckman, C.B. Degradation of the Alzheimer's Amyloid Beta Peptide by Endothelin-Converting Enzyme. *J. Biol. Chem.* **2001**, *276*, 24540–24548. [CrossRef]
257. Kurochkin, I.V.; Guarnera, E.; Berezovsky, I.N. Insulin-Degrading Enzyme in the Fight against Alzheimer's Disease. *Trends Pharmacol. Sci.* **2018**, *39*, 49–58. [CrossRef]
258. Sousa, L.; Guarda, M.; Meneses, M.J.; Macedo, M.P.; Vicente Miranda, H. Insulin-Degrading Enzyme: An Ally against Metabolic and Neurodegenerative Diseases. *J. Pathol.* **2021**, *255*, 346–361. [CrossRef]
259. Graykowski, D.; Kasparian, K.; Caniglia, J.; Gritsaeva, Y.; Cudaback, E. Neuroinflammation Drives APOE Genotype-Dependent Differential Expression of Neprilysin. *J. Neuroimmunol.* **2020**, *346*, 577315. [CrossRef]
260. Zagon, I.S.; McLaughlin, P.J. *Endogenous Opioids in the Etiology and Treatment of Multiple Sclerosis*; Exon Publications: Brisbane City, Australia, 2017; ISBN 978-0-9944381-3-3.
261. Ban, M.; McCauley, J.L.; Zuvich, R.; Baker, A.; Bergamaschi, L.; Cox, M.; Kemppinen, A.; D'Alfonso, S.; Guerini, F.R.; Lechner-Scott, J.; et al. A Non-Synonymous SNP within Membrane Metalloendopeptidase-like 1 (MMEL1) Is Associated with Multiple Sclerosis. *Genes Immun.* **2010**, *11*, 660–664. [CrossRef]

262. Bernstein, H.-G.; Keilhoff, G.; Dobrowolny, H.; Steiner, J. The Many Facets of CD26/Dipeptidyl Peptidase 4 and Its Inhibitors in Disorders of the CNS—A Critical Overview. *Rev. Neurosci.* **2022**, *34*. [CrossRef]
263. Tejera-Alhambra, M.; Casrouge, A.; de Andrés, C.; Ramos-Medina, R.; Alonso, B.; Vega, J.; Albert, M.L.; Sánchez-Ramón, S. Low DPP4 Expression and Activity in Multiple Sclerosis. *Clin. Immunol. Orlando Fla* **2014**, *150*, 170–183. [CrossRef] [PubMed]

current issues in molecular biology

MDPI

Review

Origin and Emergence of Microglia in the CNS—An Interesting (Hi)story of an Eccentric Cell

Iasonas Dermitzakis [1], Maria Eleni Manthou [1], Soultana Meditskou [1], Marie-Ève Tremblay [2], Steven Petratos [3], Lida Zoupi [4], Marina Boziki [5], Evangelia Kesidou [5,6], Constantina Simeonidou [6] and Paschalis Theotokis [1,5,*]

[1] Department of Histology-Embryology, School of Medicine, Aristotle University of Thessaloniki, 54124 Thessaloniki, Greece
[2] Division of Medical Sciences, University of Victoria, Victoria, BC V8P 5C2, Canada
[3] Department of Neuroscience, Central Clinical School, Monash University, Melbourne, VIC 3004, Australia
[4] Centre for Discovery Brain Sciences & Simons Initiative for the Developing Brain, University of Edinburgh, Edinburgh EH8 9XD, UK
[5] Laboratory of Experimental Neurology and Neuroimmunology, Second Department of Neurology, AHEPA University Hospital, 54621 Thessaloniki, Greece
[6] Laboratory of Experimental Physiology, School of Medicine, Aristotle University of Thessaloniki, 54124 Thessaloniki, Greece
* Correspondence: ptheotokis@auth.gr

Abstract: Microglia belong to tissue-resident macrophages of the central nervous system (CNS), representing the primary innate immune cells. This cell type constitutes ~7% of non-neuronal cells in the mammalian brain and has a variety of biological roles integral to homeostasis and pathophysiology from the late embryonic to adult brain. Its unique identity that distinguishes its "glial" features from tissue-resident macrophages resides in the fact that once entering the CNS, it is perennially exposed to a unique environment following the formation of the blood–brain barrier. Additionally, tissue-resident macrophage progenies derive from various peripheral sites that exhibit hematopoietic potential, and this has resulted in interpretation issues surrounding their origin. Intensive research endeavors have intended to track microglial progenitors during development and disease. The current review provides a corpus of recent evidence in an attempt to disentangle the birthplace of microglia from the progenitor state and underlies the molecular elements that drive microgliogenesis. Furthermore, it caters towards tracking the lineage spatiotemporally during embryonic development and outlining microglial repopulation in the mature CNS. This collection of data can potentially shed light on the therapeutic potential of microglia for CNS perturbations across various levels of severity.

Keywords: microglia; origin; yolk sac; progeny; molecular cues; development

1. Introduction

The central nervous system's (CNS) principal innate immune cells are tissue-resident macrophages, which include microglia [1,2]. While microglia are the parenchymal brain macrophages, the perivascular, meningeal, and choroid plexus macrophages constitute the non-parenchymal tissue-resident macrophages of the CNS [3]. Microglia have a range of biological activities in both the developing and adult mammalian brain, although this population of cells makes up the lowest percentage of non-neuronal cells in the mammalian brain [4]. The release of mediators (e.g., trophic factors, cytokines) and phagocytosis are the two main mechanisms by which microglia shape brain development and perform key functions across life [5]. These microglial activities are implicated in developmental processes such as synaptic patterning, myelinogenesis, axonal dynamics, cell positioning, and survival [6]. In the adult brain, microglial activities are central to the regulation of acute and chronic immune responses and maintenance of CNS homeostasis through the removal of viruses, bacteria, and other foreign particles, but also cellular debris and synapses, mediation of neurogenesis following CNS injury, and protection of neural tissue [7–9]. However, microglia as innate immune cells are sensitive to chronic inflammation, which can impair their beneficial functions and participate in the etiology of protracted neurodegenerative diseases such as Parkinson's and Alzheimer's diseases, multiple sclerosis, and amyotrophic lateral sclerosis (ALS) [10–12].

The term microglia—micro (small) and glia (glue)—was first introduced in 1919 by Pío del Río Hortega, who proposed that microglia adopt a malleable morphology, transforming from a resting to an activated state during disease exhibiting phagocytic properties [13]. This view was recently considered too simplistic, as microglia can adopt a wide variety of morphological and functional states [5]. Under normal physiological conditions, microglia display a ramified morphology with multiple branches and processes constantly surveilling the CNS parenchyma. Inflammatory stimuli can change microglial morphology, for instance converting microglia from a ramified to an amoeboid form characterized by an enlarged cell body and retracted processes. In contrast to the ramified state, amoeboid microglia with an amoeboid morphology are generally considered to exhibit a high phagocytic and proinflammatory phenotype. The activated microglial cells were previously categorized as: classical (M1) or alternative (M2), corresponding to either a proinflammatory and neurotoxic state or an anti-inflammatory state, respectively. However, it is now suggested that the M1/M2 phenotypes are not representative of in vivo microglia states because microglia rarely appear with a distinct M1 or M2 phenotype [5,14].

Tissue-resident macrophages are present in the CNS and across different organs, such as osteoclasts in bone, intestinal macrophages in the gastrointestinal tract, Kupffer cells in liver, alveolar macrophages in lungs, and Langerhans cells in skin [1]. Microglial cells are unique tissue-resident macrophages that differ from their hematogenous origins due to their surrounding environment, which is immune-privileged owing to the formation of the blood–brain barrier (BBB). The timing of BBB formation is vital for the invasion of microglia progenitors during embryonic development. Many studies have delineated that closure is vitally important at specific embryonic days. The permeability of BBB was found to decrease for large molecules from E12.5, and it became impermeable to small molecules as early as E14.5 [15]. This tight regulation showcases the importance of CNS master regulator elements to protect the central environment from pathogens and other harmful agents.

Each tissue-resident macrophage type has a distinct embryonic origin, as their progenitors derive from different waves of hemopoiesis. Consequently, the understanding of embryonic hematopoiesis is vital for delineating the microglial origin. Regarding hematopoiesis in embryonic life, three waves have been described in *mice*. The primitive hematopoiesis starts at E7.5 in the yolk sac (YS), generating primitive erythroid, megakaryocyte, and macrophage progenitors such as early c-MYB-independent erythro-myeloid precursors (EMPs). The second hematopoietic wave, called transient definitive hematopoiesis, originates from YS hemogenic endothelium, giving rise to late c-MYB-dependent EMPs at E8.25 and progenitors with lymphoid potentials at E9, which additionally emerge from the developing aorta-gonad-mesonephros (AGM) region. The definitive hematopoiesis occurs at E10.5 with the generation of hematopoietic stem cells (HSCs) that originate from the embryonic AGM region, colonizing slightly later the fetal liver [16–19].

The present review aims to define existing data on the origin of microglia because there has been controversy over their ontogeny. The developmental milestones that are being covered herein are the primary cues that direct microgliogenesis. The ontogeny of microglia is investigated thoroughly, as it is of prime importance considering that this cell type is involved in the pathogenesis of many diseases and is presented as a target for therapies that are being developed to control the associated phenotypes.

2. Discovery and Ontogeny of Microglia

The origin of microglia has been a debated topic for years. In the past, four main origin concepts have been proposed as a source of microglia: (i) the mesodermal-associated mater elements, (ii) the neuroectodermal matrix cells, (iii) the pericytes, and (iv) the invasion of monocytes especially during early development (Figure 1) [20]. Río Hortega was hailed as the "Father of Microglia", because their discovery supported the mesodermal origin, after observing the invasion of the pial elements within the CNS parenchyma [13, 21]. Using comparable staining methods, John Kershman agreed on the mesenchymal origin of microglia, which were found to be genetically related to histiocytes, a stationary phagocytic cell present in connective tissue [22]. With reference to Boya et al., the meningeal envelope was proposed to be the source of microglia, which sustains a mesodermal nature in agreement with the classical experiments by Río Hortega [23,24]. Later, the theory of multiple mesodermal sources of microglia depending on time and localization was posited [25]. However, another study proposed vascular pericytes as the parent cells of microglia [26,27]. The first reports on the monocytic origin of microglia came to the fore in 1933 and 1934 from Santha and Juba, respectively, who hypothesized that ramified microglia originated from circulating monocytes because the initial appearance of these cells coincided with the vascularization of the brain [28,29].

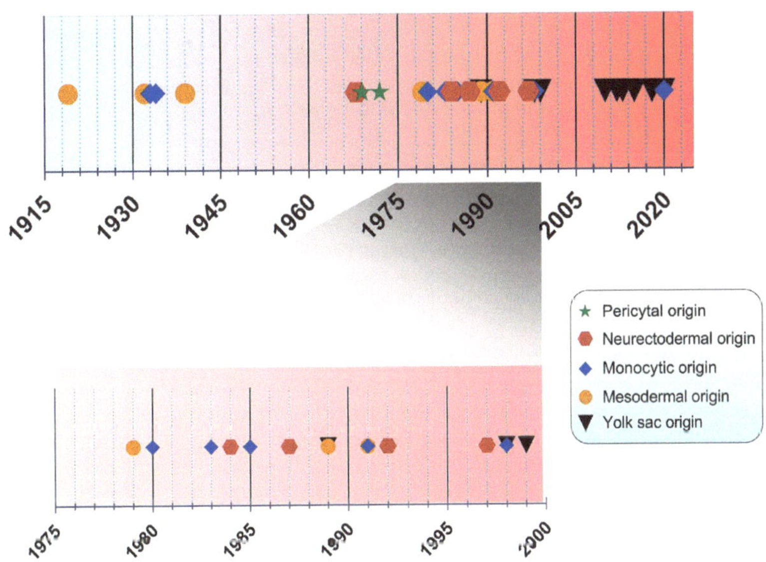

Figure 1. Timeline view of microglial origin since their discovery by Río Hortega.

In the following decades, many researchers accepted this view, demonstrating microglial monocytic identity when investigating their origin [30–33], while others rejected the possibility that microglia are derived from mononuclear blood cells [34]. In 1968, autoradiography experiments performed with tritiated thymidine were conducted in adult *rats*, showing that cells of the subependymal layer give rise to a number of glial cell types, such as astrocytes and microglia, offering a different perspective regarding microglial origin [35]. The neuroectodermal origin was also supported by Kitamura et al., implying that glioblasts are the source of both astrocytes and microglia in *mice* [36]. It was also proposed that microglia and astroglia have a common progenitor cell developing from neuroepithelial cells [37]. Performing non-radioactive in situ hybridization and immunoperoxidase techniques, only a small population of microglia were found to be derived from bone marrow progenitors, because most of the cells were shown to be generated from locally residing precursors with a neuroectodermal ontogeny [38]. The non-monocytic origin of microglia favored by Schelper and Adrian implicated that these cells are CNS intrinsic ones, enforcing the above theory of a neuroectodermal origin [39]. This perception was also put forward by other researchers, but began to lose ground from the 2000's onwards. [40,41].

The view of the origin of microglia from the YS was first introduced in 1989 [42]. A nucleoside diphosphatase histochemical study was conducted to evaluate the distribution of microglia in the developing *human* CNS, implying that mesenchymal cells with haemopoietic potential migrate into neural tissues and then give rise to cells resembling microglia [43]. Likewise, primitive macrophages of YS were found to be derived from fetal macrophages before the appearance of pro-monocytes/monocytes colonizing the embryonic tissues in *mice* [42]. In an *avian* model, microglia precursors were demonstrated to invade neural tissue from the pial surface and proliferated inside the CNS, indicating that their penetration through the embryonic CNS vessels is not possible [44]. However, a *human* embryogenesis study using lectin$^+$ and CD68$^+$ markers revealed two populations of microglia, indicating two different potential origins, specifically from the YS and bone marrow. Different routes of entry were also proposed: one through the mesenchyme and the other via the blood circulation [45]. Alliot et al., aiming to delineate the origin of microglia in *mice*, detected these cells in the brain from E8 being derived from YS progenitors, which proliferate in situ [46].

The YS origin of microglia was confirmed by Ginhoux et al. by performing a fate mapping analysis in *mice* and showing that YS primitive myeloid progenitors generated before E7.5 can contribute to the CNS microglial population [47]. Moreover, in this study, RUNX1$^+$ YS progenitors were found to migrate into the brain through blood vessels between E8.5 and E9.5 [47]. The YS origin was further supported by identifying the transcription factor MYB, which is required for the development of HSCs as well as CD11b^{high} monocytes and macrophages [48], contrary to YS-derived macrophages, which are the potential precursors of CNS microglia [49]. Specifically, primitive c-kit$^+$ EMPs detected from E8 in the YS were proposed to serve as the precursors of microglia in *mice* [50]. As the progenitors of microglia were identified to be the EMPs of YS, the vast majority of other tissue-resident macrophages arise from fetal monocytes that derive from late c-MYB$^+$ EMPs of the YS [51]. The HSC-derived hematopoiesis that takes place for monocytes at E14.5 and granulocytes at E16.5 in *mice* advocates that these progenitors only seldom replace parenchymal microglia, which mainly emanates from CSF-1R$^+$ EMPs. [52]. This view was re-evaluated by Sheng et al., who developed the Kit^{MercreMer} fate mapping *mouse* strain and suggested that all resident-tissue macrophages, except microglia and Langerhans cells of the epidermis, are derived from HSCs [53].

In 2018, De et al. identified two distinct microglial cell populations, namely canonical (non-HOXB8) and HOXB8 microglia using a transgenic strategy, fluorescence-activated cell sorting technique in YS and qRT-PCR in HOXB8 cells in the different hematopoietic tissues [54]. The HOXB8 population was suggested to be derived from the second wave of YS hematopoiesis populating the AGM and fetal liver. Besides the YS, an additional source of microglia was proposed by Fehrenbach et al., who considered the definitive hemopoiesis as responsible for microglial development and recruitment to the *mouse* CNS, especially at the post-YS phase [55]. Besides parenchymal microglia, a genetic distinct population of macrophages was identified, namely the border-associated macrophages (BAMs) residing among the meninges, choroid plexus, and perivascular spaces. Like microglia, these cells are generated by early EMPs; however, microglia require TGF-β for their development, whereas BAMs are TGF-β-independent. Additionally, in the *mouse* YS, two distinctive primitive populations were observed: the CD206$^-$ and CD206$^+$ macrophages. The differentiation of these populations after their final colonization is mediated by environmental drivers [56]. Interestingly, tamoxifen dosing in CCR2-CreER transgenic *mice* suggested that not only YS EMPs, but also fetal HSC-derived monocytes participate in the generation of IBA1$^+$TMEM119$^+$P2RY12$^+$ parenchymal microglia, IBA1$^+$, and isolectin$^+$ BAMs in the *mouse* brain [57]. Lastly, a recent study in eight aborted *human* embryos proposed that tissue-resident macrophages development is very similar to other mammalian species, highlighting the presence of two distinct waves of YS-derived macrophages. Specifically for microglia, they were found to be derived from the early first wave along with a minor contribution from the second one [58].

To recapitulate, the YS is the main site of microglial origin. The suggested microglial progenitors in *mice* are the early, c-MYB-independent, CSF-1R$^+$ EMPs of the YS. However, the definite nomenclature of the progenitors and the confirmation in *human* models are still under consideration.

3. Molecular Cues Orchestrating Microgliogenesis

Upon birth, the phenotype of microglia corresponds to an amoeboid shape, phagocytically and mitotically active, while in later developmental stages, microglia become ramified. The RUNX1, a transcription factor expressed during the first two postnatal weeks at the forebrain by amoeboid microglia, downregulates the proliferation of these cells and assists in their transformation towards a ramified morphology [59]. During embryonic development, RUNX1 controls the expression of the transcription factor PU.1 [60]. In *Irf8*-deficient YS, the number of A1 cells (CD45$^+$ c-kit^{lo} CX$_3$CR1$^-$ immature cells) remained unchanged, while the A2 population (CD45$^+$ c-kit$^-$ CX$_3$CR1$^+$ cells) decreased [50]. Additionally, *Pu.1* deficiency provoked an impairment of A1 and A2 progenitors. From A2 cells, microglia were generated and expanded in the developing brain under the influence of specific matrix metalloproteinases, such as MMP-9 and MMP-8. Factors such as MYB, BATF3, ID2, Klf4, and NR4A1 were not necessary for the development of microglia from their progenitors [50,61]. While PU.1 was essential for terminal myeloid differentiation, early myeloid genes such as *Gm-csfr*, *G-csfr*, and *Mpo* were maintained in *Pu.1*$^{-/-}$ embryos, whereas myeloid genes associated with terminal differentiation (etc. *Cd11b*, *Cd64*, and *M-csfr*) were found to be impaired [62].

The CSF-1R is a vital receptor for microglial cell development expressed on YS macrophages and microglia at E9.5 and throughout brain development. In contrast to many tissue macrophages, adult microglia can still be replenished, albeit at reduced levels in *Csf-1*$^{op/op}$ *mice*. Although the microglia presented—even in small amounts—in a null mutation model of the *Csf-1* in *Csf-1*$^{op/op}$ *mice*, microglia were fully depleted in *mice* lacking CSF-1R [47]. This was a strong clue that a second ligand of CSF-1R, namely the IL-34, was implicated in microgliogenesis. As the microglial phenotype in *Csf-1r*$^{-/-}$ *mice* was more severe than that observed in *Csf-1*$^{op/op}$ *mice*, it was evident that IL-34 plays a significant role in the regulation of microglial homeostasis. Its mRNA expression in the brain is also significantly higher than that of CSF-1 during early postnatal development [47]. In addition, in *il-34-* and *csf-1ra*-deficient *zebrafish larva*, the migration and colonization of CNS by embryonic macrophages was impaired, indicating a role for the Il34-Csf1ra pathway during microglial cell expansion throughout the CNS [63].

Microglia require TGF-β signaling to be maintained in their surveillant state, but not for their survival. The absence of TGF-β1 was found to have an impact on microglial development from E14.5, but not on microglial progenitors at E10.5 [64,65]. Other transcription factors that include SALL1, SALL3, and MEIS3 are involved in the specification of tissue-resident macrophages during organogenesis and ensure microglial function [66]. In fact, when the SALL1 locus was inducibly inactivated, microglial cells transformed from a ramified morphology to pro-inflammatory deregulating tissue homeostasis [64]. A sharp decline in the number of microglial cells was observed in postnatal *Dap12*-deficient *mice* that was comparable to the in vitro impairment of microglial cell differentiation [67]. This may be due to M-CSF's role in inducing microglial proliferation and survival via a pathway requiring DAP12 and β-catenin. However, another study showed that microglial populations remained unaffected in *Dap12*-deficient *mice* similar to young (embryonic and early postnatal) wild-type *mice*, while a reduction in their numbers was observed in specific CNS regions of deficient adult *mice* [50,68]. In *Nox2* gene deficiency, treatment with apocynin, which is a NOX2 inhibitor, or impairment of the VEGFR1 kinase resulted in microglia that could not migrate efficiently into the caudal subventricular zone (SVZ) of the cerebral cortex, suggesting that chemotaxis of microglia was under the influence of NOX2 and VEGFR1 activation (Figure 2) [69].

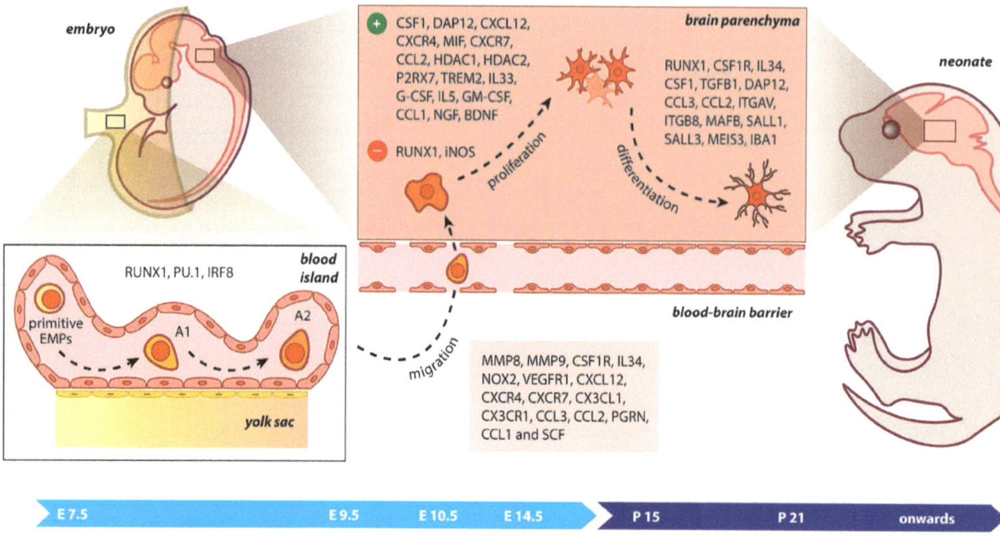

Figure 2. Microgliogenesis at a glance. The primitive erythro-myeloid progenitors (EMPs; early, c−MYB−independent, CSF−1R$^+$ EMPs) arise from the yolk sac (YS) as early as embryonic day 7.5 (E7.5). These cells give rise to CD45$^+$ c−kit$_{lo}$ CX$_3$CR1$^-$ immature (A1) cells that develop into CD45$^+$ c−kit$^-$ CX$_3$CR1$^+$ (A2) cells. The early differentiation of microglial progenitors is regulated by the expression of RUNX1, PU.1, and IRF8. The invasion of progenitors into the neural tube begins at E9.5 through blood circulation and is followed by proliferation and terminal differentiation. As the blood–brain barrier becomes impermeable to small molecules at E14.5, the microglia invasion may be prevented. The transformation of immature microglia into ramified (mature form) occurs between the second and third postnatal weeks. The migration, proliferation, and terminal differentiation of microglia are also orchestrated from the depicted molecular cues. Light blue arrow timeline represents prenatal period, dark blue arrow timeline refers to postnatal days.

The depletion of *Cxcl12* seems to block microglial cell invasion into the SVZ, whereas the ectopic *Cxcl12* expression or pharmacological impairment of CXCR4 demonstrated that the CXCL12/CXCR4 signaling is involved in microglial cell recruitment assisting cortical development. In the same context, cell death occurring in the developing forebrain stimulates microglial cell proliferation mediated via MIF activation [70]. Treatment with CXCL12 activates Erk1/2 and Akt signaling, which are necessary for microglial proliferation mediated by CXCL12. Similarly, Erk1/2 signaling was found to be important for CXCL12-depedent migration of microglial populations. Pharmacological blockade of CXCR4 or CXCR7 induced a decline in CXCL12-mediated proliferation and migration of microglial cells, suggesting that CXCR4 and CXCR7 form a receptor unit for CXCL12 in the *rodent* microglia required for the aforementioned developmental processes, both in vitro and in vivo [71]. Furthermore, CX3CL1/CX3CR1 signaling may regulate microglial invasion within CNS parenchyma during postnatal life [72]. Interestingly, the transformation of microglia from an amoeboid to a ramified morphology was proposed to be mediated by cues released from astrocytes. Utilizing time-lapse video microscopy in co-cultures of *human* fetal microglial cells and astrocytic cells, the chemokines MIP-1α and MCP-1 were identified as regulators of microglial motility and differentiation [73].

The overexpression of *miR-124* in microglia accelerated the transformation of these cells to an inactivated state through inhibition of the C/EBP-α and PU.1, while the depletion of *miR-124* led to microglial activation both in vitro and in vivo. These findings underscored the potential role of *miR-124* as a regulator of microglial surveillance in the CNS [74]. Microglial polarization is regulated by ARID1A, an epigenetic subunit of the

SWI/SNF chromatin-remodeling complex, through alterations of the chromatin state in microglia [75,76]. The migration of microglial cells also seemed to be affected by PGRN, because its knockdown resulted in a failure of microglial precursors to colonize the embryonic retina [77]. The absence of integrin αVβ8 from the CNS prevents microglial transition from immature precursors to a mature state. As αVβ8 controls TGFβ signaling to microglia, these "dysmature" microglial populations are expanded as a consequence of impaired TGFβ signaling during the perinatal period, leading to disrupted oligodendrocyte development, interneuron loss, and neuromotor dysfunction [78]. Epigenetic factors may also affect microglial development. Embryonic HDAC1 and HDAC2 absence disrupts microgliogenesis, altering the crucial acetylation marks implicated in morphology, reactivity, cell cycle, and apoptosis. Specifically, reduced proliferation and induced apoptosis were observed after ablation of the above epigenetic regulators, resulting in the hyperacetylation of specific pro-apoptotic and cell cycle genes [79].

Fate-mapping strategies remain the best way to track cells from the embryonic YS (microglia) versus bone-marrow (monocyte-derived macrophages). In terms of markers, the exact distinction between microglia and periphery-originated macrophages is challenging as they express common markers such as CD11b, CX3CR1, CD45, F4/80, and IBA-1 [80]. Nevertheless, TMEM119 has been recognized as a trans-membranous molecule that is abundantly produced only by microglia, along with P2RY12, but both markers can be downregulated in disease [5,81,82]. However, recently it was proposed that TMEM119 is neither a specific nor a reliable marker for microglial cells [83]. Siglec-H was also found to be a specific marker for microglia in *rodents*, as it was almost absent in CNS-infiltrating monocytes and CNS-associated macrophages [84]. Recently, HexB has also emerged as a promising marker, but the characterization is still largely lacking [85]. On the contrary, CD44 and CD169 are markers expressed only in peripheral-divided cells and not on resident microglia [86,87].

TREM2, as a protein involved in intracellular signals, interacts with transmembrane protein DAP12, thus activating the Wnt/β-catenin pathway and stabilizing β-catenin via blocking GSK3β activation. Thus, TREM2 promotes the survival and proliferation of primary microglial cells [88]. In addition, the transcription factor MAFB may be involved in regulating microglial cell development and homeostasis [89]. The homeostasis is further preserved by the epigenetic regulator MECP2, which controls microglial responsiveness to external stimuli [90,91]. In the postnatal developing brain, the absence of microglial EED, a Polycomb protein vital for synaptic pruning, led to the upregulation of phagocytosis-related genes [92]. Contrariwise, the deletion of microglial *Tgm2* in *mice* resulted in the downregulation of microglial phagocytic-related genes accompanied by synaptic pruning and cognitive impairment [93]. A P2RX7-induced proliferation of embryonic spinal cord microglia was proposed after comparison of wild-type and *P2rx7-/-* embryos. The ablation of *P2rx7* also affected microglial density, while *Pannexin-1-/-* embryos showed unaltered proliferation rates. Altogether, microglial proliferation may be regulated by P2RX7 receptors in a Pannexin-1-independent way during early development [94].

Another in vitro study confirmed that IL-33, which is released by astrocytes and endothelial cells, enhances the proliferation of microglial populations [95]. Similarly, in the uninjured CNS, G-CSF increased microglial numbers [96]. However, the GM-CSF was a stronger stimulus for microglial proliferation in *human* brain cultures [97]. The increasing microglial populations were correlated with a direct effect of GM-CSF upon treatment with IL-5, whereas IL-5 induced an intense cellular metabolism in contrast with GM-CSF treatment in microglial cell cultures [98]. Moreover, 1 ng/mL of CCL-1 mediated chemotaxis, while 100 ng/mL increased motility, proliferation, and phagocytosis of microglial cells in culture [99]. An induction of microglial cell proliferation was mediated in vitro by CCL2 along with *miR-10* [100]. Neurotrophins have a potential role in modulating the proliferation and survival of microglial populations in vitro. Specifically, NGF and BDNF increased microglial proliferation, contrary to NT-3 and NT-4 [101]. Lastly, SCF was identified as a promoter of microglial cell proliferation, migration, and phagocytosis in culture (Table 1) [102].

Summarizing, microgliogenesis is a complex biological process strictly regulated by multiple molecular drivers in a similar pattern to other CNS cells, such as oligodendrocytes [103].

Table 1. Molecular drivers of microglial early differentiation, migration, proliferation, and terminal differentiation.

Gene	Locus	Protein	Species	Biological Role	Ref.
BDNF	11p14.1	Brain derived neurotrophic factor	Mice	Proliferation	[101]
CCL1	17q12	C-C motif chemokine ligand 1	Mice	Migration; Proliferation	[99]
CCL2	17q12	C-C motif chemokine ligand 2	Human; Mice	Migration; Proliferation; Terminal differentiation	[73,100]
CCL3	17q12	C-C motif chemokine ligand 3	Human	Migration; Terminal differentiation	[73]
CSF1	1p13.3	Colony stimulating factor 1	Mice	Proliferation; Terminal differentiation	[47,68]
CSF1R	5q32	Colony stimulating factor 1 receptor	Mice; Zebrafish	Migration; Terminal differentiation	[47,63]
CX3CL1	16q21	C-X3-C motif chemokine ligand 1	Mice	Migration	[72]
CX3CR1	3p22.2	C-X3-C motif chemokine receptor 1	Mice	Migration	[72]
CXCL12	10q11.21	C-X-C motif chemokine ligand 12	Mice; Rat	Migration; Proliferation	[70,71]
CXCR4	2q22.1	C-X-C motif chemokine receptor 4	Mice; Rat	Migration; Proliferation	[70,71]
CXCR7	2q37.3	C-X-C chemokine receptor type 7	Rat	Migration; Proliferation	[71]
DAP12	19q13.12	DNAX-activating protein of 12 kDa	Mice	Proliferation; Terminal differentiation	[67,68]
G-CSF	17q21.1	Granulocyte colony-stimulating factor	Mice	Proliferation	[96]
GM-CSF	5q31.1	Granulocyte-macrophage colony-stimulating factor	Human	Proliferation	[97]
HDAC1	1p35.2–p35.1	Histone deacetylase 1	Mice	Proliferation	[79]
HDAC2	6q21	Histone deacetylase 2	Mice	Proliferation	[79]
IBA1	6p21.33	Ionized calcium binding adaptor molecule 1	Mice	Terminal differentiation	[104]
IL33	9p24.1	Interleukin 33	Mice	Proliferation	[95]
IL34	16q22.1	Interleukin 34	Mice; Zebrafish	Migration; Terminal differentiation	[47,63]
IL5	5q31.1	Interleukin 5	Rat	Proliferation	[98]
INOS	19p13.11	Inducible nitric oxide synthase	Mice	Proliferation	[105]
IRF8	16q24.1	Interferon regulatory factor 8	Mice	Early differentiation	[50]
ITGAV	2q32.1	Integrin subunit alpha V	Mice	Terminal differentiation	[78]
ITGB8	7p21.1	Integrin subunit beta 8	Mice	Terminal differentiation	[78]
MAFB	20q12	MAF bZIP transcription factor B	Mice	Terminal differentiation	[89]
MEIS3	19q13.32	Meis homeobox 3	Mice	Terminal differentiation	[66]
MIF	22q11.23	Macrophage migration inhibitory factor	Mice	Proliferation	[70]
MMP8	11q22.2	Matrix metallopeptidase 8	Mice	Migration	[50]
MMP9	20q13.12	Matrix metallopeptidase 9	Mice	Migration	[50]
NGF	1p13.2	Nerve growth factor	Mice	Proliferation	[101]
NOX2	Xp21.1-p11.4	NADPH oxidase 2	Mice	Migration	[69]
P2RX7	12q24.31	Purinergic receptor P2X 7	Mice	Proliferation	[94]
PGRN	17q21.31	Progranulin	Zebrafish	Migration	[77]
RUNX1	21q22.12	RUNX family transcription factor 1	Mice	Proliferation; Early and terminal differentiation	[59,60]

Table 1. *Cont.*

Gene	Locus	Protein	Species	Biological Role	Ref.
SALL1	16q12.1	Spalt like transcription factor 1	Mice	Terminal differentiation	[66]
SALL3	18q23	Spalt like transcription factor 3	Mice	Terminal differentiation	[66]
SCF	12q21.32	Stem cell factor	Mice	Migration; Proliferation	[102]
SPI1	11p11.2	Transcription factor PU.1	Mice	Early differentiation	[50]
TGFB1	19q13.2	Transforming growth factor beta 1	Mice	Terminal differentiation	[65]
TREM2	6p21.1	Triggering receptor expressed on myeloid cells 2	Mice	Proliferation	[88]
VEGFR1	13q12.3	Vascular endothelial growth factor receptor 1	Mice	Migration	[69]

Data are retrieved from "The Human Protein Atlas" [106], and "Gene" database of the National Center for Biotechnology Information [107]. Ref.: references.

4. Spatiotemporal Distribution in Various Species

In *rodents*, microglia were observed in the fetal forebrain at E11, when the telencephalic vesicles form [108]. Other studies identified E12 as the initial point of brain colonization [109,110]. Using in vivo immunohistochemistry and ex vivo time-lapse analysis of microglia, E11.5 was identified as the first day of the microglial entrance in the cortex [111]. The route includes in turn the pial surface, lateral ventricle, and cortical wall, moving over towards the cortical plate in the later embryonic phases. Three invasion phases in the cortical parenchyma have been proposed: (a) between E10.5 and E14.5, a gradual increase in the number of microglial cells takes place, succeeded by (b) a rapid phase with a significant rise in microglia from E14.5 to E15.5, followed by (c) the last slow wave of entry from E15.5 to E17.5. Before the invasion in the parenchyma, the peripheral microglia proliferates, especially at early phases [111]. Stremmel et al. demonstrated that, from E8.5, the CX_3CR1^+ pre-macrophages were detectable in the YS proliferating and preparing to enter the blood circulation for their migration to the brain parenchyma, while Kierdorf et al. suggested that E9.5 is the starting point for the migration of microglial progenitors into the neural tube [50]. The invading wave of YS progenitors to the tissue peaks around E10.5, then excessively decreases towards E12.5 and disappears at E14.5. Consequently, microglial progenitors are dependent on the vascular system for their migration [112]. Finally, the transformation of immature microglia into ramified, mature cells occurs between the second and third postnatal week (Figure 2) [113,114].

In *humans*, well-differentiated microglia were observed after 35 weeks of gestation (GW) [115]. However, Rezaie and Male suggested that colonization of the spinal cord starts around 9 GW, with the major influx of microglial cell populations estimated around 16 GW. In the second trimester, the cerebrum is colonized by microglial populations widely dispersed in the intermediate zone at 20–22 GW [116]. In the initial phase of microglial colonization between 12 and 14 GW, two cell populations were identified by Rezaie et al., namely $CD68^{++}$ $RCA\text{-}1^{+}$ MHC II^{-} amoeboid cells located in the subplate and $RCA\text{-}1^{++}$ $CD68^{-}$ MHC II^{-} progenitors first observed in the marginal layer and lower cortical plate and which ramified within the subplate [117]. In 2006, the first intracerebral microglial populations were described close to the meninges and choroid plexus, next to the di-telencephalic fissure at 5.5 GW, whereas the cortical anlagen was populated with cells starting at 10–12 GW [118]. Routes of entry were found to be different for the cerebral cortex compared with the diencephalon. Microglial cells invaded the cerebrum from the ventricular lumen and the leptomeninges, starting at 4.5 GW. From 12 GW, the intraparenchymal vascular route of entry could be determined [119]. In 2010, Verney et al. suggested that the invasion of amoeboid microglia occurred between 4.5 and 5.5 GW into the *human* forebrain; this is in accordance with the data from other animal models such as *rodents*, regarding the spatiotemporal patterns observed for microglial development. Ultimately, the meninges, choroid plexus, and ventricles were identified as the three early routes of microglial entry [120].

In *avians*, the first microglial population was found to be located within the brain independently of vascularization, reaching the nervous system parenchyma by passing through the pial basal lamina [121]. More specifically, before E9, the cerebellar anlage contained only a small number of microglial precursors. Microglial precursors cross the pial surface at the basal region of the peduncles to enter the cerebellar anlage. Then, microglia proceed radially to the various cortical layers by migrating via the white matter. Following the ultimate settlement of microglial cells, differentiation then ensues [122].

5. Proliferation in the Adult Compromised CNS

As the BBB and microglial cell maturation are established, the question arises as to how microglia are renewed in the adult brain. The participation of bone marrow-derived cells in the repopulation of microglial cell niches was proposed in various conditions, especially after bone marrow transplantation [123–128], and in diseases such as stroke [129], cerebral ischemia [130], bacterial meningitis [131], entorhinal cortex lesions [132], Parkinson's disease [133], Alzheimer's disease [134,135], multiple sclerosis [136], facial nerve axotomy and autoimmune encephalitis [137], scrapie [138], and brain and peripheral nerve injury [139–141]. During aging and the transition from plasticity to proinflammatory activation in primary neurodegeneration, the latest data also suggest that many metabolic byproducts and mitochondrial components can serve as damage-associated molecules, creating an extracellular gradient and accumulation of reactive oxygen species, which in turn propagate the inflammatory neurodegeneration [142,143]. Under acute situations such as when a stab wound inflicts damage to a brain region, the resident microglia need the contribution of circulating monocytes to efficiently respond to the extra load of detritus [144]. It has been suggested that even after recovering from severe brain inflammation, resident microglia form a remarkably stable cell pool that is seldom replenished by hematogenous cells in adult animals [145].

A physiological process that aids in the development of the adult microglial cell population is the proliferation of microglial precursors in the developing brain [146]. Lawson et al. suggested that resident microglia synthesize DNA and go on to divide in situ. Additionally, cells were found to be recruited from the circulating monocyte pool through an intact BBB and rapidly differentiated into resident microglia. These two processes contributed almost equally to the steady-state turnover of resident microglia [147]. In a *mouse* model of ALS, the local proliferation of resident microglia had the greatest contribution to the observing microgliosis, while the effects of bone marrow-derived cells were limited among the microglia populations [148]. Strong evidence for the local self-renewal of CNS microglia as the main source of repopulation of adult microglia were obtained from a model using chimeric animals obtained by parabiosis showing that these cells could be maintained independently from bone marrow–derived cells during adulthood in ALS and facial nerve axotomy [149]. However, Ly-6C^{hi}CCR2^{+} monocytes were found to be recruited to the lesioned brain differentiating into mature microglia. Remarkably, monocyte invasion during CNS pathology with an intact BBB or in non-diseased adult CNS required previous conditioning of brains, such as direct tissue irradiation [150]. Indeed, brain conditioning with lethal irradiation and alkylating agents such as busulfan was found to be vital for an efficient microglial cell repopulation after hematopoietic stem cell transplantation [151].

In 2013, Li et al. observed that after ischemic stroke, a small number of blood-derived CX3CR1$^{GFP/+}$ cells invaded the brain parenchyma; however, these cells were phenotypically different from resident microglia with distinct kinetics. This study delineated the greatest impact of local resident microglia on the repopulation of parenchymal cells compared to recruited blood-derived cells after ischemic stroke [152]. The efficiency of microglia for self-renewal arising from a CNS-resident pool independently from peripheral myeloid cells was also supported by another experimental study that investigated the repopulation of brain parenchyma using a model of conditional depletion of microglial cells [153]. During the process of cellular restoration, the proliferation of local microglia was found to be dependent on the IL-1 receptor, which was highly expressed by local cell pools.

Bone-marrow-derived macrophages populated the brain only after irradiation and bone marrow transplantation, and did not express the IL-1 receptor [153].

In *zebrafish*, using temporal-spatial resolution fate mapping analysis, embryonic microglia emerged from the rostral blood island in a RUNX1-independent and PU.1-dependent manner, while adult microglia originated from the ventral wall of the dorsal aorta in a RUNX1-dependent, c-MYB- and PU.1-independent manner [154]. The microglial self-renewal was shown to resemble a stochastic process at steady state, whereas clonal microglial expansion seems to predominate under unilateral facial nerve axotomy [155]. In another study, the partial microglial depletion resulted in the engraftment of peripherally derived macrophages independently of irradiation. These newly-engrafted cell populations differ transcriptionally from microglia [156]. Similarly, another depletion study showed that the microglial niche is filled with new cells via local proliferation of CX3CR1^{+}F4/80^{low}Clec12a^{-} microglia and invasion of CX3CR1^{+}F4/80^{hi}Clec12a^{+} macrophages derived from Ly6C^{hi} monocytes. This engraftment was associated with vascular activation and type I interferon, while it was shown to be independent of BBB integrity [157]. These peripherally engrafted cells were transcriptionally distinct from microglia, showcasing different surface marker expression, phagocytic capacity, and cytokine release [157,158].

Through additional studies, Huang et al. delineated that repopulated microglial cell populations are entirely generated from residual microglial proliferation after acute depletion [159], instead of nestin-expressing progenitors, as was argued in a CSF1R inhibitor-mediated experiment [160]. In agreement with the previous statement, Zhan et al. demonstrated that after acute ablation, the newborn adult microglia generated via self-renewal from the local CX3CR1^{+} microglia without any contribution of nestin^{+} progenitors or peripheral myeloid cells. The repopulated microglia formed stable and distinct clusters with minimum migration capacity via clonal expansion. Although these regenerated microglial cells were presented in an immature state, microglial differentiation was mediated by NF-κB and interferon pathways [161]. A fate mapping study from Chen et al. showed that after neonatal stroke, a monocyte-to-microglia transition is possible [57]. In contrast, a study conducted in 2021 showed that microglia are not replaced by bone-marrow-derived cells in Alzheimer's disease similar to the BAMs, which seldom replenished the microglial cell pool [162]. Ultimately, microglial cell manipulation is being intensely investigated in the context of immune-mediated diseases such as multiple sclerosis, where microglia are heavily implicated as pathogenic mediators of progressive disease [163–165], and targeted therapies are being developed [166,167].

Summarizing the results of the above studies, it is postulated that the greatest contribution to microglial repopulation is based upon its local self-renewal, both in steady state and disease. However, circulating monocytes may also contribute to a lesser extent, especially in disease. The final confirmation of the exact repopulation pattern necessitates further investigation.

6. Conclusions

The widely accepted, contemporary view of the origin of CNS-resident microglia is the YS. However, this was hotly debated until the early 2010s. Although this may pass unnoticed to the majority of the research community in the immune-related neuroscience field, understanding the underlying molecular development they undergo during embryogenesis may aid towards developing novel therapies that ideally could decelerate, halt, or reverse neurodegeneration by targeting the microglia-mediated repair process. A main challenge now is to elucidate the precise biological identity of each different microglial state as well as the variable microglial activity per CNS region, allowing us to perform selective interventions. Another field of application that can potentially benefit from relevant developmental research is aging, where mechanisms implicating microgliogenesis can be exploited in favor of slowing the senescent progress by, e.g., combating oxidative stress. Finally, the understanding of cellular ontogeny may enable successful lab-approached manipulations aimed at depletion of microglial cells and beneficial microglial renewal in the CNS, in both homeostasis and disorders.

Author Contributions: I.D. and P.T., writing—original draft preparation and visualization; M.E.M., S.M., M.-È.T., S.P. and L.Z., conceptualization, review and editing; M.B., E.K. and C.S., review and editing. All authors have read and agreed to the published version of the manuscript.

Funding: This research received no external funding.

Institutional Review Board Statement: Not applicable.

Informed Consent Statement: Not applicable.

Data Availability Statement: Not applicable.

Conflicts of Interest: The authors declare no conflict of interest.

Abbreviations

AGM	Aorta-gonad-mesonephros
Akt	Protein kinase B
ALS	Amyotrophic lateral sclerosis
ARID1A	AT-rich interaction domain 1A
BAMs	Border-associated macrophages
BATF3	Basic leucine zipper transcriptional factor ATF-like 3
BBB	Blood–brain barrier
BDNF	Brain-derived neurotrophic factor
C/EBP-α	CCAAT/enhancer-binding protein alpha
CCL1	Chemokine (C-C motif) ligand 1
CCL2	Chemokine (C-C motif) ligand 2
CCL3	Chemokine (C-C motif) ligand 3
CCR2	C-C chemokine receptor type 2
CD11b	Cluster of differentiation molecule 11B
CD206	Cluster of differentiation molecule 206
CD45	Cluster of differentiation molecule 45
CD64	Cluster of differentiation molecule 64
CD68	Cluster of differentiation molecule 68
CNS	Central nervous system
CSF-1	Colony stimulating factor-1
CSF1R	Colony stimulating factor 1 receptor
CX3CL1	Chemokine (C-X3-C motif) ligand 1
CX3CR1	CX3C motif chemokine receptor 1
CXCL12	C-X-C motif chemokine ligand 12
CXCR4	C-X-C chemokine receptor type 4
CXCR7	C-X-C chemokine receptor type 7
DAP12	DNAX-activating protein of 12 kDa
E	Embryonic day
EED	Embryonic ectoderm development
EMPs	Erythro-myeloid progenitors
Erk1/2	Extracellular signal-regulated kinase 1/2
G-CSF	Granulocyte colony stimulating factor
G-CSFR	Granulocyte colony stimulating factor receptor
GM-CSF	Granulocyte-macrophage colony-stimulating factor
GM-CSFR	Granulocyte-macrophage colony-stimulating factor receptor
GSK3β	Glycogen synthase kinase-3 beta
GW	Gestational week
HDAC1	Histone Deacetylase 1
HDAC2	Histone Deacetylase 2
HOXB8	Homeobox B8
HSC	Hematopoietic stem cells
IBA1	Ionized calcium binding adaptor molecule 1

ID2	Inhibitor of DNA binding 2
IL-33	Interleukin 33
IL-34	Interleukin 34
IL-5	Interleukin 5
iNOS	Inducible nitric oxide synthase
IRF8	Interferon regulatory factor 8
KLF4	Krüppel-like factor 4
M-CSF	Macrophage colony-stimulating factor
M-CSFR	Macrophage colony-stimulating factor receptor
MAFB	MAF bZIP transcription factor B
MCP-1	Monocyte chemoattractant protein-1
MECP2	Methyl-CpG binding protein 2
MEIS3	Meis homeobox 3
MHC II	Major histocompatibility complex class II
MIF	Macrophage migration inhibitory factor
MIP-1α	Macrophage inflammatory protein-1 alpha
miR-124	microRNA 124
MMP8	Matrix Metallopeptidase 8
MMP9	Matrix Metallopeptidase 9
MPO	Myeloperoxidase
MYB	MYB proto-oncogene, transcription factor
NF-kB	Nuclear factor kappa B
NGF	Nerve growth factor
NOX2	NADPH oxidase 2
NR4A1	Nuclear receptor subfamily 4 group A member 1
NT-3	Neurotrophin-3
NT-4	Neurotrophin-4
P2RX7	P2X purinoceptor 7
P2RY12	Purinergic receptor P2Y12
PGRN	Progranulin
qRT-PCR	Quantitative reverse transcriptase polymerase chain reaction
RCA-1	Ricinus communis agglutinin-1
RUNX1	Runt-related transcription factor 1
SALL1	Spalt like transcription factor 1
SALL3	Spalt like transcription factor 3
SCF	Stem cell factor
SVZ	Subventricular zone
TGF-β1	Transforming growth factor beta 1
TGM2	Transglutaminase 2
TMEM119	Transmembrane Protein 119
TREM2	Triggering receptor expressed on myeloid cells 2
VEGFR1	Vascular endothelial growth factor receptor-1
YS	Yolk sac
αVβ8 integrin	Integrin subunit alpha V and beta 8

References

1. Davies, L.C.; Jenkins, S.J.; Allen, J.E.; Taylor, P.R. Tissue-Resident Macrophages. *Nat. Immunol.* **2013**, *14*, 986–995. [CrossRef] [PubMed]
2. Soulet, D.; Rivest, S. Microglia. *Curr. Biol. CB* **2008**, *18*, R506–R508. [CrossRef] [PubMed]
3. Lee, E.; Eo, J.-C.; Lee, C.; Yu, J.-W. Distinct Features of Brain-Resident Macrophages: Microglia and Non-Parenchymal Brain Macrophages. *Mol. Cells* **2021**, *44*, 281–291. [CrossRef] [PubMed]
4. Dos Santos, S.E.; Medeiros, M.; Porfirio, J.; Tavares, W.; Pessôa, L.; Grinberg, L.; Leite, R.E.P.; Ferretti-Rebustini, R.E.L.; Suemoto, C.K.; Filho, W.J.; et al. Similar Microglial Cell Densities across Brain Structures and Mammalian Species: Implications for Brain Tissue Function. *J. Neurosci.* **2020**, *40*, 4622–4643. [CrossRef] [PubMed]
5. Paolicelli, R.C.; Sierra, A.; Stevens, B.; Tremblay, M.-E.; Aguzzi, A.; Ajami, B.; Amit, I.; Audinat, E.; Bechmann, I.; Bennett, M.; et al. Microglia States and Nomenclature: A Field at Its Crossroads. *Neuron* **2022**, *110*, 3458–3483. [CrossRef]
6. Lenz, K.M.; Nelson, L.H. Microglia and Beyond: Innate Immune Cells As Regulators of Brain Development and Behavioral Function. *Front. Immunol.* **2018**, *9*, 698. [CrossRef]

7. Tremblay, M.-È.; Stevens, B.; Sierra, A.; Wake, H.; Bessis, A.; Nimmerjahn, A. The Role of Microglia in the Healthy Brain. *J. Neurosci.* **2011**, *31*, 16064–16069. [CrossRef]
8. Neurons and Neuroglia-ClinicalKey. Available online: https://www.clinicalkey.com/#!/content/book/3-s2.0-B978032328782100438X (accessed on 28 December 2022).
9. Chen, Z.; Trapp, B.D. Microglia and Neuroprotection. *J. Neurochem.* **2016**, *136* (Suppl. 1), 10–17. [CrossRef]
10. Bachiller, S.; Jiménez-Ferrer, I.; Paulus, A.; Yang, Y.; Swanberg, M.; Deierborg, T.; Boza-Serrano, A. Microglia in Neurological Diseases: A Road Map to Brain-Disease Dependent-Inflammatory Response. *Front. Cell. Neurosci.* **2018**, *12*, 488. [CrossRef]
11. Guerrero, B.L.; Sicotte, N.L. Microglia in Multiple Sclerosis: Friend or Foe? *Front. Immunol.* **2020**, *11*, 374. [CrossRef]
12. Clarke, B.E.; Patani, R. The Microglial Component of Amyotrophic Lateral Sclerosis. *Brain J. Neurol.* **2020**, *143*, 3526–3539. [CrossRef]
13. Sierra, A.; de Castro, F.; Del Río-Hortega, J.; Rafael Iglesias-Rozas, J.; Garrosa, M.; Kettenmann, H. The "Big-Bang" for Modern Glial Biology: Translation and Comments on Pío Del Río-Hortega 1919 Series of Papers on Microglia. *Glia* **2016**, *64*, 1801–1840. [CrossRef]
14. Colonna, M.; Butovsky, O. Microglia Function in the Central Nervous System During Health and Neurodegeneration. *Annu. Rev. Immunol.* **2017**, *35*, 441–468. [CrossRef]
15. Sohet, F.; Lin, C.; Munji, R.N.; Lee, S.Y.; Ruderisch, N.; Soung, A.; Arnold, T.D.; Derugin, N.; Vexler, Z.S.; Yen, F.T.; et al. LSR/Angulin-1 Is a Tricellular Tight Junction Protein Involved in Blood–Brain Barrier Formation. *J. Cell Biol.* **2015**, *208*, 703–711. [CrossRef]
16. Hoeffel, G.; Ginhoux, F. Ontogeny of Tissue-Resident Macrophages. *Front. Immunol.* **2015**, *6*, 486. [CrossRef]
17. Wu, Y.; Hirschi, K.K. Tissue-Resident Macrophage Development and Function. *Front. Cell Dev. Biol.* **2020**, *8*, 617879. [CrossRef]
18. Vink, C.S.; Mariani, S.A.; Dzierzak, E. Embryonic Origins of the Hematopoietic System: Hierarchies and Heterogeneity. *HemaSphere* **2022**, *6*, e737. [CrossRef]
19. Yoder, M.C. Inducing Definitive Hematopoiesis in a Dish. *Nat. Biotechnol.* **2014**, *32*, 539–541. [CrossRef]
20. Ling, E.A. Transformation of Monocytes into Amoeboid Microglia in the Corpus Callosum of Postnatal Rats, as Shown by Labelling Monocytes by Carbon Particles. *J. Anat.* **1979**, *128*, 847–858.
21. Rio-Hortega, P. The Microglia. *Lancet* **1939**, *233*, 1023–1026. [CrossRef]
22. Kershman, J. Genesis of Microglia in the Human Brain. *Arch. Neurol. Psychiatry* **1939**, *41*, 24–50. [CrossRef]
23. Boya, J.; Calvo, J.; Prado, A. The Origin of Microglial Cells. *J. Anat.* **1979**, *129*, 177–186. [PubMed]
24. Boya, J.; Calvo, J.L.; Carbonell, A.L.; Borregon, A. A Lectin Histochemistry Study on the Development of Rat Microglial Cells. *J. Anat.* **1991**, *175*, 229–236. [PubMed]
25. Dalmau, I.; Finsen, B.; Tønder, N.; Zimmer, J.; González, B.; Castellano, B. Development of Microglia in the Prenatal Rat Hippocampus. *J. Comp. Neurol.* **1997**, *377*, 70–84. [CrossRef]
26. Barón, M.; Gallego, A. The Relation of the Microglia with the Pericytes in the Cat Cerebral Cortex. *Z. Zellforsch. Mikrosk. Anat.* **1972**, *128*, 42–57. [CrossRef]
27. Mori, S.; Leblond, C.P. Identification of Microglia in Light and Electron Microscopy. *J. Comp. Neurol.* **1969**, *135*, 57–80. [CrossRef]
28. Juba, A. Untersuchungen Über Die Entwicklung Der Hortegaschen Microglia Des Menschen. *Arch. Psychiat. Nervenkr.* **1933**, *101*, 577–592. [CrossRef]
29. Santha, K.; Juba, A. Weitere Untersuchungen Über Die Entwicklung Der Hortegaschen Mikroglia. *Arch. Psychiat. Nervenkr.* **1933**, *98*, 598–613. [CrossRef]
30. Perry, V.H.; Hume, D.A.; Gordon, S. Immunohistochemical Localization of Macrophages and Microglia in the Adult and Developing Mouse Brain. *Neuroscience* **1985**, *15*, 313–326. [CrossRef]
31. Ling, E.A.; Penney, D.; Leblond, C.P. Use of Carbon Labeling to Demonstrate the Role of Blood Monocytes as Precursors of the "ameboid Cells" Present in the Corpus Callosum of Postnatal Rats. *J. Comp. Neurol.* **1980**, *193*, 631–657. [CrossRef]
32. Murabe, Y.; Sano, Y. Morphological Studies on Neuroglia. VII. Distribution of "Brain Macrophages" in Brains of Neonatal and Adult Rats, as Determined by Means of Immunohistochemistry. *Cell Tissue Res.* **1983**, *229*, 85–95. [CrossRef]
33. Ling, E.A.; Kaur, C.; Wong, W.C. Expression of Major Histocompatibility Complex and Leukocyte Common Antigens in Amoeboid Microglia in Postnatal Rats. *J. Anat.* **1991**, *177*, 117–126.
34. Oehmichen, M.; Wiethölter, H.; Greaves, M.F. Immunological Analysis of Human Microglia: Lack of Monocytic and Lymphoid Membrane Differentiation Antigens. *J. Neuropathol. Exp. Neurol.* **1979**, *38*, 99–103. [CrossRef]
35. Lewis, P.D. The Fate of the Subependymal Cell in the Adult Rat Brain, with a Note on the Origin of Microglia. *Brain J. Neurol.* **1968**, *91*, 721–736. [CrossRef]
36. Kitamura, T.; Miyake, T.; Fujita, S. Genesis of Resting Microglia in the Gray Matter of Mouse Hippocampus. *J. Comp. Neurol.* **1984**, *226*, 421–433. [CrossRef]
37. Fedoroff, S.; Zhai, R.; Novak, J.P. Microglia and Astroglia Have a Common Progenitor Cell. *J. Neurosci. Res.* **1997**, *50*, 477–486. [CrossRef]
38. de Groot, C.J.; Huppes, W.; Sminia, T.; Kraal, G.; Dijkstra, C.D. Determination of the Origin and Nature of Brain Macrophages and Microglial Cells in Mouse Central Nervous System, Using Non-Radioactive in Situ Hybridization and Immunoperoxidase Techniques. *Glia* **1992**, *6*, 301–309. [CrossRef]

39. Schelper, R.L.; Adrian, E.K. Monocytes Become Macrophages; They Do Not Become Microglia: A Light and Electron Microscopic Autoradiographic Study Using 125-Iododeoxyuridine. *J. Neuropathol. Exp. Neurol.* **1986**, *45*, 1–19. [CrossRef]
40. Matsumoto, Y.; Fujiwara, M. Absence of Donor-Type Major Histocompatibility Complex Class I Antigen-Bearing Microglia in the Rat Central Nervous System of Radiation Bone Marrow Chimeras. *J. Neuroimmunol.* **1987**, *17*, 71–82. [CrossRef]
41. Hutchins, K.D.; Dickson, D.W.; Rashbaum, W.K.; Lyman, W.D. Localization of Morphologically Distinct Microglial Populations in the Developing Human Fetal Brain: Implications for Ontogeny. *Brain Res. Dev. Brain Res.* **1990**, *55*, 95–102. [CrossRef]
42. Takahashi, K.; Yamamura, F.; Naito, M. Differentiation, Maturation, and Proliferation of Macrophages in the Mouse Yolk Sac: A Light-Microscopic, Enzyme-Cytochemical, Immunohistochemical, and Ultrastructural Study. *J. Leukoc. Biol.* **1989**, *45*, 87–96. [CrossRef] [PubMed]
43. Fujimoto, E.; Miki, A.; Mizoguti, H. Histochemical Study of the Differentiation of Microglial Cells in the Developing Human Cerebral Hemispheres. *J. Anat.* **1989**, *166*, 253–264. [PubMed]
44. Kurz, H.; Christ, B. Embryonic CNS Macrophages and Microglia Do Not Stem from Circulating, but from Extravascular Precursors. *Glia* **1998**, *22*, 98–102. [CrossRef]
45. Andjelkovic, A.V.; Nikolic, B.; Pachter, J.S.; Zecevic, N. Macrophages/Microglial Cells in Human Central Nervous System during Development: An Immunohistochemical Study. *Brain Res.* **1998**, *814*, 13–25. [CrossRef]
46. Alliot, F.; Godin, I.; Pessac, B. Microglia Derive from Progenitors, Originating from the Yolk Sac, and Which Proliferate in the Brain. *Brain Res. Dev. Brain Res.* **1999**, *117*, 145–152. [CrossRef]
47. Ginhoux, F.; Greter, M.; Leboeuf, M.; Nandi, S.; See, P.; Gokhan, S.; Mehler, M.F.; Conway, S.J.; Ng, L.G.; Stanley, E.R.; et al. Fate Mapping Analysis Reveals That Adult Microglia Derive from Primitive Macrophages. *Science* **2010**, *330*, 841–845. [CrossRef]
48. Mizutani, M.; Pino, P.A.; Saederup, N.; Charo, I.F.; Ransohoff, R.M.; Cardona, A.E. The Fractalkine Receptor but Not CCR2 Is Present on Microglia from Embryonic Development throughout Adulthood. *J. Immunol.* **2012**, *188*, 29–36. [CrossRef]
49. Schulz, C.; Gomez Perdiguero, E.; Chorro, L.; Szabo-Rogers, H.; Cagnard, N.; Kierdorf, K.; Prinz, M.; Wu, B.; Jacobsen, S.E.W.; Pollard, J.W.; et al. A Lineage of Myeloid Cells Independent of Myb and Hematopoietic Stem Cells. *Science* **2012**, *336*, 86–90. [CrossRef]
50. Kierdorf, K.; Erny, D.; Goldmann, T.; Sander, V.; Schulz, C.; Perdiguero, E.G.; Wieghofer, P.; Heinrich, A.; Riemke, P.; Hölscher, C.; et al. Microglia Emerge from Erythromyeloid Precursors via Pu.1- and Irf8-Dependent Pathways. *Nat. Neurosci.* **2013**, *16*, 273–280. [CrossRef]
51. Hoeffel, G.; Chen, J.; Lavin, Y.; Low, D.; Almeida, F.F.; See, P.; Beaudin, A.E.; Lum, J.; Low, I.; Forsberg, E.C.; et al. C-Myb(+) Erythro-Myeloid Progenitor-Derived Fetal Monocytes Give Rise to Adult Tissue-Resident Macrophages. *Immunity* **2015**, *42*, 665–678. [CrossRef]
52. Gomez Perdiguero, E.; Klapproth, K.; Schulz, C.; Busch, K.; Azzoni, E.; Crozet, L.; Garner, H.; Trouillet, C.; de Bruijn, M.F.; Geissmann, F.; et al. Tissue-Resident Macrophages Originate from Yolk-Sac-Derived Erythro-Myeloid Progenitors. *Nature* **2015**, *518*, 547–551. [CrossRef]
53. Sheng, J.; Ruedl, C.; Karjalainen, K. Most Tissue-Resident Macrophages Except Microglia Are Derived from Fetal Hematopoietic Stem Cells. *Immunity* **2015**, *43*, 382–393. [CrossRef]
54. De, S.; Van Deren, D.; Peden, E.; Hockin, M.; Boulet, A.; Titen, S.; Capecchi, M.R. Two Distinct Ontogenies Confer Heterogeneity to Mouse Brain Microglia. *Dev. Camb. Engl.* **2018**, *145*, dev152306. [CrossRef]
55. Fehrenbach, M.K.; Tjwa, M.; Bechmann, I.; Krueger, M. Decreased Microglial Numbers in Vav1-Cre+:Dicer Knock-out Mice Suggest a Second Source of Microglia beyond Yolk Sac Macrophages. *Ann. Anat. Anat. Anz.* **2018**, *218*, 190–198. [CrossRef]
56. Utz, S.G.; See, P.; Mildenberger, W.; Thion, M.S.; Silvin, A.; Lutz, M.; Ingelfinger, F.; Rayan, N.A.; Lelios, I.; Buttgereit, A.; et al. Early Fate Defines Microglia and Non-Parenchymal Brain Macrophage Development. *Cell* **2020**, *181*, 557–573.e18. [CrossRef]
57. Chen, H.-R.; Sun, Y.-Y.; Chen, C.-W.; Kuo, Y.-M.; Kuan, I.S.; Li, Z.-R.T.; Short-Miller, J.C.; Smucker, M.R.; Kuan, C.-Y. Fate Mapping via CCR2-CreER Mice Reveals Monocyte-to-Microglia Transition in Development and Neonatal Stroke. *Sci. Adv.* **2020**, *6*, eabb2119. [CrossRef]
58. Bian, Z.; Gong, Y.; Huang, T.; Lee, C.Z.W.; Bian, L.; Bai, Z.; Shi, H.; Zeng, Y.; Liu, C.; He, J.; et al. Deciphering Human Macrophage Development at Single-Cell Resolution. *Nature* **2020**, *582*, 571–576. [CrossRef]
59. Zusso, M.; Methot, L.; Lo, R.; Greenhalgh, A.D.; David, S.; Stifani, S. Regulation of Postnatal Forebrain Amoeboid Microglial Cell Proliferation and Development by the Transcription Factor Runx1. *J. Neurosci.* **2012**, *32*, 11285–11298. [CrossRef]
60. Huang, G.; Zhang, P.; Hirai, H.; Elf, S.; Yan, X.; Chen, Z.; Koschmieder, S.; Okuno, Y.; Dayaram, T.; Growney, J.D.; et al. PU. 1 Is a Major Downstream Target of AML1 (RUNX1) in Adult Mouse Hematopoiesis. *Nat. Genet.* **2008**, *40*, 51–60. [CrossRef]
61. Goldmann, T.; Wieghofer, P.; Jordão, M.J.C.; Prutek, F.; Hagemeyer, N.; Frenzel, K.; Amann, L.; Staszewski, O.; Kierdorf, K.; Krueger, M.; et al. Origin, Fate and Dynamics of Macrophages at Central Nervous System Interfaces. *Nat. Immunol.* **2016**, *17*, 797–805. [CrossRef]
62. Olson, M.C.; Scott, E.W.; Hack, A.A.; Su, G.H.; Tenen, D.G.; Singh, H.; Simon, M.C. PU. 1 Is Not Essential for Early Myeloid Gene Expression but Is Required for Terminal Myeloid Differentiation. *Immunity* **1995**, *3*, 703–714. [CrossRef] [PubMed]
63. Wu, S.; Xue, R.; Hassan, S.; Nguyen, T.M.L.; Wang, T.; Pan, H.; Xu, J.; Liu, Q.; Zhang, W.; Wen, Z. Il34-Csf1r Pathway Regulates the Migration and Colonization of Microglial Precursors. *Dev. Cell* **2018**, *46*, 552–563.e4. [CrossRef] [PubMed]
64. Buttgereit, A.; Lelios, I.; Yu, X.; Vrohlings, M.; Krakoski, N.R.; Gautier, E.L.; Nishinakamura, R.; Becher, B.; Greter, M. Sall1 Is a Transcriptional Regulator Defining Microglia Identity and Function. *Nat. Immunol.* **2016**, *17*, 1397–1406. [CrossRef] [PubMed]

65. Butovsky, O.; Jedrychowski, M.P.; Moore, C.S.; Cialic, R.; Lanser, A.J.; Gabriely, G.; Koeglsperger, T.; Dake, B.; Wu, P.M.; Doykan, C.E.; et al. Identification of a Unique TGF-β–Dependent Molecular and Functional Signature in Microglia. *Nat. Neurosci.* **2014**, *17*, 131–143. [CrossRef] [PubMed]
66. Mass, E.; Ballesteros, I.; Farlik, M.; Halbritter, F.; Günther, P.; Crozet, L.; Jacome-Galarza, C.E.; Händler, K.; Klughammer, J.; Kobayashi, Y.; et al. Specification of Tissue-Resident Macrophages during Organogenesis. *Science* **2016**, *353*, aaf4238. [CrossRef]
67. Nataf, S.; Anginot, A.; Vuaillat, C.; Malaval, L.; Fodil, N.; Chereul, E.; Langlois, J.-B.; Dumontel, C.; Cavillon, G.; Confavreux, C.; et al. Brain and Bone Damage in KARAP/DAP12 Loss-of-Function Mice Correlate with Alterations in Microglia and Osteoclast Lineages. *Am. J. Pathol.* **2005**, *166*, 275–286. [CrossRef]
68. Otero, K.; Turnbull, I.R.; Poliani, P.L.; Vermi, W.; Cerutti, E.; Aoshi, T.; Tassi, I.; Takai, T.; Stanley, S.L.; Miller, M.; et al. Macrophage Colony-Stimulating Factor Induces the Proliferation and Survival of Macrophages via a Pathway Involving DAP12 and Beta-Catenin. *Nat. Immunol.* **2009**, *10*, 734–743. [CrossRef]
69. Lelli, A.; Gervais, A.; Colin, C.; Chéret, C.; de Almodovar, C.R.; Carmeliet, P.; Krause, K.-H.; Boillée, S.; Mallat, M. The NADPH Oxidase Nox2 Regulates VEGFR1/CSF-1R-Mediated Microglial Chemotaxis and Promotes Early Postnatal Infiltration of Phagocytes in the Subventricular Zone of the Mouse Cerebral Cortex. *Glia* **2013**, *61*, 1542–1555. [CrossRef]
70. Arnò, B.; Grassivaro, F.; Rossi, C.; Bergamaschi, A.; Castiglioni, V.; Furlan, R.; Greter, M.; Favaro, R.; Comi, G.; Becher, B.; et al. Neural Progenitor Cells Orchestrate Microglia Migration and Positioning into the Developing Cortex. *Nat. Commun.* **2014**, *5*, 5611. [CrossRef]
71. Lipfert, J.; Ödemis, V.; Wagner, D.-C.; Boltze, J.; Engele, J. CXCR4 and CXCR7 Form a Functional Receptor Unit for SDF-1/CXCL12 in Primary Rodent Microglia. *Neuropathol. Appl. Neurobiol.* **2013**, *39*, 667–680. [CrossRef]
72. Hoshiko, M.; Arnoux, I.; Avignone, E.; Yamamoto, N.; Audinat, E. Deficiency of the Microglial Receptor CX3CR1 Impairs Postnatal Functional Development of Thalamocortical Synapses in the Barrel Cortex. *J. Neurosci.* **2012**, *32*, 15106–15111. [CrossRef]
73. Rezaie, P.; Trillo-Pazos, G.; Greenwood, J.; Everall, I.P.; Male, D.K. Motility and Ramification of Human Fetal Microglia in Culture: An Investigation Using Time-Lapse Video Microscopy and Image Analysis. *Exp. Cell Res.* **2002**, *274*, 68–82. [CrossRef]
74. Ponomarev, E.D.; Veremeyko, T.; Barteneva, N.; Krichevsky, A.M.; Weiner, H.L. MicroRNA-124 Promotes Microglia Quiescence and Suppresses EAE by Deactivating Macrophages via the C/EBP-α-PU.1 Pathway. *Nat. Med.* **2011**, *17*, 64–70. [CrossRef]
75. Gong, M.; Shi, R.; Liu, Y.; Ke, J.; Liu, X.; Du, H.-Z.; Liu, C.-M. Abnormal Microglial Polarization Induced by Arid1a Deletion Leads to Neuronal Differentiation Deficits. *Cell Prolif.* **2022**, *55*, e13314. [CrossRef]
76. Su, L.; Zhang, M.; Ji, F.; Zhao, J.; Wang, Y.; Wang, W.; Zhang, S.; Ma, H.; Wang, Y.; Jiao, J. Microglia Homeostasis Mediated by Epigenetic ARID1A Regulates Neural Progenitor Cells Response and Leads to Autism-like Behaviors. *Mol. Psychiatry* **2022**, *5*, 1–5. [CrossRef]
77. Walsh, C.E.; Hitchcock, P.F. Progranulin Regulates Neurogenesis in the Developing Vertebrate Retina. *Dev. Neurobiol.* **2017**, *77*, 1114–1129. [CrossRef]
78. Arnold, T.D.; Lizama, C.O.; Cautivo, K.M.; Santander, N.; Lin, L.; Qiu, H.; Huang, E.J.; Liu, C.; Mukouyama, Y.; Reichardt, L.F.; et al. Impaired AVβ8 and TGFβ Signaling Lead to Microglial Dysmaturation and Neuromotor Dysfunction. *J. Exp. Med.* **2019**, *216*, 900–915. [CrossRef]
79. Datta, M.; Staszewski, O.; Raschi, E.; Frosch, M.; Hagemeyer, N.; Tay, T.L.; Blank, T.; Kreutzfeldt, M.; Merkler, D.; Ziegler-Waldkirch, S.; et al. Histone Deacetylases 1 and 2 Regulate Microglia Function during Development, Homeostasis, and Neurodegeneration in a Context-Dependent Manner. *Immunity* **2018**, *48*, 514–529.e6. [CrossRef]
80. Jurga, A.M.; Paleczna, M.; Kuter, K.Z. Overview of General and Discriminating Markers of Differential Microglia Phenotypes. *Front. Cell. Neurosci.* **2020**, *14*, 198. [CrossRef]
81. Bohnert, S.; Seiffert, A.; Trella, S.; Bohnert, M.; Distel, L.; Ondruschka, B.; Monoranu, C.-M. TMEM119 as a Specific Marker of Microglia Reaction in Traumatic Brain Injury in Postmortem Examination. *Int. J. Leg. Med.* **2020**, *134*, 2167–2176. [CrossRef]
82. van Wageningen, T.A.; Vlaar, E.; Kooij, G.; Jongenelen, C.A.M.; Geurts, J.J.G.; van Dam, A.-M. Regulation of Microglial TMEM119 and P2RY12 Immunoreactivity in Multiple Sclerosis White and Grey Matter Lesions Is Dependent on Their Inflammatory Environment. *Acta Neuropathol. Commun.* **2019**, *7*, 206. [CrossRef] [PubMed]
83. Vankriekelsvenne, E.; Chrzanowski, U.; Manzhula, K.; Greiner, T.; Wree, A.; Hawlitschka, A.; Llovera, G.; Zhan, J.; Joost, S.; Schmitz, C.; et al. Transmembrane Protein 119 Is Neither a Specific nor a Reliable Marker for Microglia. *Glia* **2022**, *70*, 1170–1190. [CrossRef] [PubMed]
84. Konishi, H.; Kobayashi, M.; Kunisawa, T.; Imai, K.; Sayo, A.; Malissen, B.; Crocker, P.R.; Sato, K.; Kiyama, H. Siglec-H Is a Microglia-Specific Marker That Discriminates Microglia from CNS-Associated Macrophages and CNS-Infiltrating Monocytes. *Glia* **2017**, *65*, 1927–1943. [CrossRef] [PubMed]
85. Masuda, T.; Amann, L.; Sankowski, R.; Staszewski, O.; Lenz, M.; Errico, P.D.; Snaidero, N.; Costa Jordão, M.J.; Böttcher, C.; Kierdorf, K.; et al. Novel Hexb-Based Tools for Studying Microglia in the CNS. *Nat. Immunol.* **2020**, *21*, 802–815. [CrossRef] [PubMed]
86. Bennett, M.L.; Bennett, F.C.; Liddelow, S.A.; Ajami, B.; Zamanian, J.L.; Fernhoff, N.B.; Mulinyawe, S.B.; Bohlen, C.J.; Adil, A.; Tucker, A.; et al. New Tools for Studying Microglia in the Mouse and Human CNS. *Proc. Natl. Acad. Sci. USA* **2016**, *113*, E1738–E1746. [CrossRef]

87. Butovsky, O.; Siddiqui, S.; Gabriely, G.; Lanser, A.J.; Dake, B.; Murugaiyan, G.; Doykan, C.E.; Wu, P.M.; Gali, R.R.; Iyer, L.K.; et al. Modulating Inflammatory Monocytes with a Unique MicroRNA Gene Signature Ameliorates Murine ALS. *J. Clin. Investig.* **2012**, *122*, 3063–3087. [CrossRef]
88. Zheng, H.; Jia, L.; Liu, C.-C.; Rong, Z.; Zhong, L.; Yang, L.; Chen, X.-F.; Fryer, J.D.; Wang, X.; Zhang, Y.-W.; et al. TREM2 Promotes Microglial Survival by Activating Wnt/β-Catenin Pathway. *J. Neurosci.* **2017**, *37*, 1772–1784. [CrossRef]
89. Matcovitch-Natan, O.; Winter, D.R.; Giladi, A.; Vargas Aguilar, S.; Spinrad, A.; Sarrazin, S.; Ben-Yehuda, H.; David, E.; Zelada González, F.; Perrin, P.; et al. Microglia Development Follows a Stepwise Program to Regulate Brain Homeostasis. *Science* **2016**, *353*, aad8670. [CrossRef]
90. Wittrahm, R.; Takalo, M.; Marttinen, M.; Kuulasmaa, T.; Mäkinen, P.; Kemppainen, S.; Martiskainen, H.; Rauramaa, T.; Pike, I.; Leinonen, V.; et al. MECP2 Increases the Pro-Inflammatory Response of Microglial Cells and Phosphorylation at Serine 423 Regulates Neuronal Gene Expression upon Neuroinflammation. *Cells* **2021**, *10*, 860. [CrossRef]
91. Cronk, J.C.; Derecki, N.C.; Ji, E.; Xu, Y.; Lampano, A.E.; Smirnov, I.; Baker, W.; Norris, G.T.; Marin, I.; Coddington, N.; et al. Methyl-CpG Binding Protein 2 Regulates Microglia and Macrophage Gene Expression in Response to Inflammatory Stimuli. *Immunity* **2015**, *42*, 679–691. [CrossRef]
92. Wang, Y.-Y.; Deng, Y.-S.; Dai, S.-K.; Mi, T.-W.; Li, R.-Y.; Liu, P.-P.; Liu, C.; He, B.-D.; He, X.-C.; Du, H.-Z.; et al. Loss of Microglial EED Impairs Synapse Density, Learning, and Memory. *Mol. Psychiatry* **2022**, *27*, 2999–3009. [CrossRef]
93. Liu, C.; Gao, X.; Shi, R.-X.; Wang, Y.-Y.; He, X.-C.; Du, H.-Z.; Hu, B.; Jiao, J.; Liu, C.-M.; Teng, Z.-Q. Microglial Transglutaminase 2 Deficiency Causes Impaired Synaptic Remodelling and Cognitive Deficits in Mice. *Cell Prolif.* **2023**, e13439. [CrossRef]
94. Rigato, C.; Swinnen, N.; Buckinx, R.; Couillin, I.; Mangin, J.-M.; Rigo, J.-M.; Legendre, P.; Le Corronc, H. Microglia Proliferation Is Controlled by P2X7 Receptors in a Pannexin-1-Independent Manner during Early Embryonic Spinal Cord Invasion. *J. Neurosci.* **2012**, *32*, 11559–11573. [CrossRef]
95. Yasuoka, S.; Kawanokuchi, J.; Parajuli, B.; Jin, S.; Doi, Y.; Noda, M.; Sonobe, Y.; Takeuchi, H.; Mizuno, T.; Suzumura, A. Production and Functions of IL-33 in the Central Nervous System. *Brain Res.* **2011**, *1385*, 8–17. [CrossRef]
96. Bartolini, A.; Vigliani, M.-C.; Magrassi, L.; Vercelli, A.; Rossi, F. G-CSF Administration to Adult Mice Stimulates the Proliferation of Microglia but Does Not Modify the Outcome of Ischemic Injury. *Neurobiol. Dis.* **2011**, *41*, 640–649. [CrossRef]
97. Lee, S.C.; Liu, W.; Brosnan, C.F.; Dickson, D.W. GM-CSF Promotes Proliferation of Human Fetal and Adult Microglia in Primary Cultures. *Glia* **1994**, *12*, 309–318. [CrossRef]
98. Liva, S.M.; de Vellis, J. IL-5 Induces Proliferation and Activation of Microglia via an Unknown Receptor. *Neurochem. Res.* **2001**, *26*, 629–637. [CrossRef]
99. Akimoto, N.; Ifuku, M.; Mori, Y.; Noda, M. Effects of Chemokine (C–C Motif) Ligand 1 on Microglial Function. *Biochem. Biophys. Res. Commun.* **2013**, *436*, 455–461. [CrossRef]
100. Zhang, L.; Ma, P.; Guan, Q.; Meng, L.; Su, L.; Wang, L.; Yuan, B. Effect of Chemokine CC Ligand 2 (CCL2) on A-synuclein-induced Microglia Proliferation and Neuronal Apoptosis. *Mol. Med. Rep.* **2018**, *18*, 4213–4218. [CrossRef]
101. Zhang, J.; Geula, C.; Lu, C.; Koziel, H.; Hatcher, L.M.; Roisen, F.J. Neurotrophins Regulate Proliferation and Survival of Two Microglial Cell Lines in Vitro. *Exp. Neurol.* **2003**, *183*, 469–481. [CrossRef]
102. Terashima, T.; Nakae, Y.; Katagi, M.; Okano, J.; Suzuki, Y.; Kojima, H. Stem Cell Factor Induces Polarization of Microglia to the Neuroprotective Phenotype in Vitro. *Heliyon* **2018**, *4*, e00837. [CrossRef] [PubMed]
103. Dermitzakis, I.; Manthou, M.E.; Meditskou, S.; Miliaras, D.; Kesidou, E.; Boziki, M.; Petratos, S.; Grigoriadis, N.; Theotokis, P. Developmental Cues and Molecular Drivers in Myelinogenesis: Revisiting Early Life to Re-Evaluate the Integrity of CNS Myelin. *Curr. Issues Mol. Biol.* **2022**, *44*, 3208–3237. [CrossRef] [PubMed]
104. Lituma, P.J.; Woo, E.; O'Hara, B.F.; Castillo, P.E.; Sibinga, N.E.S.; Nandi, S. Altered Synaptic Connectivity and Brain Function in Mice Lacking Microglial Adapter Protein Iba1. *Proc. Natl. Acad. Sci. USA* **2021**, *118*, e2115539118. [CrossRef] [PubMed]
105. Maksoud, M.J.E.; Tellios, V.; Lu, W.-Y. Nitric Oxide Attenuates Microglia Proliferation by Sequentially Facilitating Calcium Influx through TRPV2 Channels, Activating NFATC2, and Increasing P21 Transcription. *Cell Cycle* **2021**, *20*, 417–433. [CrossRef] [PubMed]
106. The Human Protein Atlas. Available online: https://www.proteinatlas.org/ (accessed on 15 January 2023).
107. Home-Gene-NCBI. Available online: https://www.ncbi.nlm.nih.gov/gene/ (accessed on 15 January 2023).
108. Ashwell, K. The Distribution of Microglia and Cell Death in the Fetal Rat Forebrain. *Brain Res. Dev. Brain Res.* **1991**, *58*, 1–12. [CrossRef]
109. Sorokin, S.P.; Hoyt, R.F.; Blunt, D.G.; McNelly, N.A. Macrophage Development: II. Early Ontogeny of Macrophage Populations in Brain, Liver, and Lungs of Rat Embryos as Revealed by a Lectin Marker. *Anat. Rec.* **1992**, *232*, 527–550. [CrossRef]
110. Wang, C.C.; Wu, C.H.; Shieh, J.Y.; Wen, C.Y.; Ling, E.A. Immunohistochemical Study of Amoeboid Microglial Cells in Fetal Rat Brain. *J. Anat.* **1996**, *189*, 567–574.
111. Swinnen, N.; Smolders, S.; Avila, A.; Notelaers, K.; Paesen, R.; Ameloot, M.; Brône, B.; Legendre, P.; Rigo, J.-M. Complex Invasion Pattern of the Cerebral Cortex Bymicroglial Cells during Development of the Mouse Embryo. *Glia* **2013**, *61*, 150–163. [CrossRef]
112. Stremmel, C.; Schuchert, R.; Wagner, F.; Thaler, R.; Weinberger, T.; Pick, R.; Mass, E.; Ishikawa-Ankerhold, H.C.; Margraf, A.; Hutter, S.; et al. Yolk Sac Macrophage Progenitors Traffic to the Embryo during Defined Stages of Development. *Nat. Commun.* **2018**, *9*, 75. [CrossRef]

113. Kaur, C.; Rathnasamy, G.; Ling, E.-A. Biology of Microglia in the Developing Brain. *J. Neuropathol. Exp. Neurol.* **2017**, *76*, 736–753. [CrossRef]
114. Ling, E.A.; Wong, W.C. The Origin and Nature of Ramified and Amoeboid Microglia: A Historical Review and Current Concepts. *Glia* **1993**, *7*, 9–18. [CrossRef]
115. Esiri, M.M.; al Izzi, M.S.; Reading, M.C. Macrophages, Microglial Cells, and HLA-DR Antigens in Fetal and Infant Brain. *J. Clin. Pathol.* **1991**, *44*, 102–106. [CrossRef]
116. Rezaie, P.; Male, D. Colonisation of the Developing Human Brain and Spinal Cord by Microglia: A Review. *Microsc. Res. Tech.* **1999**, *45*, 359–382. [CrossRef]
117. Rezaie, P.; Dean, A.; Male, D.; Ulfig, N. Microglia in the Cerebral Wall of the Human Telencephalon at Second Trimester. *Cereb. Cortex* **2005**, *15*, 938–949. [CrossRef]
118. Monier, A.; Evrard, P.; Gressens, P.; Verney, C. Distribution and Differentiation of Microglia in the Human Encephalon during the First Two Trimesters of Gestation. *J. Comp. Neurol.* **2006**, *499*, 565–582. [CrossRef]
119. Monier, A.; Adle-Biassette, H.; Delezoide, A.-L.; Evrard, P.; Gressens, P.; Verney, C. Entry and Distribution of Microglial Cells in Human Embryonic and Fetal Cerebral Cortex. *J. Neuropathol. Exp. Neurol.* **2007**, *66*, 372–382. [CrossRef]
120. Verney, C.; Monier, A.; Fallet-Bianco, C.; Gressens, P. Early Microglial Colonization of the Human Forebrain and Possible Involvement in Periventricular White-Matter Injury of Preterm Infants. *J. Anat.* **2010**, *217*, 436–448. [CrossRef]
121. Cuadros, M.A.; Martin, C.; Coltey, P.; Almendros, A.; Navascués, J. First Appearance, Distribution, and Origin of Macrophages in the Early Development of the Avian Central Nervous System. *J. Comp. Neurol.* **1993**, *330*, 113–129. [CrossRef]
122. Cuadros, M.A.; Rodríguez-Ruiz, J.; Calvente, R.; Almendros, A.; Marín-Teva, J.L.; Navascués, J. Microglia Development in the Quail Cerebellum. *J. Comp. Neurol.* **1997**, *389*, 390–401. [CrossRef]
123. Krall, W.J.; Challita, P.M.; Perlmutter, L.S.; Skelton, D.C.; Kohn, D.B. Cells Expressing Human Glucocerebrosidase from a Retroviral Vector Repopulate Macrophages and Central Nervous System Microglia after Murine Bone Marrow Transplantation. *Blood* **1994**, *83*, 2737–2748. [CrossRef]
124. Kennedy, D.W.; Abkowitz, J.L. Kinetics of Central Nervous System Microglial and Macrophage Engraftment: Analysis Using a Transgenic Bone Marrow Transplantation Model. *Blood* **1997**, *90*, 986–993. [CrossRef] [PubMed]
125. Eglitis, M.A.; Mezey, É. Hematopoietic Cells Differentiate into Both Microglia and Macroglia in the Brains of Adult Mice. *Proc. Natl. Acad. Sci. USA* **1997**, *94*, 4080–4085. [CrossRef] [PubMed]
126. Priller, J.; Flügel, A.; Wehner, T.; Boentert, M.; Haas, C.A.; Prinz, M.; Fernández-Klett, F.; Prass, K.; Bechmann, I.; de Boer, B.A.; et al. Targeting Gene-Modified Hematopoietic Cells to the Central Nervous System: Use of Green Fluorescent Protein Uncovers Microglial Engraftment. *Nat. Med.* **2001**, *7*, 1356–1361. [CrossRef] [PubMed]
127. Simard, A.R.; Rivest, S. Bone Marrow Stem Cells Have the Ability to Populate the Entire Central Nervous System into Fully Differentiated Parenchymal Microglia. *FASEB J.* **2004**, *18*, 998–1000. [CrossRef]
128. Asheuer, M.; Pflumio, F.; Benhamida, S.; Dubart-Kupperschmitt, A.; Fouquet, F.; Imai, Y.; Aubourg, P.; Cartier, N. Human CD34+ Cells Differentiate into Microglia and Express Recombinant Therapeutic Protein. *Proc. Natl. Acad. Sci. USA* **2004**, *101*, 3557–3562. [CrossRef]
129. Beck, H.; Voswinckel, R.; Wagner, S.; Ziegelhoeffer, T.; Heil, M.; Helisch, A.; Schaper, W.; Acker, T.; Hatzopoulos, A.K.; Plate, K.H. Participation of Bone Marrow-Derived Cells in Long-Term Repair Processes after Experimental Stroke. *J. Cereb. Blood Flow Metab.* **2003**, *23*, 709–717. [CrossRef]
130. Hess, D.C.; Abe, T.; Hill, W.D.; Studdard, A.M.; Carothers, J.; Masuya, M.; Fleming, P.A.; Drake, C.J.; Ogawa, M. Hematopoietic Origin of Microglial and Perivascular Cells in Brain. *Exp. Neurol.* **2004**, *186*, 134–144. [CrossRef]
131. Djukic, M.; Mildner, A.; Schmidt, H.; Czesnik, D.; Brück, W.; Priller, J.; Nau, R.; Prinz, M. Circulating Monocytes Engraft in the Brain, Differentiate into Microglia and Contribute to the Pathology Following Meningitis in Mice. *Brain J. Neurol.* **2006**, *129*, 2394–2403. [CrossRef]
132. Bechmann, I.; Goldmann, J.; Kovac, A.D.; Kwidzinski, E.; Simbürger, E.; Naftolin, F.; Dirnagl, U.; Nitsch, R.; Priller, J. Circulating Monocytic Cells Infiltrate Layers of Anterograde Axonal Degeneration Where They Transform into Microglia. *FASEB J.* **2005**, *19*, 647–649. [CrossRef]
133. Rodriguez, M.; Alvarez-Erviti, L.; Blesa, F.J.; Rodríguez-Oroz, M.C.; Arina, A.; Melero, I.; Ramos, L.I.; Obeso, J.A. Bone-Marrow-Derived Cell Differentiation into Microglia: A Study in a Progressive Mouse Model of Parkinson's Disease. *Neurobiol. Dis.* **2007**, *28*, 316–325. [CrossRef]
134. Malm, T.M.; Koistinaho, M.; Pärepalo, M.; Vatanen, T.; Ooka, A.; Karlsson, S.; Koistinaho, J. Bone-Marrow-Derived Cells Contribute to the Recruitment of Microglial Cells in Response to Beta-Amyloid Deposition in APP/PS1 Double Transgenic Alzheimer Mice. *Neurobiol. Dis.* **2005**, *18*, 134–142. [CrossRef]
135. Simard, A.R.; Soulet, D.; Gowing, G.; Julien, J.-P.; Rivest, S. Bone Marrow-Derived Microglia Play a Critical Role in Restricting Senile Plaque Formation in Alzheimer's Disease. *Neuron* **2006**, *49*, 489–502. [CrossRef]
136. Ye, S.; Theotokis, P.; Lee, J.Y.; Kim, M.J.; Nheu, D.; Ellen, O.; Bedford, T.; Ramanujam, P.; Wright, D.K.; McDonald, S.J.; et al. NgR-Fc Delivered by Hematopoietic Cells Enhances Neurorepair in a Multiple Sclerosis Model. *Brain Commun.* **2023**, in press.
137. Flügel, A.; Bradl, M.; Kreutzberg, G.W.; Graeber, M.B. Transformation of Donor-Derived Bone Marrow Precursors into Host Microglia during Autoimmune CNS Inflammation and during the Retrograde Response to Axotomy. *J. Neurosci. Res.* **2001**, *66*, 74–82. [CrossRef]

138. Priller, J.; Prinz, M.; Heikenwalder, M.; Zeller, N.; Schwarz, P.; Heppner, F.L.; Aguzzi, A. Early and Rapid Engraftment of Bone Marrow-Derived Microglia in Scrapie. *J. Neurosci.* **2006**, *26*, 11753–11762. [CrossRef]
139. Vallières, L.; Sawchenko, P.E. Bone Marrow-Derived Cells That Populate the Adult Mouse Brain Preserve Their Hematopoietic Identity. *J. Neurosci.* **2003**, *23*, 5197–5207. [CrossRef]
140. Massengale, M.; Wagers, A.J.; Vogel, H.; Weissman, I.L. Hematopoietic Cells Maintain Hematopoietic Fates upon Entering the Brain. *J. Exp. Med.* **2005**, *201*, 1579–1589. [CrossRef]
141. Zhang, J.; Shi, X.Q.; Echeverry, S.; Mogil, J.S.; De Koninck, Y.; Rivest, S. Expression of CCR2 in Both Resident and Bone Marrow-Derived Microglia Plays a Critical Role in Neuropathic Pain. *J. Neurosci.* **2007**, *27*, 12396–12406. [CrossRef]
142. Marchi, S.; Guilbaud, E.; Tait, S.W.G.; Yamazaki, T.; Galluzzi, L. Mitochondrial Control of Inflammation. *Nat. Rev. Immunol.* **2023**, *23*, 159–173. [CrossRef]
143. Joshi, A.U.; Minhas, P.S.; Liddelow, S.A.; Haileselassie, B.; Andreasson, K.I.; Dorn, G.W.; Mochly-Rosen, D. Fragmented Mitochondria Released from Microglia Trigger A1 Astrocytic Response and Propagate Inflammatory Neurodegeneration. *Nat. Neurosci.* **2019**, *22*, 1635–1648. [CrossRef]
144. Leong, S.K.; Ling, E.A. Amoeboid and Ramified Microglia: Their Interrelationship and Response to Brain Injury. *Glia* **1992**, *6*, 39–47. [CrossRef] [PubMed]
145. Lassmann, H.; Schmied, M.; Vass, K.; Hickey, W.F. Bone Marrow Derived Elements and Resident Microglia in Brain Inflammation. *Glia* **1993**, *7*, 19–24. [CrossRef] [PubMed]
146. Dalmau, I.; Vela, J.M.; González, B.; Finsen, B.; Castellano, B. Dynamics of Microglia in the Developing Rat Brain. *J. Comp. Neurol.* **2003**, *458*, 144–157. [CrossRef]
147. Lawson, L.J.; Perry, V.H.; Gordon, S. Turnover of Resident Microglia in the Normal Adult Mouse Brain. *Neuroscience* **1992**, *48*, 405–415. [CrossRef] [PubMed]
148. Solomon, J.N.; Lewis, C.-A.B.; Ajami, B.; Corbel, S.Y.; Rossi, F.M.V.; Krieger, C. Origin and Distribution of Bone Marrow-Derived Cells in the Central Nervous System in a Mouse Model of Amyotrophic Lateral Sclerosis. *Glia* **2006**, *53*, 744–753. [CrossRef]
149. Ajami, B.; Bennett, J.L.; Krieger, C.; Tetzlaff, W.; Rossi, F.M.V. Local Self-Renewal Can Sustain CNS Microglia Maintenance and Function throughout Adult Life. *Nat. Neurosci.* **2007**, *10*, 1538–1543. [CrossRef]
150. Mildner, A.; Schmidt, H.; Nitsche, M.; Merkler, D.; Hanisch, U.-K.; Mack, M.; Heikenwalder, M.; Brück, W.; Priller, J.; Prinz, M. Microglia in the Adult Brain Arise from Ly-6ChiCCR2+ Monocytes Only under Defined Host Conditions. *Nat. Neurosci.* **2007**, *10*, 1544–1553. [CrossRef]
151. Capotondo, A.; Milazzo, R.; Politi, L.S.; Quattrini, A.; Palini, A.; Plati, T.; Merella, S.; Nonis, A.; di Serio, C.; Montini, E.; et al. Brain Conditioning Is Instrumental for Successful Microglia Reconstitution Following Hematopoietic Stem Cell Transplantation. *Proc. Natl. Acad. Sci. USA* **2012**, *109*, 15018–15023. [CrossRef]
152. Li, T.; Pang, S.; Yu, Y.; Wu, X.; Guo, J.; Zhang, S. Proliferation of Parenchymal Microglia Is the Main Source of Microgliosis after Ischaemic Stroke. *Brain J. Neurol.* **2013**, *136*, 3578–3588. [CrossRef]
153. Bruttger, J.; Karram, K.; Wörtge, S.; Regen, T.; Marini, F.; Hoppmann, N.; Klein, M.; Blank, T.; Yona, S.; Wolf, Y.; et al. Genetic Cell Ablation Reveals Clusters of Local Self-Renewing Microglia in the Mammalian Central Nervous System. *Immunity* **2015**, *43*, 92–106. [CrossRef]
154. Xu, J.; Zhu, L.; He, S.; Wu, Y.; Jin, W.; Yu, T.; Qu, J.Y.; Wen, Z. Temporal-Spatial Resolution Fate Mapping Reveals Distinct Origins for Embryonic and Adult Microglia in Zebrafish. *Dev. Cell* **2015**, *34*, 632–641. [CrossRef]
155. Tay, T.L.; Mai, D.; Dautzenberg, J.; Fernández-Klett, F.; Lin, G.; Sagar, N.; Datta, M.; Drougard, A.; Stempfl, T.; Ardura-Fabregat, A.; et al. A New Fate Mapping System Reveals Context-Dependent Random or Clonal Expansion of Microglia. *Nat. Neurosci.* **2017**, *20*, 793–803. [CrossRef]
156. Cronk, J.C.; Filiano, A.J.; Louveau, A.; Marin, I.; Marsh, R.; Ji, E.; Goldman, D.H.; Smirnov, I.; Geraci, N.; Acton, S.; et al. Peripherally Derived Macrophages Can Engraft the Brain Independent of Irradiation and Maintain an Identity Distinct from Microglia. *J. Exp. Med.* **2018**, *215*, 1627–1647. [CrossRef]
157. Lund, H.; Pieber, M.; Parsa, R.; Han, J.; Grommisch, D.; Ewing, E.; Kular, L.; Needhamsen, M.; Espinosa, A.; Nilsson, E.; et al. Competitive Repopulation of an Empty Microglial Niche Yields Functionally Distinct Subsets of Microglia-like Cells. *Nat. Commun.* **2018**, *9*, 4845. [CrossRef]
158. Shemer, A.; Grozovski, J.; Tay, T.L.; Tao, J.; Volaski, A.; Süß, P.; Ardura-Fabregat, A.; Gross-Vered, M.; Kim, J.-S.; David, E.; et al. Engrafted Parenchymal Brain Macrophages Differ from Microglia in Transcriptome, Chromatin Landscape and Response to Challenge. *Nat. Commun.* **2018**, *9*, 5206. [CrossRef]
159. Huang, Y.; Xu, Z.; Xiong, S.; Sun, F.; Qin, G.; Hu, G.; Wang, J.; Zhao, L.; Liang, Y.-X.; Wu, T.; et al. Repopulated Microglia Are Solely Derived from the Proliferation of Residual Microglia after Acute Depletion. *Nat. Neurosci.* **2018**, *21*, 530–540. [CrossRef]
160. Elmore, M.R.P.; Najafi, A.R.; Koike, M.A.; Dagher, N.N.; Spangenberg, E.E.; Rice, R.A.; Kitazawa, M.; Matusow, B.; Nguyen, H.; West, B.L.; et al. Colony-Stimulating Factor 1 Receptor Signaling Is Necessary for Microglia Viability, Unmasking a Microglia Progenitor Cell in the Adult Brain. *Neuron* **2014**, *82*, 380–397. [CrossRef]
161. Zhan, L.; Krabbe, G.; Du, F.; Jones, I.; Reichert, M.C.; Telpoukhovskaia, M.; Kodama, L.; Wang, C.; Cho, S.-H.; Sayed, F.; et al. Proximal Recolonization by Self-Renewing Microglia Re-Establishes Microglial Homeostasis in the Adult Mouse Brain. *PLoS Biol.* **2019**, *17*, e3000134. [CrossRef]

162. Wu, X.; Saito, T.; Saido, T.C.; Barron, A.M.; Ruedl, C. Microglia and CD206+ Border-Associated Mouse Macrophages Maintain Their Embryonic Origin during Alzheimer's Disease. *eLife* **2021**, *10*, e71879. [CrossRef]
163. Luo, C.; Jian, C.; Liao, Y.; Huang, Q.; Wu, Y.; Liu, X.; Zou, D.; Wu, Y. The Role of Microglia in Multiple Sclerosis. *Neuropsychiatr. Dis. Treat.* **2017**, *13*, 1661–1667. [CrossRef]
164. Schetters, S.T.T.; Gomez-Nicola, D.; Garcia-Vallejo, J.J.; Van Kooyk, Y. Neuroinflammation: Microglia and T Cells Get Ready to Tango. *Front. Immunol.* **2018**, *8*, 1905. [CrossRef] [PubMed]
165. Goddery, E.N.; Fain, C.E.; Lipovsky, C.G.; Ayasoufi, K.; Yokanovich, L.T.; Malo, C.S.; Khadka, R.H.; Tritz, Z.P.; Jin, F.; Hansen, M.J.; et al. Microglia and Perivascular Macrophages Act as Antigen Presenting Cells to Promote CD8 T Cell Infiltration of the Brain. *Front. Immunol.* **2021**, *12*, 726421. [CrossRef] [PubMed]
166. O'Loughlin, E.; Madore, C.; Lassmann, H.; Butovsky, O. Microglial Phenotypes and Functions in Multiple Sclerosis. *Cold Spring Harb. Perspect. Med.* **2018**, *8*, a028993. [CrossRef] [PubMed]
167. Nheu, D.; Ellen, O.; Ye, S.; Ozturk, E.; Pagnin, M.; Kertadjaja, S.; Theotokis, P.; Grigoriadis, N.; McLean, C.; Petratos, S. Modulation of the Microglial Nogo-A/NgR Signaling Pathway as a Therapeutic Target for Multiple Sclerosis. *Cells* **2022**, *11*, 3768. [CrossRef]

current issues in molecular biology

MDPI

Article

Overexpression of *OLIG2* and *MYT1L* Transcription Factors Enhance the Differentiation Potential of Human Mesenchymal Stem Cells into Oligodendrocytes

Ifrah Fahim [1], Aisha Ishaque [1], Faiza Ramzan [1], Shamsul Azlin Bin Ahmad Shamsuddin [2], Anwar Ali [3], Asmat Salim [1] and Irfan Khan [1,*]

[1] Dr. Panjwani Center for Molecular Medicine and Drug Research, International Center for Chemical and Biological Sciences, University of Karachi, Karachi 75270, Pakistan

[2] Institute of Biological Sciences, Faculty of Sciences, Universiti Malaya, Kuala Lumpur 50603, Malaysia

[3] Department of Physiology, University of Karachi, Karachi 75270, Pakistan

* Correspondence: khan@iccs.edu; Tel.: +92-21-99261671

Abstract: Background: Demyelinating diseases represent a broad spectrum of disorders and are characterized by the loss of specialized glial cells (oligodendrocytes), which eventually leads to neuronal degeneration. Stem cell-based regenerative approaches provide therapeutic options to regenerate demyelination-induced neurodegeneration. Objectives: The current study aims to explore the role of oligodendrocyte-specific transcription factors (*OLIG2* and *MYT1L*) under suitable media composition to facilitate human umbilical-cord-derived mesenchymal stem cells (hUC-MSCs) differentiation toward oligodendrocyte for their potential use to treat demyelinating disorders. Methodology: hUC-MSCs were isolated, cultured, and characterized based on their morphological and phenotypic characteristics. hUC-MSCs were transfected with *OLIG2* and *MYT1L* transcription factors individually and in synergistic (*OLIG2* + *MYT1L*) groups using a lipofectamine-based transfection method and incubated under two different media compositions (normal and oligo induction media). Transfected hUC-MSCs were assessed for lineage specification and differentiation using qPCR. Differentiation was also analyzed via immunocytochemistry by determining the expression of oligodendrocyte-specific proteins. Results: All the transfected groups showed significant upregulation of *GFAP* and *OLIG2* with downregulation of *NES*, demonstrating the MSC commitment toward the glial lineage. Transfected groups also presented significant overexpression of oligodendrocyte-specific markers (*SOX10*, *NKX2.2*, *GALC*, *CNP*, *CSPG4*, *MBP*, and *PLP1*). Immunocytochemical analysis showed intense expression of OLIG2, MYT1L, and NG2 proteins in both normal and oligo induction media after 3 and 7 days. Conclusions: The study concludes that *OLIG2* and *MYT1L* have the potential to differentiate hUC-MSCs into oligodendrocyte-like cells, which is greatly facilitated by the oligo induction medium. The study may serve as a promising cell-based therapeutic strategy against demyelination-induced neuronal degeneration.

Keywords: mesenchymal stem cells; fate specification; oligodendrocytes; differentiation; gene expression

1. Introduction

Demyelinating diseases are associated with the gradual and progressive loss of myelin which ultimately results in the impairment of axonal conduction velocity and gives rise to various neurological complications [1]. Such disorders are further characterized by neuronal degeneration [2]. The most representative primary demyelinating disease includes multiple sclerosis (MS). It is a chronic autoimmune disorder of the CNS that is characterized by the formation of demyelinating plaques within the white matter. It is strongly associated with the initiation of inflammatory cascades, and the ultimate damage to the neuronal axons. Worldwide prevalence of MS is expected to be 2.8 million by the year 2020, affecting 1 out of every 2786 individuals and diagnosed at an average age of 32 years [3,4].

Although continuous advances have been made over time for pharmacological therapies, these approaches provide transient treatment and only offer symptom management [5]. The majority of medications focus on one of the two strategies, i.e., minimizing disease progression or treating a specific symptom. However, these medications are frequently associated with undesirable side effects with a limited therapeutic window because of the protective role of the blood–brain barrier [6]. Immunomodulatory therapies are most successful in the early disease phase but are not effective for relapsing remitting MS [7]. Consequently, researchers have been working to develop more effective treatments by introducing gene-therapy approaches by following three steps: (i) prevention of specific symptoms, (ii) reversing disease progression, and (iii) healing CNS damage through facilitating remyelination and axonal repair [6]. Recently, clinically relevant biomarkers for MS, such as miRNAs, have emerged and can be utilized to evaluate the efficacy of ongoing treatment, detect pathophysiological processes, and develop personalized treatment plans [8].

One of the emerging and effective approaches for the treatment of various degenerative anomalies is regenerative medicine. Cell-based therapy is an important aspect of regenerative medicine and is the most applicable treatment modality [2,3,9,10]. Stem cell-based treatment is a promising therapeutic strategy that effectively facilitates tissue repair and performs cellular replacement of the damaged area. Mesenchymal stem cells (MSCs) are adult, multipotent stem cells that have been reported to treat various degenerative pathologies, including neurodegenerative and demyelinating disorders [10–14]. A study previously conducted by our group has shown the differentiation potential of MSCs toward neuronal lineage [15]. MSCs have also been reported to induce oligodendrocyte differentiation under the influence of various factors. A study conducted by Oppliger et al. reported that Wharton's jelly-derived MSCs secrete proangiogenic and neuroprotective factors, which regulate oligodendrocyte differentiation [14]. MSCs have also been found to be effective in reducing the myelin sheath damage caused by spinal cord injury when co-transplanted with neural stem cells [16]. Zhang et al. demonstrated that hBM-MSCs treatment in experimental autoimmune encephalomyelitis (EAE) mice greatly reduced the area of demyelination and facilitated the increase in BDNF+ cells [17]. Phases 1 and 2 of the clinical trials are also being conducted using MSCs to analyze their therapeutic effect in MS patients. A study submitted to clinicaltrials.gov indicated the safety and feasibility of MSCs injection (both intrathecally and intravenously) in patients with MS [18]. Genetic manipulation of MSCs is a potential strategy for enhancing their therapeutic potential and induction of fate specification by the overexpression of certain transcription factors or genes [19–21]. *OLIG2* belongs to the basic helix-loop-helix transcription factor family and is a key regulatory gene for oligodendrocyte lineage specification and regulates crucial phases of early oligodendrocyte development. It has also been documented as an upstream *SOX10* regulator, which also plays a key role to regulate oligodendrocyte development [20,22]. *MYT1L* belongs to the family of myelin transcription factors and is involved in the proliferation and differentiation of oligodendrocyte precursor cells, which essentially performs myelination and remyelination of the central nervous system. It has also been reported to play an important role in neurogenesis and neural differentiation. *MYT1L* significantly improves myelination [19], suggesting a possible therapeutic target for myelin repair.

Keeping in consideration the potential role of *OLIG2* and *MYT1L* in oligodendrocyte differentiation and myelination, respectively, this study was designed to induce hUC-MSC differentiation toward oligodendrocyte by their genetic modification, both in normal and oligo induction media. The study may provide a promising cell-based treatment option for demyelination-induced neurodegenerative diseases.

2. Materials and Methods

2.1. Ethical Consent and Umbilical Cord Sample Collection

Human umbilical cord samples (n = 10) were collected in a sterile glass bottle containing PBS and 0.5% EDTA (Sigma-Aldrich Chemie, GmbH, Taufkirchen, Germany) from Zainab Panjwani Memorial Hospital, following the cesarean section delivery of healthy donors. Informed consent was taken from the donors' parents. The study protocol regarding the human participants was approved by the independent ethical committee (reference no. IEC-009-UCB-2015) of the Dr. Panjwani Center for Molecular Medicine and Drug Research, International Center for Chemical and Biological Sciences, University of Karachi.

2.2. Isolation and Propagation of hUC-MSCs

The cord tissue was washed thoroughly with PBS to remove blood clots and was cut into small pieces of about 1–3 mm^2. The cord explants were transferred into T-75 tissue culture flasks (Cat. No. 708003, Nest, Wuxi, China) containing Dulbecco's modified Eagle's medium (DMEM) (Cat. No. 11965-092, Gibco, Paisley, UK) supplemented with 10% fetal bovine serum (FBS) (Cat. No. 10500-64, Gibco, Paisley, UK), 1 mM sodium pyruvate (Cat. No. 11360-070, Gibco, UK), 1 mM L-glutamine (Cat. No. 25030681, Gibco, Paisley, UK), and 100 U antibiotic (penicillin–streptomycin) (Cat. No. 15070-063, Gibco, Paisley, UK). The flasks were incubated at 37 °C in a 5% humidified CO_2 incubator (ESCO, Singapore). The non-adherent hematopoietic cells were removed from the flasks by replacing the media with fresh DMEM after every 3 days. The cells migrated out from the explants, adhered to the flask surface, and started to proliferate. At this stage, MSCs were termed as passage 0 (P0) cells. When the cells reached 80–90% confluence, they were subcultured to subsequent passages using 0.25% trypsin–EDTA solution (Cat. No. 25200-056, Gibco, Paisley, UK). Passages 2–4 hUC-MSCs were used for all the experimental work.

2.3. Characterization of hUC-MSCs

hUC-MSCs were characterized based on their morphological features, surface-specific markers by immunocytochemistry and flow cytometry, and by assessing their multilineage differentiation potential as described in our previous studies [23,24].

2.3.1. Morphological Features of hUC-MSCs

To assess morphological features, hUC-MSCs were maintained for 3–5 subsequent passages and routinely examined under phase contrast microscope. Images were captured from each passage using a charge-coupled device (CCD) camera (Nikon Eclipse Ts2, Tokyo, Japan).

2.3.2. Immunocytochemistry

Passage 2 hUC-MSCs were seeded on coverslips placed in a 24-well plate (CLS3526, Corning, Corning, NY, USA) at a density of about 3000–5000 cells/well. Complete DMEM was added in each well and the plate was incubated at 37 °C in a humidified CO_2 incubator. The next day, the media were removed and cells were washed twice with PBS. Cells were fixed with 4% paraformaldehyde (PFA) (Cat. No. 30525894 Carl Roth, Karlsruhe, Germany) and permeabilized with 0.1% Triton-X 100 (Cat. No. 9036195, Sigma-Aldrich, Taufkirchen, Germany) for 10 min each at room temperature. Non-specific binding sites were blocked using 2% blocking solution (2% BSA with 0.1% Tween 20 in PBS). Primary antibodies against MSC positive markers (CD29, CD105, Vimentin, CD117, Lin28, and Stro1) and negative markers (CD45 and HLA-DR) at a dilution of 1:200 were added in the designated wells and incubated overnight at 4 °C. The next day, antibody solutions were removed and cells were washed gently five times with PBS. Alexa fluor-546 conjugated secondary antibody at a dilution of 1:200 and Alexa fluor-488 phalloidin was added in each well and incubated for 1 h at 37 °C. Nuclei were stained with DAPI (0.5 µg/mL) for 15 min at room temperature. Cells were washed five times with PBS and coverslips were mounted on glass slides with Fluoromount aqueous mounting medium (F4680, Sigma, St. Louis, MI,

USA). Images were captured under a fluorescence microscope (NiE, Nikon, Tokyo, Japan). Antibody details are mentioned in Table 1.

Table 1. List of antibodies used for MSC characterization and oligodendrocyte differentiation.

S. No.	Primary Antibody	Function/ Binding to	Working Dilution	Catalog Number	Manufacturer
		MSC Characterization Markers			
1.	CD29	Membrane glycoprotein	1:100	MAB-1981	Chemicon International, Katy, TX, USA
2.	CD105	Endoglin	1:100	560839	BD Pharmingen, San Diego, CA, USA
3.	Vimentin	Epithelial–mesenchymal transition	1:100	V6389	Sigma-Aldrich, Inc., St. Louis, MI, USA
4.	C-Kit (CD117)	Stem cell factor receptor	1:100	32–9000	Zymed Laboratories, Inc., South San Francisco, CA, USA
5.	Lin28	Cell surface *MSC marker*	1:100	PA1-096	Molecular Probes, Invitrogen, Eugene, OR, USA
6.	Stro-1	Mesenchymal precursor cell marker	1:100	14-6688-82	Molecular Probes, Invitrogen, Eugene, OR, USA
7.	HLA-DR	MHC class II immunogenic marker	1:100	14-9956-82	Molecular Probes, Invitrogen, Eugene, OR, USA
8.	CD45	Lymphocyte antigen	1:100	CBL415	BD Pharmingen, Diego, CA, USA
		Oligodendrocyte-specific Markers			
9.	OLIG2	Oligodendrocyte lineage-specific marker	1:100	PA5-85734	Molecular Probes, Invitrogen, Eugene, OR, USA
10.	Myt1L	Myelin transcription factor 1-like	1:50	PA5-34468	Molecular Probes, Invitrogen, Eugene, OR, USA
11.	NG2	Neural/Glial antigen 2	1:100	PA5-100235	Molecular Probes, Invitrogen, Eugene, OR, USA
12.	MBP	Myelin basic protein	1:100	MA1-24990	Molecular Probes, Invitrogen, Eugene, OR, USA
		Secondary Antibodies			
13.	Goat Anti-rabbit	Alexa Fluor 546	1:200	A-11010	Molecular Probes, Invitrogen, Eugene, OR, USA
14.	Anti-Rat IgG Isotype	Alexa Fluor 488	1:200	012-090-003	Jackson Immuno Research, Inc., West Grove, PA, USA

2.3.3. Immunophenotyping

hUC-MSCs were cultured in T-75 flask and trypsinized when 80–90% confluence was attained. Pellet was washed with PBS and incubated with blocking solution (1% BSA, 1 mM EDTA, and 0.1% sodium azide) for 30 min. The suspension was centrifuged at 400 g for 5 min and primary antibodies for MSC-specific markers (anti CD90, CD105, CD44, and CD73) were added for 2 h at 37 °C. The cell suspension was centrifuged at 400 g for 5 min, washed 3 times with ice-cold FACS solution, and incubated with Alexa flour 546 conjugated secondary antibody for an hour at 37 °C. Finally, the suspension was centrifuged again and washed three times. The pellet was resuspended in ice-cold FACS solution and analyzed by flow cytometer (BD FACS Calibur, Becton Dickinson, Franklin Lakes, NJ, USA).

2.3.4. Trilineage Differentiation

To assess trilineage differentiation potential, hUC-MSCs were seeded in a 6-well plate and nourished with DMEM. Once the cells reached 70–80% confluence, DMEM was replaced with lineage-specific induction media, i.e., osteogenic (0.1 μM dexamethasone (Cat. No. D4902, Sigma-Aldrich, Taufkirchen, Germany), 10 μM β-glycerophosphate (Sigma-Aldrich; Cat. No. G6376), and 50 μM L-ascorbate 2-phosphate (Cat. No. A8960, Sigma-Aldrich, Taufkirchen, Germany), adipogenic (1 μM dexamethasone, 10 μM insulin (Cat. No. 11070738, Sigma-Aldrich, Taufkirchen, Germany), 200 μM indomethacin (Cat. No. 190217, MP Biomedical, Burlingame, CA, USA), chondrogenic (100 nM dexamethasone, 20 ng TGFβ1 (Cat. No. RPA124Hu01, Claud Clone, Wuhan, China), 10 ng insulin, and 100 μM ascorbic acid (Sigma-Aldrich; Cat. No. 50817). The induction media were changed after every 3 days. After 21 days of incubation, cells were washed with PBS and fixed with 4% PFA. MSC differentiation was analyzed by staining the cells with Alizarin red (Cat. No. 155984, MP Biomedical, Burlingame, CA, USA), Oil red O (Cat. No. 130223, Sigma-Aldrich, Taufkirchen, Germany) and Alcian blue (Cat. No. 74240, Carl Roth, Karlsruhe, Germany) stains for the presence of calcium deposits, oil droplets, and proteoglycans, respectively. Stained cells were observed under bright-field microscope (Eclipse TE 2000-S, Nikon, Tokyo, Japan).

2.4. Isolation of Plasmid Vectors

E. coli stab cultures of *OLIG2* and *MYT1L* plasmid constructs were obtained from Addgene (www.addgene.org, accessed on 13 March 2023); *OLIG2* plasmid ID # 32933 and *Myt1L* plasmid ID # 32926). *E.coli* were grown on Luria broth and plasmid DNA was isolated by using GeneJET™ Plasmid Maxiprep Kit (Thermo Scientific, Waltham, MA, USA) according to the instructions provided by the manufacturer. Isolated plasmids were quantified via spectrophotometric analysis and electrophoresed on 1% agarose gel to evaluate their purity.

2.5. Experimental Groups

The study comprised four experimental groups, i.e., control (non-transfected hUC-MSCs), *OLIG2*-transfected, *MYT1L*-transfected, and synergistic (*OLIG2* + *MYT1L*)-transfected groups. All the groups were incubated under two different media compositions, i.e., normal DMEM and oligo induction medium (5% FBS supplemented OPTI-MEM, 0.1 mM β-mercaptoethanol, and B-27 supplement-2x). The experimental details have been mentioned in Table 2.

Table 2. Experimental setup details of the hUC-MSC genetic modification.

Experimental Groups	Transcription Factor(s) Inserted
Normal Medium	
Control	–
OLIG2-transfected	*OLIG2*
MYT1L-transfected	*MYT1L*
Synergistic	*OLIG2* + *MYT1L*
Oligo Induction Medium	
Control	–
OLIG2-transfected	*OLIG2*
MYT1L-transfected	*MYT1L*
Synergistic	*OLIG2* + *MYT1L*

2.6. Transfection of hUC-MSCs

Lipofectamine-based transfection technique was used to transfect hUC-MSCs with the desired transcription factors (*OLIG2* and *MYT1L*). Briefly, Lipofectamine® 3000 transfection reagent (Cat. No. L3000-008, Thermo Fisher Scientific, Waltham, MA, USA) and master mix of each plasmid DNA were diluted individually in OPTI-MEM. Diluted plasmids were mixed with lipofectamine (1:1 ratio) and incubated for 15 min at room temperature. This DNA/lipid mixture was added dropwise in 80–90% confluent T-75 flasks individually and in combination. The control group was not transfected with any of the transcription factors. Each transfected group was incubated under standard cell culture conditions for 3 and 7 days in two different media compositions, as mentioned in Table 2.

2.7. Morphological Examination of Transfected hUC-MSCs

Transfected hUC-MSCs were incubated in normal and oligo induction media for 3 and 7 days and monitored regularly for the induction of differentiation by observing their morphological features under phase contrast microscope.

2.8. Gene Expression Analysis

RNA was extracted from control and transfected groups using Trizol reagent (15596026, Invitrogen) reagent and quantified via spectrophotometer. RNA yield equivalent to 1 μg was reverse-transcribed into cDNA using RevertAid First Strand cDNA Synthesis Kit (K1622, Thermo Scientific, USA) according to the manufacturer's instructions. Real-time PCR was performed to analyze the expression of oligodendrocyte-specific genes in the transfected groups. Each sample was run in triplicates and GAPDH was used as a standard internal control. Primer sequences specific to each gene have been provided in Table 3.

Table 3. Primer sequences of the targeted genes used for qPCR analysis.

<table>
<tr><th></th><th>Genes</th><th>Primer Sequences (5′-3′)</th><th>Annealing Temperature</th></tr>
<tr><td rowspan="3">Lineage-specific Genes</td><td>NES (F)
NES (R)</td><td>TTCCAGACTCCACTCCCCTG
CTCAGTCCCCAGGTCCTCAA</td><td>55 °C</td></tr>
<tr><td>GFAP (F)
GFAP (R)</td><td>ATGCTGGCTTCAAGGAGACC
GGTGGCTTCATCTGCTTCCT</td><td>55 °C</td></tr>
<tr><td>OLIG2 (F)
OLIG2 (R)</td><td>TCAAGTCATCCTCGTCCAGC
TCACCAGTCGCTTCATCTCC</td><td>55 °C</td></tr>
<tr><td rowspan="8">Oligodendrocyte-specific Gene</td><td>MYT1L (F)
MYT1L (R)</td><td>GACTGCGGAACAGGATTTGG
CGACCAGGGTTTGAAGATGC</td><td>55 °C</td></tr>
<tr><td>NKX2.2 (F)
NKX2.2 (R)</td><td>TTCCTCGCCACCAGCC
TTCGGCCACAGAGCCC</td><td>55 °C</td></tr>
<tr><td>SOX10 (F)
SOX10 (R)</td><td>ACGTCAAGCGGCCCAT
TCCCACCTTGCTCGGC</td><td>55 °C</td></tr>
<tr><td>GALC (F)
GALC (R)</td><td>GAATTTTCCAAAGAATGGCTGGG
CAGTGATGATCAAGTTACT-
GCCA</td><td>55 °C</td></tr>
<tr><td>CNP (F)
CNP (R)</td><td>CCTTCAAGAAGGAGCTGCGA
AGCTTGTCCACATCACTCGG</td><td>55 °C</td></tr>
<tr><td>CSPG4 (F)
CSPG4 (R)</td><td>GGATGCCACCCTACAAGTGA
TTTTGCGCCTCTAGTGGGAT</td><td>55 °C</td></tr>
<tr><td>PLP1 (F)
PLP1 (R)</td><td>ATTCTTTGGAGCGGGTGTGT
GAAGGTGAGCAGGGAAACCA</td><td>55 °C</td></tr>
<tr><td>MBP (F)
MBP (R)</td><td>GCGGCCCCTGTCTCC
GCGGCTCCCTGGGTC</td><td>55 °C</td></tr>
</table>

2.9. Protein Expression Analysis of Transfected MSCs

Normal and transfected MSCs incubated in both normal and oligo induction media were analyzed for the expression of oligodendrocyte-specific proteins (OLIG2, MYT1L, NG2, and MBP) by immunocytochemistry as mentioned above. Images were captured under fluorescent microscope (Nikon, Tokyo, Japan). The fluorescent intensity of each group was quantified via ImageJ software.

2.10. Statistical Analysis

Statistical analysis was performed using IBM SPSS Statistics software (version 21; SPSS Inc, Armonk, NY, USA) to establish statistical significance at the accepted level; $p \leq 0.05$ ($p < 0.05$ = *, $p < 0.01$ = **, and $p < 0.001$ = ***). Each experiment was run in triplicates and acquired data were analyzed through an independent sample *t*-test. The results have been presented as mean ± SEM.

3. Results

3.1. Umbilical Cord Processing; Isolation, Propagation, and Morphological Features of hUC-MSCs

Umbilical cord tissue was processed under the sterile environment of a biosafety cabinet (Figure 1A). After about 2 weeks of explant culture, MSCs migrated out of the tissues, adhered to the flask surface, and started to form colonies. The cells proliferated further and adopted fibroblast like morphology, which is the typical characteristic of MSCs. At this stage, hUC-MSC culture was termed P0. On reaching 80–90% confluence, they were subcultured to subsequent passages (P1 and P2) for experimental work (Figure 1B–F).

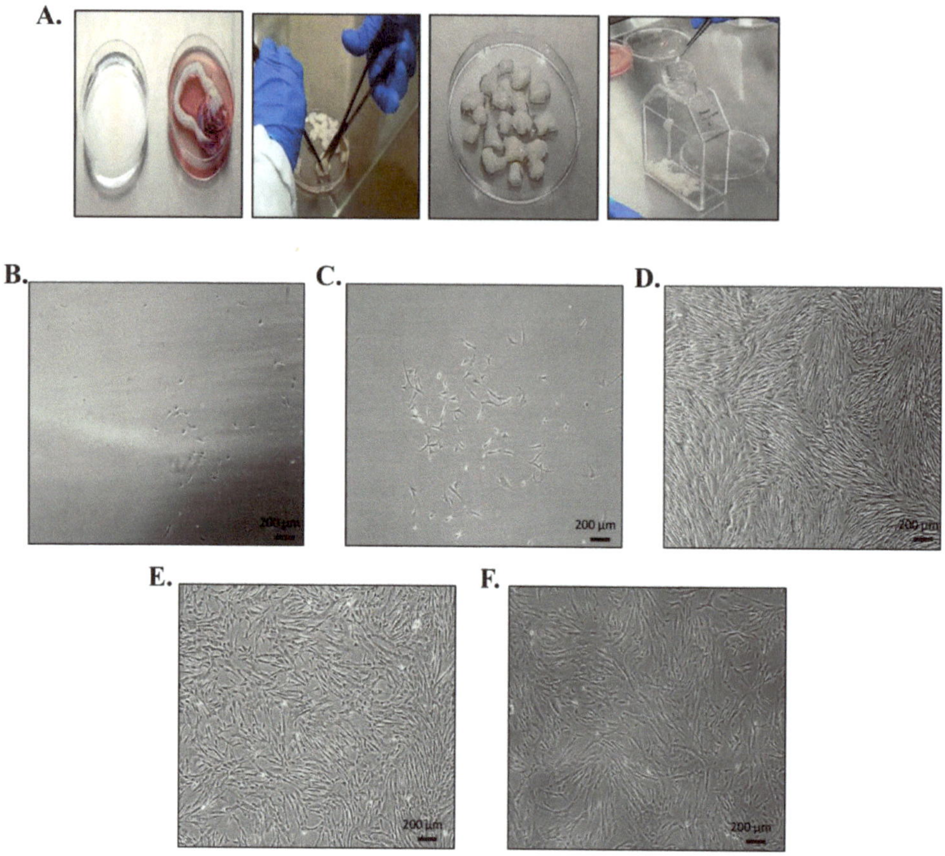

Figure 1. Umbilical cord processing; hUC-MSC isolation and propagation: hUC-MSCs were isolated from human umbilical cord. (**A**) Cord tissue was washed thoroughly, minced into small pieces (explant) and transferred to T-75 tissue culture flasks for incubation. (**B**) Cord tissue shows cell outgrowth after about 2 weeks of explant culture and (**C**) proliferating colonies of hUC-MSCs. (**D**) P0 confluent hUC-MSCs presenting fibroblast like morphology, which were subcultured to (**E**,**F**) passage 1 and passage 2, respectively.

3.2. Characterization of hUC-MSCs

hUC-MSCs characterization was performed via immunocytochemistry, flow cytometry, and trilineage differentiation potential. Immunocytochemical analysis indicated the positive expression of MSC-specific markers (CD29, CD105, Vimentin, CD117, Lin28, and Stro1) and negative expression of hematopoietic markers (CD45 and HLA-DR) as shown in Figure 2A. hUC-MSCs also showed prominent features of trilineage differentiation, i.e., mineral deposits in case of osteogenic differentiation, oil droplet formation, and proteoglycan content in case of adipogenic and chondrogenic differentiation after staining with Alizarin red, Oil red O and Alcian blue stains, respectively (Figure 2B). Flow cytometry also revealed the positive expression of MSC surface antigens (CD90, CD105, CD44, and CD73) as shown in Figure 2C.

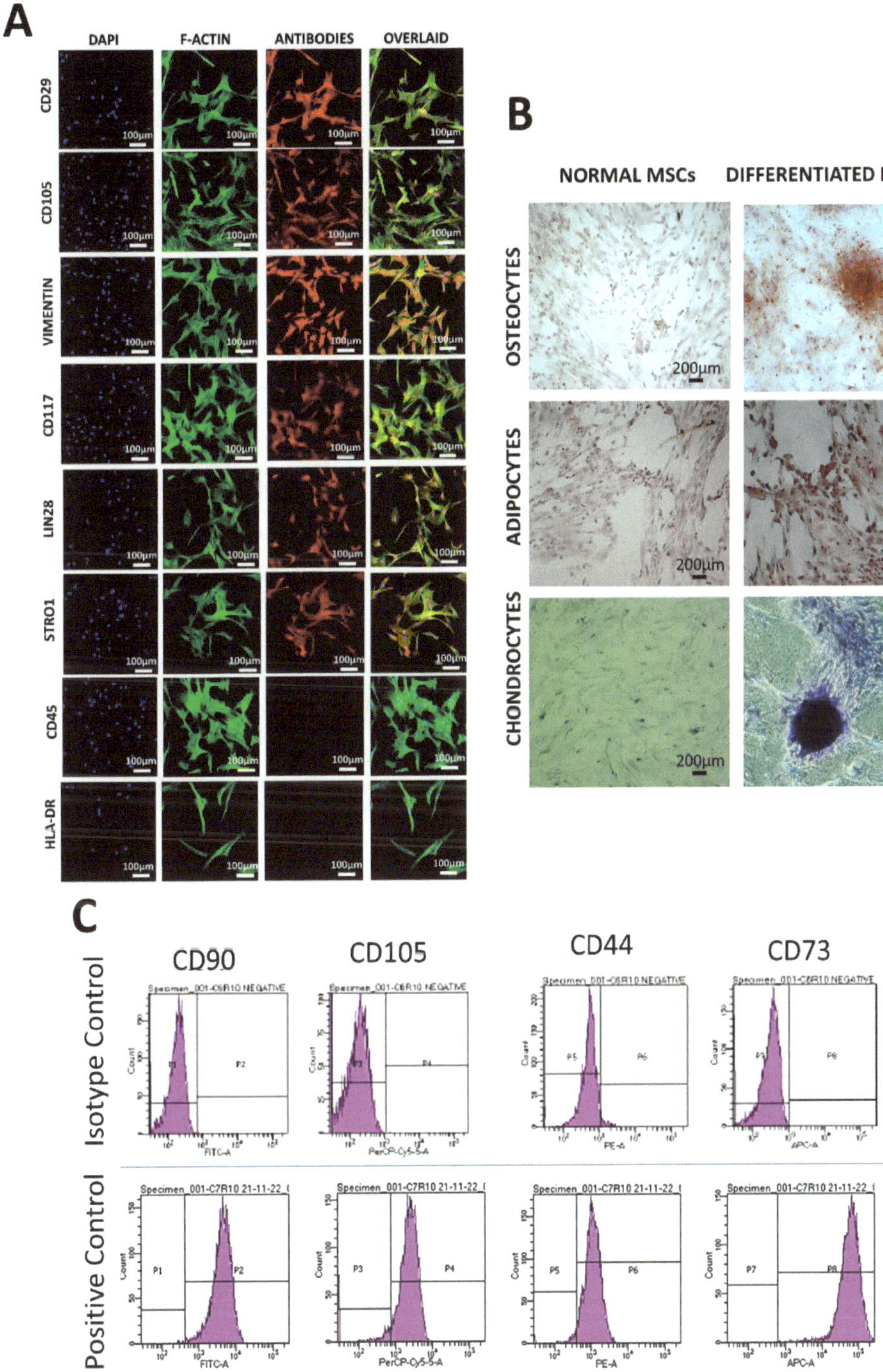

Figure 2. Characterization of mesenchymal stem cells: (**A**) hUC-MSCs showing positive expression of surface-specific markers, i.e., CD29, CD105, Vimentin, CD117, Lin28, and Stro1 and negative expression of hematopoietic markers, i.e., CD45 and HLA-DR. (**B**) Bright field images showing hUC-MSC

differentiation toward osteogenic, adipogenic, and chondrogenic lineages indicated by the presence of mineral deposits, oil droplets, and proteoglycan content, stained with Alizarin red, Oil red O, and Alcian blue stain, respectively. (**C**) Flow cytometry analysis presenting the positive expression of MSC-specific markers, i.e., CD44, CD73, CD90, and CD105.

3.3. *Transfection, Differentiation, and Morphological Assessment of hUC-MSCs*

hUC-MSCs were transfected with *OLIG2* and *MYT1L* transcription factors individually and in synergistic (*OLIG2* + *MYT1L*) groups. Transfected cells started to show slight morphological features of oligodendrocyte-like cells after 3 days of incubation in the oligo induction medium. On the seventh day of incubation, hUC-MSCs showed pronounced differentiation toward oligodendrocyte-like cells, as indicated by their morphological characteristics. Differentiation was more evident in transfected hUC-MSCs incubated in the oligo induction medium compared to normal medium.

3.4. *Gene Expression Analysis of Transfected hUC-MSCs Incubated in Normal Medium*

Gene expression analysis of the *OLIG2*, *MYT1L*, and their synergistic *(OLIG2* + *MYT1L)* transfected groups showed significant transcriptional activation of *OLIG2* and *MYT1L* genes in their respective groups compared to non-transfected control after 3 days of incubation in the normal medium. Lineage specification analysis indicated significant downregulation of *NES* and upregulation of *GFAP* and *OLIG2* genes, showing the commitment of transfected hUC-MSCs toward glial lineage. Transcriptional analysis of oligodendrocyte-specific genes revealed the substantial overexpression of *SOX10*, *NKX2.2*, *GALC*, *CNP*, *CSPG4*, *MBP*, and *PLP1*, indicating the differentiation and fate specification of hUC-MSCs toward oligodendrocyte-like cells. However, *NKX2.2* was found to be downregulated in the synergistic group (Figure 3).

3.5. *Gene Expression Analysis of Transfected hUC-MSCs Incubated in Oligo Induction Medium*

Gene expression analysis of the *OLIG2*, *MYT1L*, and their synergistic *(OLIG2* + *MYT1L)* transfected groups showed significant transcriptional activation of *OLIG2* and *MYT1L* genes in their respective groups compared to non-transfected control, after 3 days of incubation in the oligo induction medium. Lineage specification analysis of all the transfected groups indicated significant downregulation of *NES*; however, *GFAP* and *OLIG2* genes were significantly overexpressed, showing the commitment of transfected hUC-MSCs toward glial lineage. Transcriptional analysis of oligodendrocyte-specific genes revealed the upregulation of *SOX10*, *NKX2.2*, *GALC*, *CNP*, *CSPG4*, *MBP*, and *PLP1*, demonstrating the fate specification and differentiation of hUC-MSCs toward oligodendrocyte-like cells. However, *CSPG4* exhibited reduced expression in the synergistic *(OLIG2* + *MYT1L)* group as compared to the control group (Figure 4).

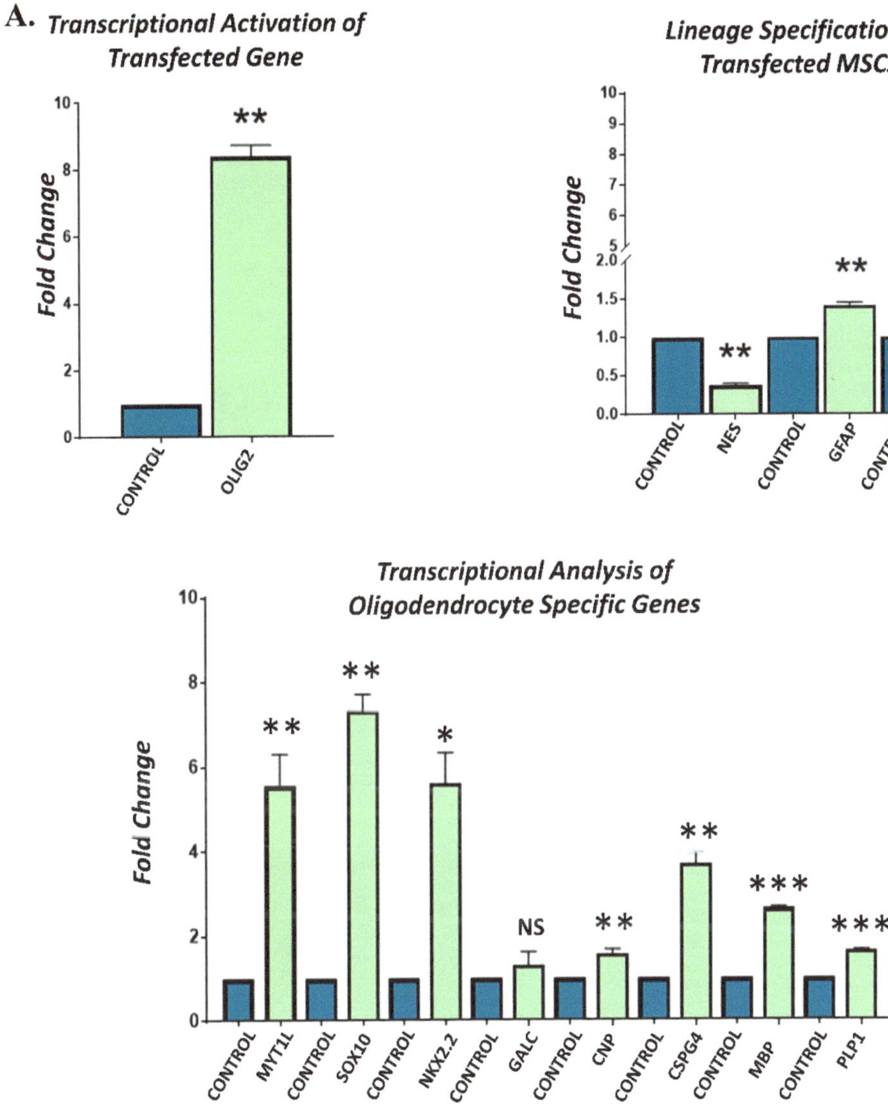

Figure 3. *Cont.*

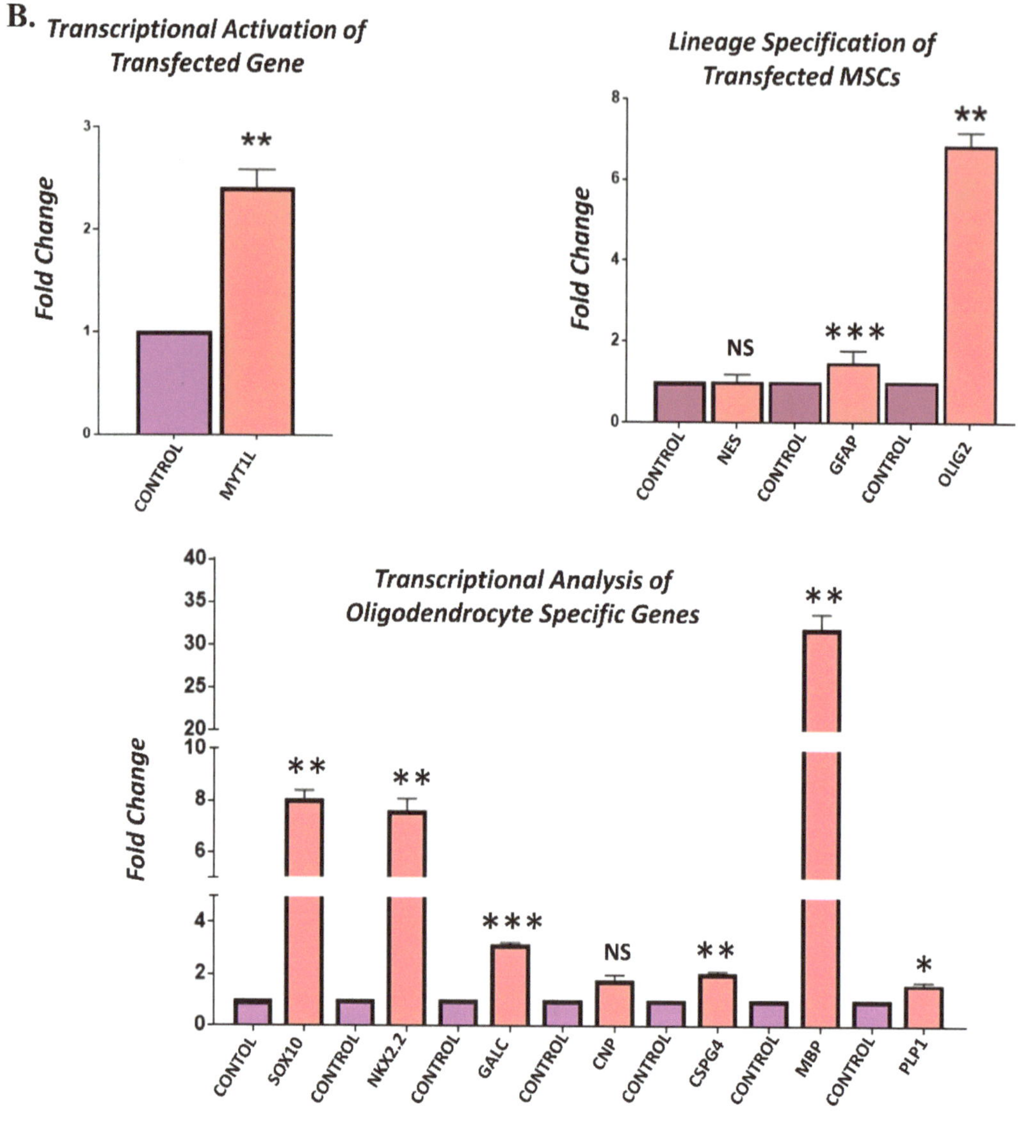

Figure 3. *Cont.*

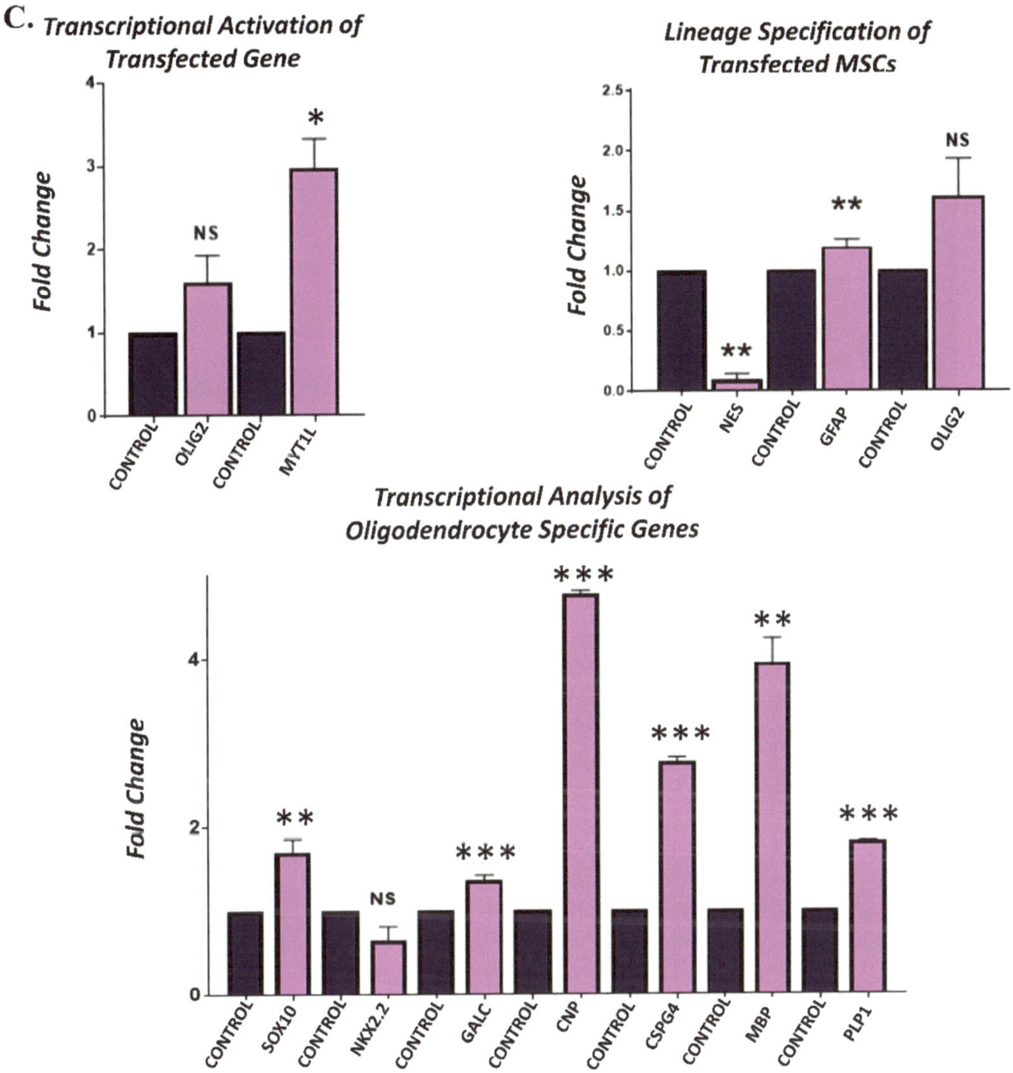

Figure 3. Gene expression analysis of transfected hUC-MSCs incubated in normal medium: qPCR analysis indicating the transcriptional activation of *OLIG2* and *MYT1L* genes in (**A**) *OLIG2*, (**B**) *MYT1L*, and (**C**) synergistic (*OLIG2* + *MYT1L*) transfected groups. Lineage specification analysis presented higher expression levels of *GFAP* and *OLIG2* in comparison to *NES*, demonstrating the glial fate specification. Transcriptional analysis of oligodendrocyte-specific genes, i.e., *SOX10*, *NKX2.2*, *GALC*, *CNP*, *CSPG4*, *MBP*, and *PLP1*, presenting their significant overexpression compared to the non-transfected control group after 3 days of incubation in normal medium. Each experiment was run in triplicates and acquired data were analyzed through an independent sample *t*-test at statistical significance level; $p \leq 0.05$ ($p < 0.05$ = *, $p < 0.01$ = **, and $p < 0.001$ = ***). NS = not significant.

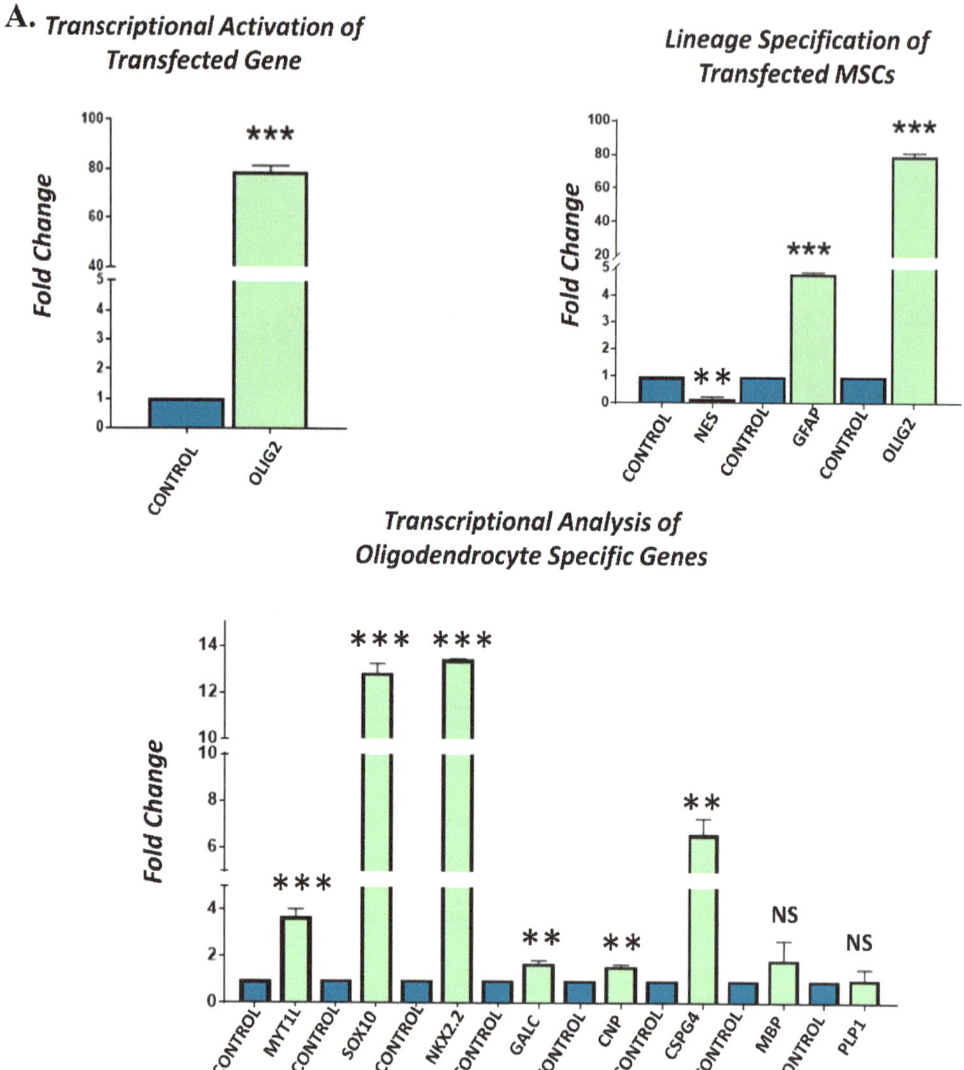

Figure 4. *Cont.*

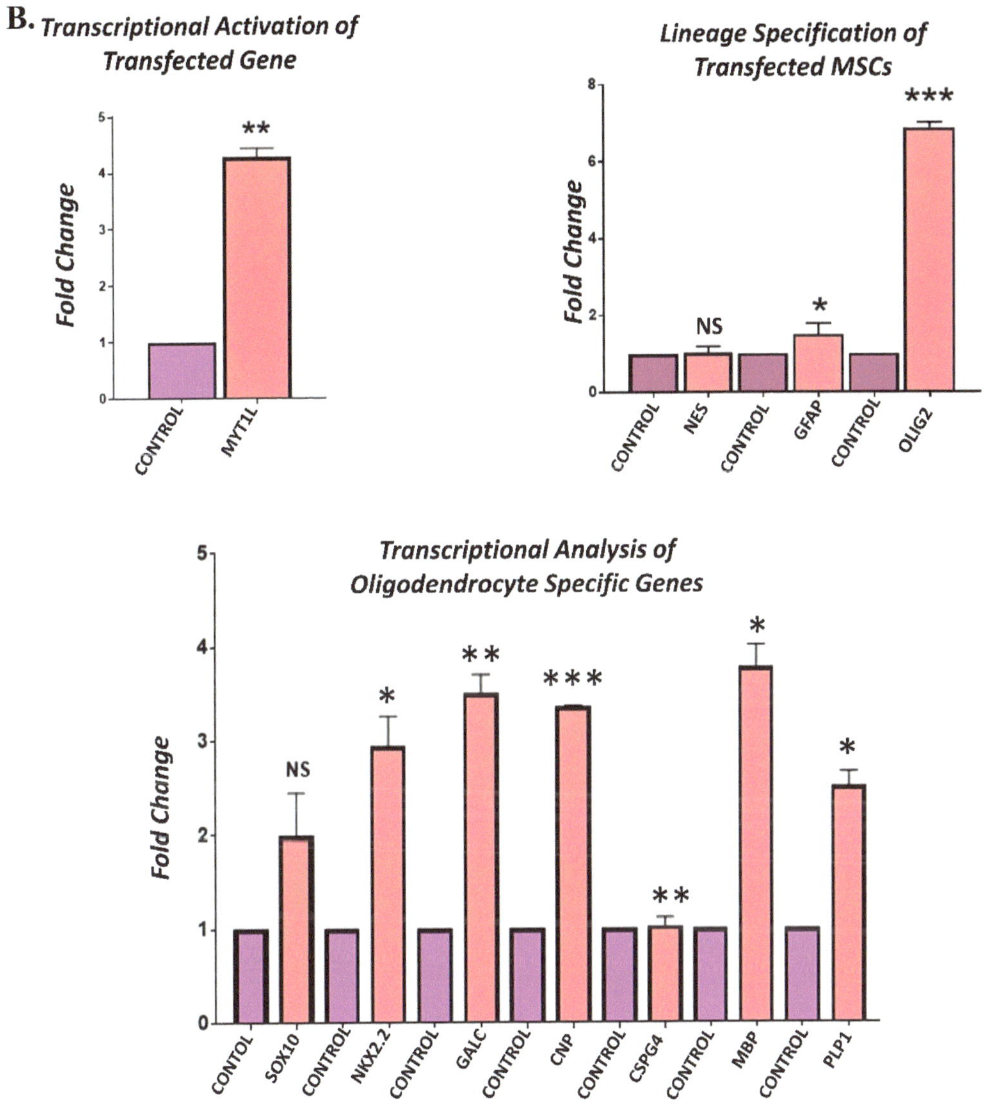

Figure 4. *Cont.*

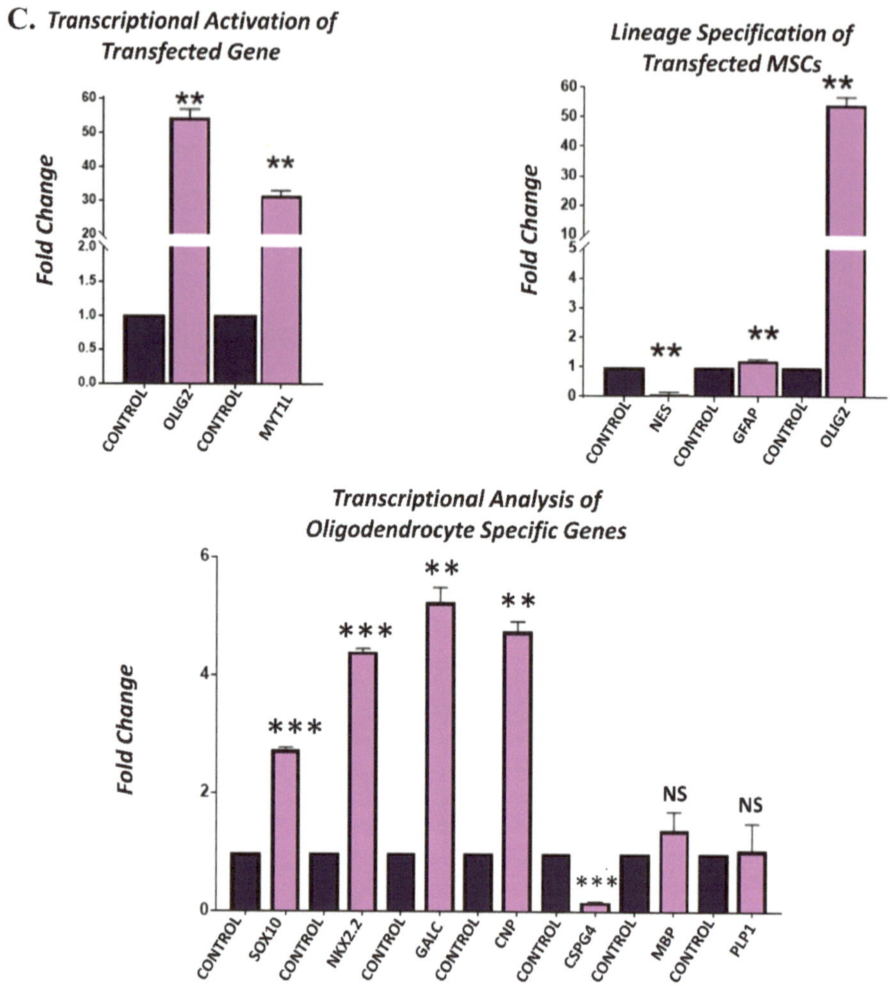

Figure 4. Gene expression analysis of transfected hUC-MSCs incubated in oligo induction medium: qPCR analysis showing the transcriptional activation of *OLIG2* and *MYT1L* genes in (**A**) *OLIG2*, (**B**) *MYT1L*, and (**C**) synergistic (*OLIG2* + *MYT1L*) transfected groups. Lineage specification analysis indicated higher expression level of *GFAP* and *OLIG2* compared to *NES*, demonstrating the glial fate specification. Transcriptional analysis of oligodendrocyte-specific genes, i.e., *SOX10*, *NKX2.2*, *GALC*, *CNP*, *CSPG4*, *MBP*, and *PLP1*, presenting their significant overexpression compared to the control group after 3 days of incubation in oligo induction medium. Each experiment was run in triplicates and acquired data were analyzed through an independent sample *t*-test at statistical significance level; $p \leq 0.05$ ($p < 0.05$ = *, $p < 0.01$ = **, and $p < 0.001$ = ***). NS = not significant.

3.6. Protein Expression Analysis of Transfected hUC-MSCs in Normal and Oligo Induction Media after 3 Days of Incubation

Immunocytochemical analysis indicated the positive expression of MYT1L, OLIG2, and NG2 and negative expression of MBP proteins in *OLIG2*, *MYT1L*, and their synergistic (*OLIG2* + *MYT1L*) transfected groups after 3 days of incubation in both normal and oligo induction media as shown in Figure 5A. Fluorescent signal exhibited by MYT1L, OLIG2, and NG2 proteins also showed a significant increase in intensities in all the transfected groups incubated in the normal medium after 3 days. However, MBP showed reduced intensity compared to the control group (Figure 5B). *OLIG2*, *MYT1L*, and their synergistic (*OLIG2* + *MYT1L*) transfected groups also showed intense fluorescent signal of MYT1L, OLIG2, and NG2 and reduced signals for MBP proteins after 3 days of incubation in the oligo induction medium compared to control group (Figure 5C).

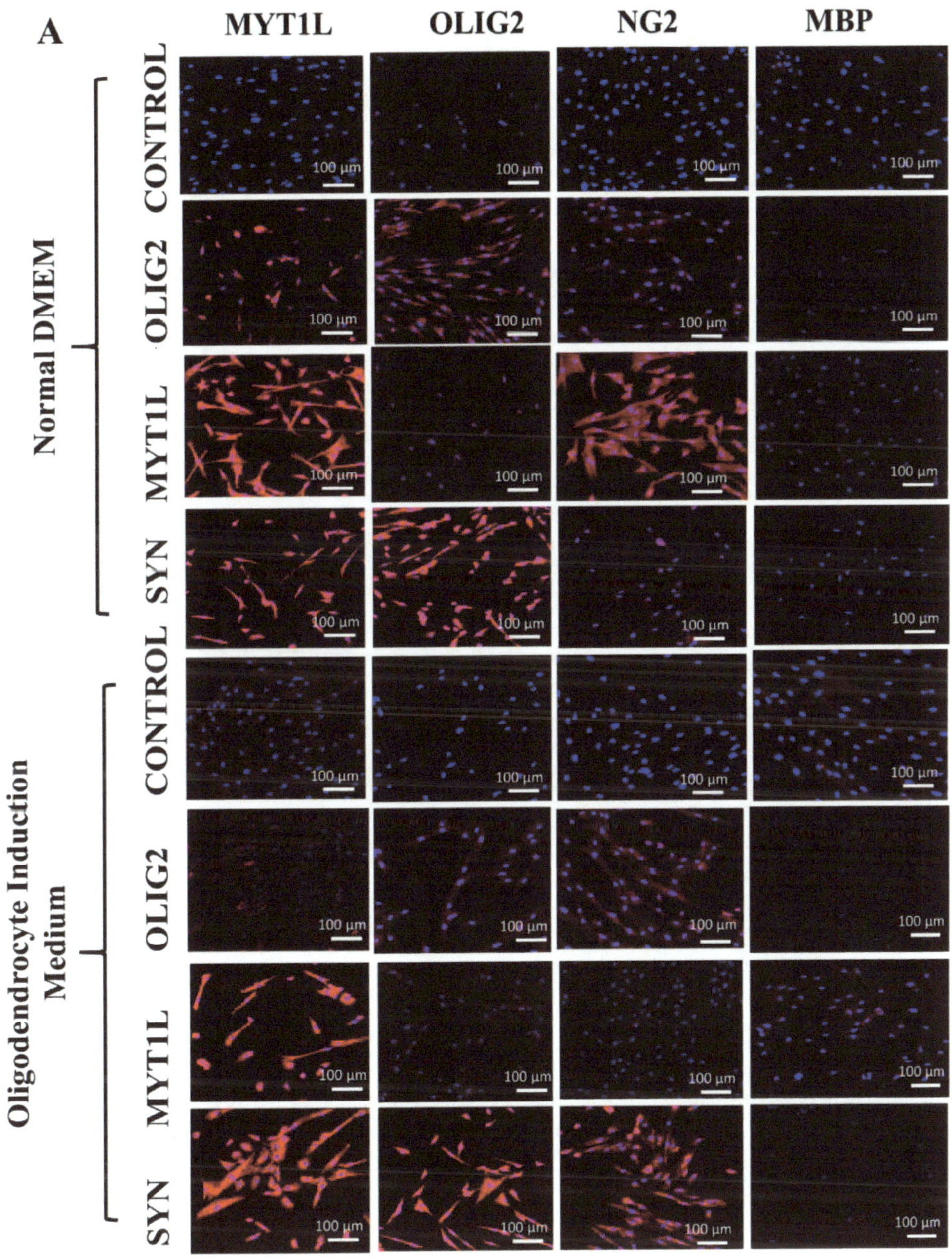

Figure 5. *Cont.*

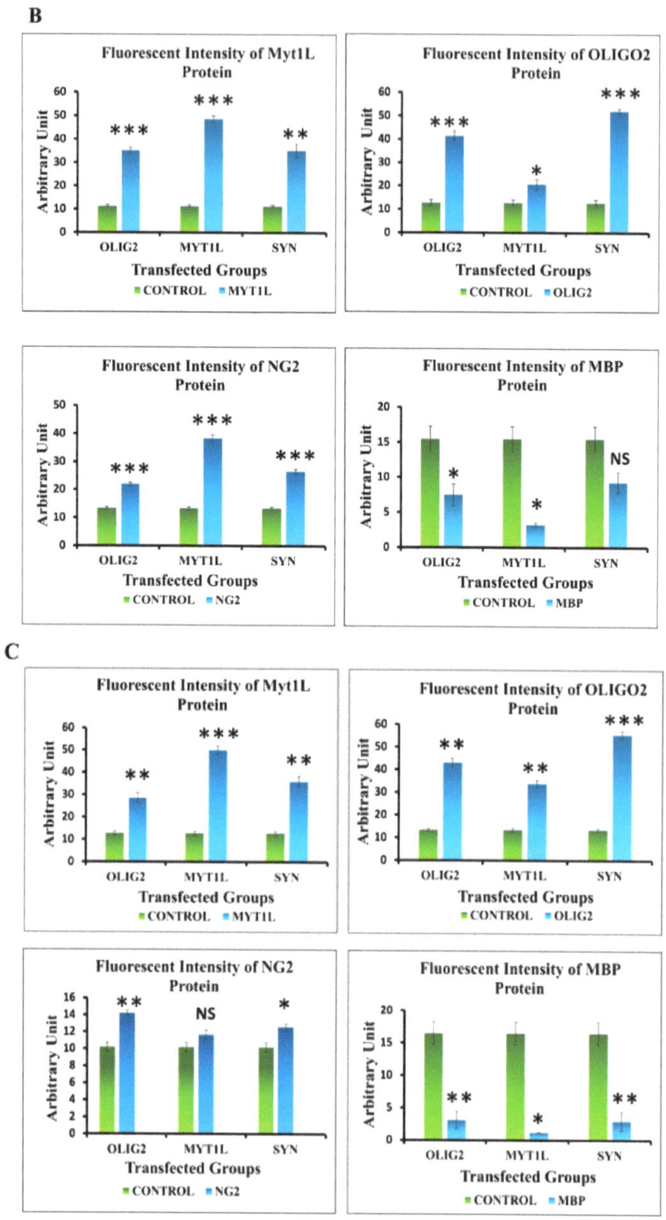

Figure 5. Protein expression/immunocytochemical analysis of transfected hUC-MSCs in normal and oligo induction media after 3 days: (**A**) Immunocytochemical analysis of *OLIG2*, *MYT1L*, and synergistic (*OLIG2* + *MYT1L*) transfected groups showing intense expression of MYT1L, OLIG2, and NG2, and a reduced expression of MBP proteins, incubated in both normal and oligo induction media. (**B**,**C**) Fluorescent intensities showing intense expression of *MYT1L*, *OLIG2*, and NG2 proteins, whereas MBP was found to exhibit reduced intensity in all the transfected groups compared to the non-transfected control group after 3 days of incubation in both normal and oligo induction media. The fluorescent values (n = 30) were analyzed through an independent sample t-test at statistical significance level; $p \leq 0.05$ ($p < 0.05$ = *, $p < 0.01$ = **, and $p < 0.001$ = ***). NS = not significant.

3.7. Protein Expression Analysis of Transfected hUC-MSCs in Normal and Oligo Induction Media after 7 Days of Incubation

Immunocytochemical analysis indicated the positive expression of oligodendrocyte-specific proteins, i.e., MYT1L, OLIG2, NG2, and MBP by differentiated hUC-MSCs in all the transfected, i.e., *OLIG2, MYT1L,* and synergistic (*OLIG2 + MYT1L*) groups after 7 days of incubation in normal and oligo induction media, as shown in Figure 6A. Fluorescent signals of MYT1L, OLIG2, NG2, and MBP proteins also showed a significant increase in intensities in all the transfected groups in the normal medium after 7 days of incubation, except the *OLIG2*-transfected group, which showed a reduced MBP intensity (Figure 6B). *OLIG2, MYT1L,* and their synergistic (*OLIG2 + MYT1L*) transfected groups showed an intense expression of MYT1L, OLIG2, NG2, and MBP proteins after 7 days of incubation compared to the control group in the oligo induction medium (Figure 6C).

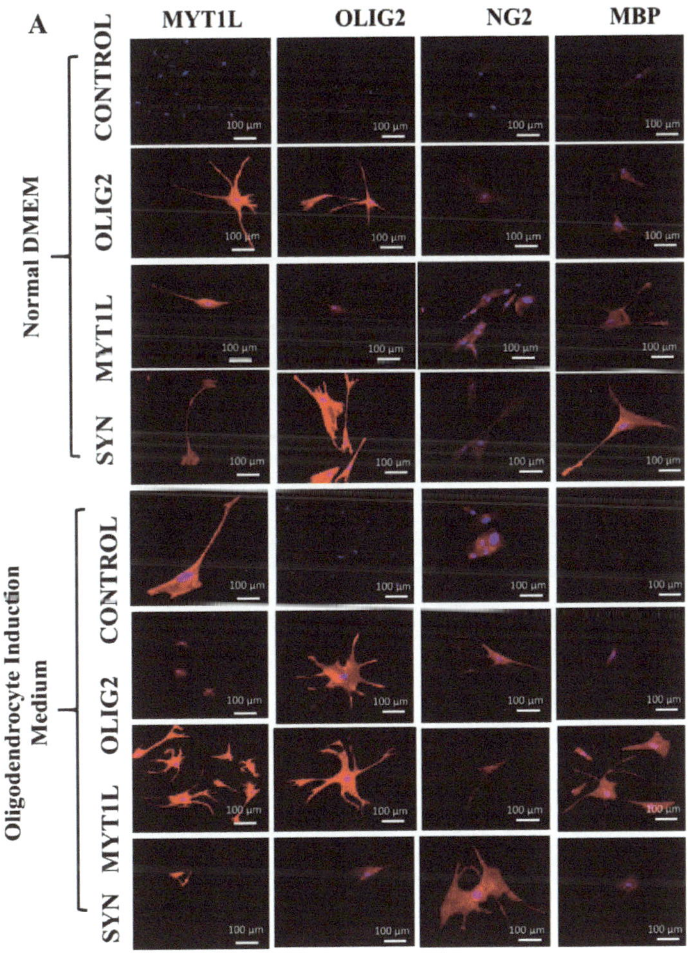

Figure 6. *Cont.*

B.

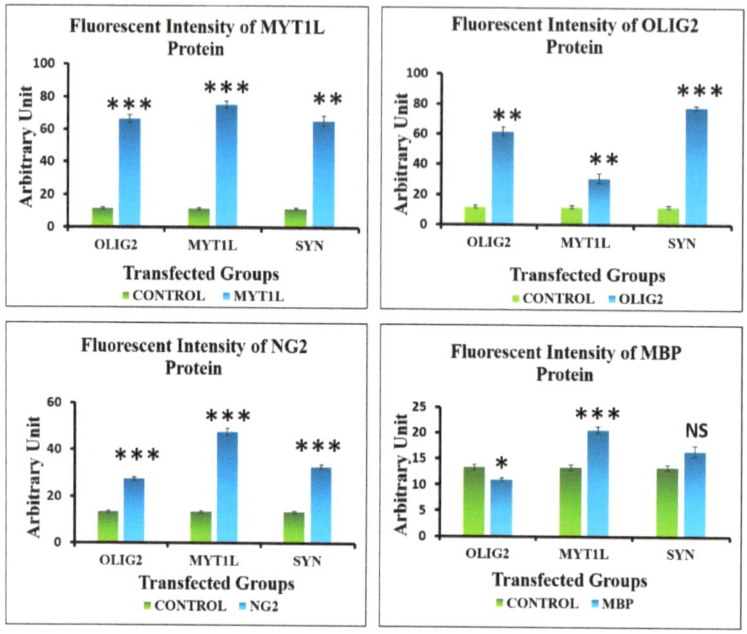

C.

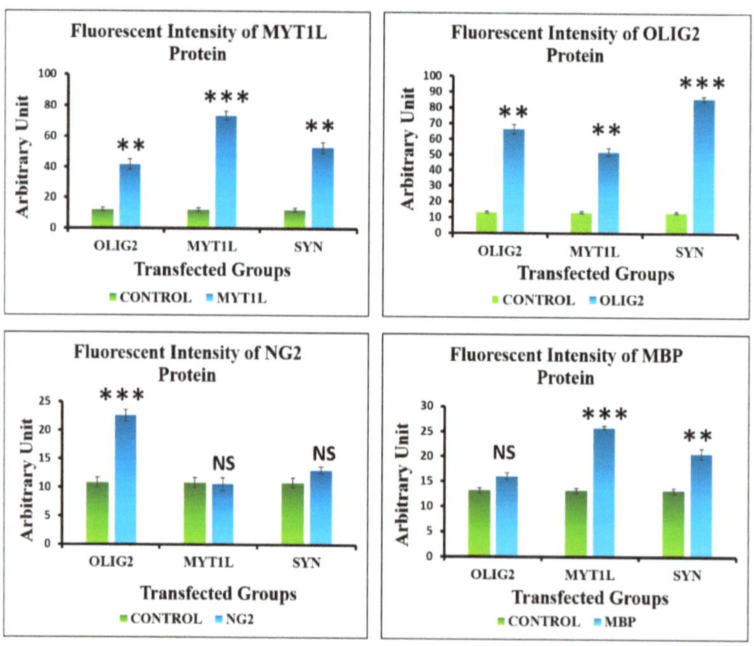

Figure 6. Protein expression/immunocytochemical analysis of transfected hUC-MSCs in normal and oligo induction media after 7 days: (**A**) Immunocytochemical analysis of *OLIG2*, *MYT1L*, and synergistic (*OLIG2* + *MYT1L*) transfected groups, indicating positive expression of MYT1L, OLIG2, NG2, and MBP proteins. (**B**,**C**) Fluorescent intensities showing intense expression of oligodendrocyte-

specific proteins, i.e., MYT1L, OLIG2, NG2, and MBP in all the transfected groups as compared to the non-transfected control group after 7 days of incubation in both normal and oligo induction media. However, the OLIG2-transfected group exhibited reduced fluorescence signals of MBP in the normal medium. The fluorescent values (n = 30) were analyzed through an independent sample t-test at statistical significance level; $p \leq 0.05$ ($p < 0.05$ = *, $p < 0.01$ = **, and $p < 0.001$ = ***). NS = not significant.

4. Discussion

The current study demonstrates the effective role of transcriptional regulators (*OLIG2* and *MYT1L*) as a remarkable tool for stimulating myelin repair in lethal demyelinating disorders using cell-based therapeutic approach. Such disorders are often characterized by the loss of oligodendrocytes (OLs). These cells play a fundamental role to provide metabolic support to axons and are responsible for the appropriate conduction of nerve impulse; therefore, an injury or damage to OLs result in neurodegeneration [1]. OLs and their progenitor cells (OPC) are the potential promising targets for cell-based regenerative applications due to their less diversified functional features and greater region/subtype specificity compared to neurons [3,25].

Presently, there is no effective treatment available for MS. Current pharmacological therapies only offer symptom management and slow down the disease progression by modulating the immune response or inflammatory cascades [26].

Therefore, there is a need to find treatment strategies that can facilitate endogenous myelination, thus favoring neuroprotection. Recent studies have reported the effective role of cell-based therapies for neurological and demyelinating disorders. In this context, mesenchymal stem cells are the attractive candidate due to their multilineage differentiation toward cells of all lineages, i.e., ectoderm, endoderm, and mesoderm. MSCs have also been reported to exhibit remarkable regeneration potential, self-renewal capabilities, and immunomodulatory features [2,12]. MSCs are also effective to treat neurological disorders and exhibit neuroprotective features which make them an attractive candidate for cell-based therapies [20,26].

A study conducted on BM-MSCs-derived oligodendrocyte precursor cells (OPCs) was found to boost remyelination and reduce demyelination after their differentiation into mature oligodendrocytes in animal models [27]. hUC-MSCs have also been shown to improve behavioral functions and reduce the histopathological deficits in EAE mice over a long term (i.e., 50 days) by inhibiting perivascular immune cell infiltrations and reducing demyelination and axonal injury in the spinal cord [28]. A recently conducted study on Wharton's jelly-derived MSCs has shown their enhanced remyelination potential and increased oligodendrocyte count in a cuprizone-induced MS model [29].

In the present study, hUC-MSCs were isolated from the human umbilical cord and characterized based on their native features, i.e., presence of surface-specific markers and trilineage differentiation potential. Our preliminary study was categorized into two main parts to assess the effect of two different media compositions, i.e., normal and oligo induction media (5% FBS-supplemented OPTI-MEM, 0.1 mM β- mercaptoethanol, and B-27 supplement-2x) on MSC fate specification and differentiation via their genetic modification by inserting oligodendrocyte-specific transcription factors, i.e., *OLIG2* and *MYT1L*. To achieve this ultimate objective, *OLIG2* and *MYT1L* plasmids were used to transfect hUC-MSCs individually and in synergistic (*OLIG2* + *MYT1L*) groups, through a non-viral gene transfer method, using Lipofectamine® 3000 transfection reagent. Non-viral gene expression of the transcription factors has been reported to serve as a powerful transfection strategy that facilitates the stable delivery of transcription factors and allows their transcriptional activation [18].

Transfected cells were incubated in normal and oligo induction media and observed for differentiation by examining their morphological features. We observed the induction of differentiation on day 3 with no apparent change in morphology; however, hUC-MSCs after 7 days of incubation in the oligo induction medium indicated prominent cell differentiation with characteristic morphological features of oligodendrocyte-like cells. The differentiation potential of MSCs toward oligodendrocytes has also been reported previously by other studies [22].

Gene expression profile of transfected hUC-MSCs showed transcriptional activation of *OLIG2* and *MYT1L* genes in their respective transfected groups, indicating the induction of differentiation. To assess the fate specification of transfected hUC-MSCs, lineage-specific markers were analyzed, which revealed the downregulation of neuronal stem cell marker (*NES)* and upregulation of glial lineage markers, i.e., *GFAP* and *OLIG2*. Higher expression of *OLIG2* gene compared to *GFAP* demonstrates the fate specification of MSCs toward oligodendrocytes.

MSC differentiation was further assessed by analyzing the expression of oligodendrocyte-specific markers (*SOX10, NKX2.2, GALC, CNP, CSPG4, MBP*, and *PLP*1). Expression of these genes was found to be significantly upregulated in all the transfected groups and it was more pronounced in the oligo induction medium in comparison to the normal medium, demonstrating the differentiation and fate specification of MSCs toward oligodendrocytes. Expression of these OL markers demonstrates the differentiated state of transfected cells. Overexpression of *SOX10* and *OLIG2* has also been reported previously to induce oligodendrocyte differentiation, thereby acting as the master regulatory genes. *OLIG2* and *NKX2.2* have also been shown to support the development of OPC lineage, and *Myt1L* expression by mature oligodendrocytes is associated with myelination and remyelination [30,31].

We also determined the protein expression by immunocytochemistry. The differentiated hUC-MSCs significantly expressed oligodendrocyte-specific proteins, i.e., OLIG2, MYT1L, and NG2 after 3 and 7 days of incubation in normal and oligo induction media, as indicated by their fluorescent intensities. Fluorescent signals were found to be significantly higher in the oligo induction medium as compared to the normal medium. Taken together these findings, our study demonstrates the fundamental role of *OLIG2* and *MYT1L* transcription factors in hUC-MSCs differentiation toward oligodendrocyte-like cells, which were greatly facilitated by the oligo induction medium, emphasizing the significance of transcriptional regulators as a remarkable tool for stimulating myelin repair in lethal demyelinating disorders. Further studies are required to explore the mechanism behind oligodendrocyte differentiation and to analyze their myelination potential in animal models of demyelinating disorder. The findings of the study may serve as a promising cell-based therapeutic modality in treating demyelinating and neurodegenerative ailments.

5. Conclusions

The overall findings of our study conclude that *OLIG2* and *MYT1L* play a crucial role to induce hUC-MSC differentiation toward oligodendrocyte-like cells in both normal and oligo induction media at gene and protein levels. However, hUC-MSC differentiation and fate specification were greatly facilitated by the oligo induction medium. The study emphasizes the role of the transcription regulator as a remarkable tool for stimulating myelin repair in lethal demyelinating disorders. These findings may help to develop cell-based therapeutic strategies for demyelinating diseases and their use in future clinical studies.

Author Contributions: I.F.: Conducted experiments and wrote the original manuscript. A.I.: Evaluated and analyzed the data, and reviewed the manuscript. F.R.: Helped in manuscript preparation and evaluation. S.A.B.A.S.: Evaluated and analyzed the data. A.A.: Helped in data analysis and writing and secured the funding. A.S.: Analyzed and evaluated the data and helped in manuscript finalization. I.K.: Conceived and designed the study, evaluated and analyzed the data, and finalized the manuscript. All authors have read and agreed to the published version of the manuscript.

Funding: The study was partially supported by the Higher Education Commission Pakistan, NRPU. Grant no. 6573.

Institutional Review Board Statement: The study was approved with reference no. IEC-009-UCB-2015.

Informed Consent Statement: Formal written consent was obtained.

Data Availability Statement: No additional data to provide.

Acknowledgments: Authors acknowledge the imaging facility of Dr. Panjwani Center for Molecular Medicine and Drug Research.

Conflicts of Interest: Authors declare no conflict of Interest.

References

1. Cruz-Martinez, P.; González-Granero, S.; Molina-Navarro, M.M.; Pacheco-Torres, J.; García-Verdugo, J.M.; Geijo-Barrientos, E.; Jones, J.; Martinez, S. Intraventricular Injections of Mesenchymal Stem Cells Activate Endogenous Functional Remyelination in a Chronic Demyelinating Murine Model. *Cell Death Dis.* **2016**, *7*, e2223. [CrossRef] [PubMed]
2. Dulamea, A.O. The Contribution of Oligodendrocytes and Oligodendrocyte Progenitor Cells to Central Nervous System Repair in Multiple Sclerosis: Perspectives for Remyelination Therapeutic Strategies. *Neural Regen. Res.* **2017**, *12*, 1939–1944. [CrossRef] [PubMed]
3. Lopez, J.A.; Denkova, M.; Ramanathan, S.; Dale, R.C.; Brilot, F. Pathogenesis of Autoimmune Demyelination: From Multiple Sclerosis to Neuromyelitis Optica Spectrum Disorders and Myelin Oligodendrocyte Glycoprotein Antibody-Associated Disease. *Clin. Transl. Immunol.* **2021**, *10*, e1316. [CrossRef] [PubMed]
4. Wang, F.; Tang, H.; Zhu, J.; Zhang, J.H. Transplanting Mesenchymal Stem Cells for Treatment of Ischemic Stroke. *Cell Transplant.* **2018**, *27*, 1825–1834. [CrossRef] [PubMed]
5. Ishaque, A.; Salim, A.; Simjee, S.U.; Khan, I.; Adli, D.S.H. Alpha Terpineol Directs Bone Marrow Mesenchymal Stem Cells toward Neuronal Lineage through Regulation of Wnt Signaling Pathway. *Cell Biochem. Funct.* **2023**, *41*, 223–233. [CrossRef]
6. Islam, M.A.; Kundu, S.; Hassan, R. Gene Therapy Approaches in an Autoimmune Demyelinating Disease: Multiple Sclerosis. *Curr. Gene Ther.* **2020**, *19*, 376–385. [CrossRef]
7. Stangel, M.; Penner, I.K.; Kallmann, B.A.; Lukas, C.; Kieseier, B.C. Towards the Implementation of 'no Evidence of Disease Activity' in Multiple Sclerosis Treatment: The Multiple Sclerosis Decision Model. *Ther. Adv. Neurol. Disord.* **2015**, *8*, 3–13. [CrossRef]
8. Harris, V.K.; Sadiq, S.A. Biomarkers of Therapeutic Response in Multiple Sclerosis: Current Status. *Mol. Diagn. Ther.* **2014**, *18*, 605–617. [CrossRef]
9. Aslam, S.; Khan, I.; Jameel, F.; Zaidi, M.B.; Salim, A. Umbilical Cord-Derived Mesenchymal Stem Cells Preconditioned with Isorhamnetin: Potential Therapy for Burn Wounds. *World J. Stem Cells* **2020**, *12*, 1652–1666. [CrossRef]
10. Scopetti, M.; Santurro, A.; Gatto, V.; Russa, R.L.; Manetti, F.; Errico, S.D.; Frati, P.; Fineschi, V. Mesenchymal Stem Cells in Neurodegenerative Diseases: Opinion Review on Ethical Dilemmas. *World J. Stem Cells* **2020**, *12*, 168–177. [CrossRef]
11. Khanabdali, R.; Saadat, A.; Fazilah, M.; Bazli, K.F.K.; Qazi, R.e.M.; Khalid, R.S.; Hasan Adli, D.S.; Moghadamtousi, S.Z.; Naeem, N.; Khan, I.; et al. Promoting Effect of Small Molecules in Cardiomyogenic and Neurogenic Differentiation of Rat Bone Marrow-Derived Mesenchymal Stem Cells. *Drug Des. Devel. Ther.* **2016**, *10*, 81–91. [CrossRef] [PubMed]
12. Alanazi, A.; Alassiri, M.; Jawdat, D.; Almalik, Y. Mesenchymal Stem Cell Therapy: A Review of Clinical Trials for Multiple Sclerosis. *Regen. Ther.* **2022**, *21*, 201–209. [CrossRef] [PubMed]
13. Turano, E.; Scambi, I.; Virla, F.; Bonetti, B.; Mariotti, R. Extracellular Vesicles from Mesenchymal Stem Cells: Towards Novel Therapeutic Strategies for Neurodegenerative Diseases. *Int. J. Mol. Sci.* **2023**, *24*, 2917. [CrossRef] [PubMed]
14. Oppliger, B.; Joerger-Messerli, M.S.; Simillion, C.; Mueller, M.; Surbek, D.V.; Schoeberlein, A. Mesenchymal Stromal Cells from Umbilical Cord Wharton's Jelly Trigger Oligodendroglial Differentiation in Neural Progenitor Cells through Cell-to-Cell Contact. *Cytotherapy* **2017**, *19*, 829–838. [CrossRef] [PubMed]
15. Ishaque, A.; Khan, I.; Salim, A.; Qazi, R.E.M.; Malick, T.S.; Adli, D.S.H. Effect of α-Pinene and Thymoquinone on the Differentiation of Bone Marrow Mesenchymal Stem Cells into Neuroprogenitor Cells. *BioImpacts* **2022**, *12*, 147–154. [CrossRef]
16. Sun, L.; Wang, F.; Chen, H.; Liu, D.; Qu, T.; Li, X.; Xu, D.; Liu, F.; Yin, Z.; Chen, Y. Co-Transplantation of Human Umbilical Cord Mesenchymal Stem Cells and Human Neural Stem Cells Improves the Outcome in Rats with Spinal Cord Injury. *Cell Transplant.* **2019**, *28*, 147–154. [CrossRef]
17. Zhang, J.; Li, Y.; Chen, J.; Cui, Y.; Lu, M.; Elias, S.B.; Mitchell, J.B.; Hammill, L.; Vanguri, P.; Chopp, M. Human Bone Marrow Stromal Cell Treatment Improves Neurological Functional Recovery in EAE Mice. *Exp. Neurol.* **2005**, *195*, 16–26. [CrossRef]
18. Shiri, E.; Pasbakhsh, P.; Borhani-Haghighi, M.; Alizadeh, Z.; Nekoonam, S.; Mojaverrostami, S.; Pirhajati Mahabadi, V.; Mehdi, A.; Zibara, K.; Kashani, I.R. Mesenchymal Stem Cells Ameliorate Cuprizone-Induced Demyelination by Targeting Oxidative Stress and Mitochondrial Dysfunction. *Cell. Mol. Neurobiol.* **2021**, *41*, 1467–1481. [CrossRef]
19. Coursimault, J.; Guerrot, A.M.; Morrow, M.M.; Schramm, C.; Zamora, F.M.; Shanmugham, A.; Liu, S.; Zou, F.; Bilan, F.; Le Guyader, G.; et al. MYT1L-Associated Neurodevelopmental Disorder: Description of 40 New Cases and Literature Review of Clinical and Molecular Aspects. *Hum. Genet.* **2022**, *141*, 65–80. [CrossRef]
20. Tahmasebi, F.; Pasbakhsh, P.; Barati, S.; Madadi, S.; Kashani, I.R. The Effect of Microglial Ablation and Mesenchymal Stem Cell Transplantation on a Cuprizone-Induced Demyelination Model. *J. Cell. Physiol.* **2021**, *236*, 3552–3564. [CrossRef]
21. Popescu, B.F.G.; Lucchinetti, C.F. Pathology of Demyelinating Diseases. *Annu. Rev. Pathol. Mech. Dis.* **2012**, *7*, 185–217. [CrossRef] [PubMed]

22. Matjusaitis, M.; Wagstaff, L.J.; Martella, A.; Baranowski, B.; Blin, C.; Gogolok, S.; Williams, A.; Pollard, S.M. Reprogramming of Fibroblasts to Oligodendrocyte Progenitor-like Cells Using CRISPR/Cas9-Based Synthetic Transcription Factors. *Stem Cell Rep.* **2019**, *13*, 1053–1067. [CrossRef]
23. Khalid, S.; Ekram, S.; Salim, A.; Chaudhry, G.R.; Khan, I. Transcription Regulators Differentiate Mesenchymal Stem Cells into Chondroprogenitors, and Their in Vivo Implantation Regenerated the Intervertebral Disc Degeneration. *World J. Stem Cells* **2022**, *14*, 163–182. [CrossRef] [PubMed]
24. Ekram, S.; Khalid, S.; Bashir, I.; Salim, A.; Khan, I. Human Umbilical Cord-Derived Mesenchymal Stem Cells and Their Chondroprogenitor Derivatives Reduced Pain and Inflammation Signaling and Promote Regeneration in a Rat Intervertebral Disc Degeneration Model. *Mol. Cell. Biochem.* **2021**, *476*, 3191–3205. [CrossRef]
25. Stadelmann, C.; Timmler, S.; Barrantes-Freer, A.; Simons, M. Myelin in the Central Nervous System: Structure, Function, and Pathology. *Physiol. Rev.* **2019**, *99*, 1381–1431. [CrossRef] [PubMed]
26. Mojaverrostami, S.; Khadivi, F.; Zarini, D.; Mohammadi, A. Combination Effects of Mesenchymal Stem Cells Transplantation and Anodal Transcranial Direct Current Stimulation on a Cuprizone-Induced Mouse Model of Multiple Sclerosis. *J. Mol. Histol.* **2022**, *53*, 817–831. [CrossRef]
27. Bojnordi, M.N.; Ghasemi, H.H.; Akbari, E. Remyelination after Lysophosphatidyl Choline-Induced Demyelination Is Stimulated by Bone Marrow Stromal Cell-Derived Oligoprogenitor Cell Transplantation. *Cells Tissues Organs* **2015**, *200*, 300–306. [CrossRef]
28. Liu, R.; Zhang, Z.; Lu, Z.; Borlongan, C.; Pan, J.; Chen, J.; Qian, L.; Liu, Z.; Zhu, L.; Zhang, J.; et al. Human Umbilical Cord Stem Cells Ameliorate Experimental Autoimmune Encephalomyelitis by Regulating Immunoinflammation and Remyelination. *Stem Cells Dev.* **2013**, *22*, 1053–1062. [CrossRef]
29. Zhang, K.; Chen, S.; Yang, Q.; Guo, S.; Chen, Q.; Liu, Z.; Li, L.; Jiang, M.; Li, H.; Hu, J.; et al. The Oligodendrocyte Transcription Factor 2 OLIG2 Regulates Transcriptional Repression during Myelinogenesis in Rodents. *Nat. Commun.* **2022**, *13*, 1423. [CrossRef]
30. Xing, L.; Chai, R.; Wang, J.; Lin, J.; Li, H.; Wang, Y.; Lai, B.; Sun, J.; Chen, G. Expression of Myelin Transcription Factor 1 and Lamin B Receptor Mediate Neural Progenitor Fate Transition in the Zebrafish Spinal Cord PMN Domain. *J. Biol. Chem.* **2022**, *298*, 102452. [CrossRef]
31. Shi, Y.; Shao, Q.; Li, Z.; Gonzalez, G.A.; Lu, F.; Wang, D.; Pu, Y.; Huang, A.; Zhao, C.; He, C.; et al. Myt1L Promotes Differentiation of Oligodendrocyte Precursor Cells and Is Necessary for Remyelination After Lysolecithin-Induced Demyelination. *Neurosci. Bull.* **2018**, *34*, 247–260. [CrossRef] [PubMed]

current issues in molecular biology

Review

Therapeutic Plasma Exchange and Multiple Sclerosis Dysregulations: Focus on the Removal of Pathogenic Circulatory Factors and Altering Nerve Growth Factor and Sphingosine-1-Phosphate Plasma Levels

Dimitar Tonev [1,*] and Albena Momchilova [2]

1 Department of Anesthesiology and Intensive Care, University Hospital "Tzaritza Yoanna—ISUL", Medical University of Sofia, 1527 Sofia, Bulgaria
2 Institute of Biophysics and Biomedical Engineering, Bulgarian Academy of Science, 1113 Sofia, Bulgaria; albena_momchilova@abv.bg
* Correspondence: dgtsofia@abv.bg

Abstract: Multiple sclerosis (MS) is predominantly an immune-mediated disease of the central nervous system (CNS) of unknown etiology with a possible genetic predisposition and effect of certain environmental factors. It is generally accepted that the disease begins with an autoimmune inflammatory reaction targeting oligodendrocytes followed by a rapid depletion of their regenerative capacity with subsequent permanent neurodegenerative changes and disability. Recent research highlights the central role of B lymphocytes and the corresponding IgG and IgM autoantibodies in newly forming MS lesions. Thus, their removal along with the modulation of certain bioactive molecules to improve neuroprotection using therapeutic plasma exchange (TPE) becomes of utmost importance. Recently, it has been proposed to determine the levels and precise effects of both beneficial and harmful components in the serum of MS patients undergoing TPE to serve as markers for appropriate TPE protocols. In this review we discuss some relevant examples, focusing on the removal of pathogenic circulating factors and altering the plasma levels of nerve growth factor and sphingosine-1-phosphate by TPE. Altered plasma levels of the reviewed molecular compounds in response to TPE reflect a successful reduction of the pro-inflammatory burden at the expense of an increase in anti-inflammatory potential in the circulatory and CNS compartments.

Keywords: multiple sclerosis; immune pathophysiology; autoantibodies; nerve growth factor; sphingosine-1-phosphate; therapeutic plasma exchange; neuroprotection

1. Introduction

Multiple sclerosis (MS) is an autoimmune multifocal central nervous system (CNS) inflammatory disease, characterized by chronic inflammation, demyelination, axonal damage, and subsequent gliosis. The disease is of unknown etiology with a possible genetic predisposition and effect of certain environmental factors [1,2]. Although there is no complete consensus regarding the pathological processes leading to MS, it is generally accepted that the disease begins with an autoimmune inflammatory reaction targeting oligodendrocytes (OLs) followed by a rapid depletion of OLs regenerative capacity with subsequent permanent neurodegenerative changes and disability [3]. Therefore, the therapeutic efforts should be focused with priority on the first stage of demyelination, when the damage is not yet irreversible. The most efficient treatment modality for neurodegeneration remains an early and aggressive anti-inflammatory intervention, because the prevention of tissue injury may best control the escalating T-cell-driven and bystander B-cell activation, ongoing breakdown of blood–brain barrier (BBB) and epitope spreading, that may perpetuate neuroaxonal damage [4]. After the impressive efficacy of anti-CD20 antibody therapy for patients with a relapsing–remitting form of the disease, there is renewed attention to B cells in the pathogenesis of MS [5]. Recent research highlights the central role of B lymphocytes in the development of MS lesions, in particular the main role of IgG and IgM in newly forming lesions [6]. Thus, early and aggressive control of antibodies contributing to oligodendrocyte and axonal damage in MS becomes of utmost importance. However, the questionable efficacy of anti-CD20 therapy in reducing the antibody levels [7], along with its delayed onset of action compared to the rapid action of therapeutic apheresis, raised issues of combination therapies in general [8] and between apheresis and anti-CD20 antibody therapy in particular [9]. On the other hand, although pathogenetically justified, the role of apheresis (or therapeutic plasma exchange (TPE), a term used interchangeably) in MS patients still has a limited and even questioned application [7,10]. As usually happens, the latter critical review could pave the way for searching for new answers. It was suggested that further studies should be undertaken to determine the levels and precise effects of both beneficial and harmful components in sera of MS patients during different phases of the disease in terms of their capability to serve as markers for appropriate TPE protocols [10]. The aim of our review is to discuss some relevant examples of the proposed field of new research, focusing on the removal of pathogenic circulating factors and altering the plasma levels of nerve growth factor (NGF) and sphingosine-1-phosphate (S1P) by TPE and their impact on MS dysregulations.

In this focus review, after the short summary of the pathogenesis, we explore the relevant data on autoantibodies, NGF, S1P, and TPE regarding MS, from both detrimental and beneficial points of view.

2. Methodology

A literature search was conducted through June 2023 of MEDLINE, EMBASE, and Cochrane Library, based on Medical Subject Heading (MeSH) of "therapeutic plasma exchange", "nanomembrane-based", "plasmapheresis", "apheresis", immuno-mediated", "autoimmune", "neurological", "disorders", "diseases", "Multiple Sclerosis", "MS", "acute", "chronic", "relapsing remitting", "secondary progressive", "primary progressive", "aggressive", "attacks", "exacerbations", "relapses", "Central Nervous System", "CNS", "dysregulations", "inflammation", "neuro-inflammation", "degeneration", "neuro-degeneration", "demyelination", "myelination", "remyelination", "neuroprotection", "immunomodulation", "oxidative stress", "axons", "neurons", "conductivity", "T cell", "B cells", "activation", "glia", "microglia", "oligodendrocytes", "OLs", "oligodendrocyte progenitor cells", "OPCs", "astrocytes", "polarization", "cytokines", "chemokines", "pro-inflammatory", "anti-inflammatory", "autoantibodies", "pathogenic", "antigens", "epitopes", "complement", "immune complexes", "Nerve Growth Factor", "NGF", "neurotrophins", "receptors", "tropomyosin receptor kinase A", "TrkA", "p75 neurotrophin receptor", "p75NTR", "Sphingosine-1-Phosphate", "S1P", "S1P receptor", "S1PR", "S1PR1", "S1PR2", "S1PR3", "S1PR4", "S1PR5", "plasma levels", as well as by manual search in the local database. The search had no language restrictions.

3. Pathogenesis of MS

3.1. Between Space and Time Axes

MS is an autoimmune multifocal CNS inflammatory disease, characterized by chronic inflammation, demyelination, axonal damage, and subsequent gliosis. The most affected CNS regions by the disease are the periventricular area, subcortical area, optic nerve, spinal cord, brainstem, and cerebellum. MS is categorized as relapsing–remitting (RR), secondary progressive (SP), and primary progressive (PP) [11]. The pathogenesis of MS suggests that in genetically susceptible subjects, independent populations of T lymphocytes are activated in the immune system, migrate across the BBB, and trigger CNS tissue damage. They release pro-inflammatory cytokines, initiate cytotoxic activities of microglia with the release of nitrous oxide and other superoxide radicals, stimulate B cells and macrophages, and activate the complement system [12]. Autoantibodies against myelin basic protein and myelin OLs glycoprotein have been detected in MS patients. These antibodies may mediate injury by complement fixation or linking with innate effector cells such as CNS resident macrophages [12]. Despite the specific clinical form, the initial stage of the disease is characterized by an autoimmune inflammatory response mainly against the OLs in the CNS, resulting in demyelination (inflammatory component). Soon after the regenerative capacity of the OLs is exhausted, the inflammatory processes attack the neurons themselves, leading to the permanent injury and dysfunction of the CNS (neurodegenerative component). Both inflammatory and neurodegenerative components of MS pathogenesis are believed to be involved from the very beginning of the disease, giving different clinical presentations in the context of spatial and temporal pathological changes) (Figure 1) [13].

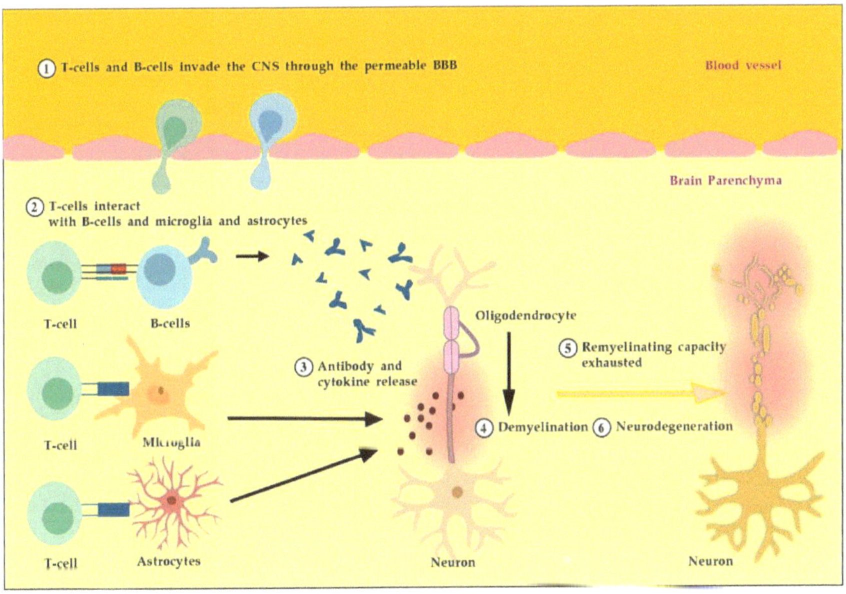

Figure 1. Pathogenesis of MS. Described processes 1 to 6 occur consecutively and in parallel in terms of the spatial (peripheral vs. CNS inflammation) and temporal (acute vs. chronic inflammation) axes. Adapted from [3] and modified.

3.2. *Between Detrimental and Beneficial Neuro-Inflammatory Responses*

3.2.1. The Role of Peripheral Immune Cells

MS neuro-inflammation is characterized by pathogenic immune responses involving T cells (CD4+ and CD8+ T cells), B cells, and myeloid cells along with the reduced function of regulatory T cells [14]. In the early inflammatory phase of MS, peripheral adaptive immune cells infiltrate the CNS through a compromised BBB (Figure 2A). These activated cells interact with each other and with CNS resident cells. They secrete cytokines such as IFN-γ by Th1, IL-6, IL-17 by Th17, GM-CSF, IL-6, TNF-α by B cells, and cytotoxic molecules such as granzyme B by CD8+ T cells. B cells can further evolve into pathogenic autoantibody-producing plasma cells. As a result, T and B cells activate macrophages and microglia that produce cytokines, nitric oxide, and reactive oxygen species (ROS). This cytotoxic pro-inflammatory environment causes oligodendrocyte and axonal damage through direct cell contact-dependent processes and the release of neurotoxic mediators [13]. It destroys the myelin sheaths around axons and causes energy failure in the axon. Yet, macrophages and microglia can still clear the myelin debris, allowing for the recruitment of oligodendrocyte progenitor cells (OPCs) that will partially remyelinate the lesion [13,15].

In the progressive phase of MS, the inflammation is restricted within the CNS due to the persistence of activated immune cells in situ, despite the absence of infiltrating T and B lymphocytes from the periphery (Figure 2B). This chronic inflammatory process affects the whole brain parenchyma, even at sites distant from the underlying focal demyelinating lesions. Diffuse chronic CNS inflammation is thought to be more common in patients with progressive forms of MS [16,17]. Notably, plasmablasts and plasma B cells form tertiary follicle-like structures in the meninges. Their location in the leptomeninges contributes to the demyelination of subpial gray matter and highlights the importance of B lymphocytes in the pathogenesis of the progressive form of MS. The BBB is closed and the inflammation is maintained by innate resident CNS cells, i.e., microglia and astrocytes. They produce cytokines (TNF-α, IL-6) and release ROS, causing damage to myelin [18].

Recent data suggest that neuro-inflammation may be beneficial to some extent [19]. In experimental autoimmune encephalomyelitis (EAE) models, the treatment of mice with IFN-γ, classically considered a pro-inflammatory cytokine, leads to reduced morbidity and mortality [20]. Evidence also supports the protective role of tumor necrosis factor alpha (TNF-α) in EAE. Mice lacking TNF-α and its related receptors showed a significant delay in remyelination [21]. This could be related to the missing TNF-α induction of neurotrophins expression as well, such as NGF and brain-derived neurotrophic factor (BDNF) [22]. TNF-α treatment significantly reduced the severity of the disease in immunized TNF-deficient mice [23]. The results suggest that some pro-inflammatory cytokines may also play an indirect rather than direct role in disease control and remyelination [20,21,23]. Anti-inflammatory cytokines, such as IL-4 and IL-10, may have a direct protective effect instead [24,25].

Immune cells also exert a neuroprotective effect in MS via the production and local secretion of neurotrophins, such as NGF and BDNF [26]. In addition, after suppressing B cell cytokines BAFF and APRIL with atacicept (cytokines important for B cell survival and function), adversely increased clinical activity in MS was observed. The latter provides indirect evidence for the anti-inflammatory functions of certain B cells [27].

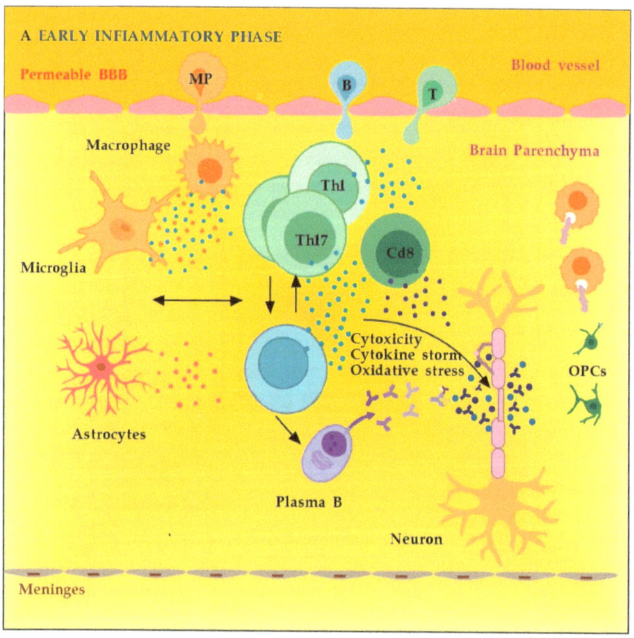

Figure 2. *Cont.*

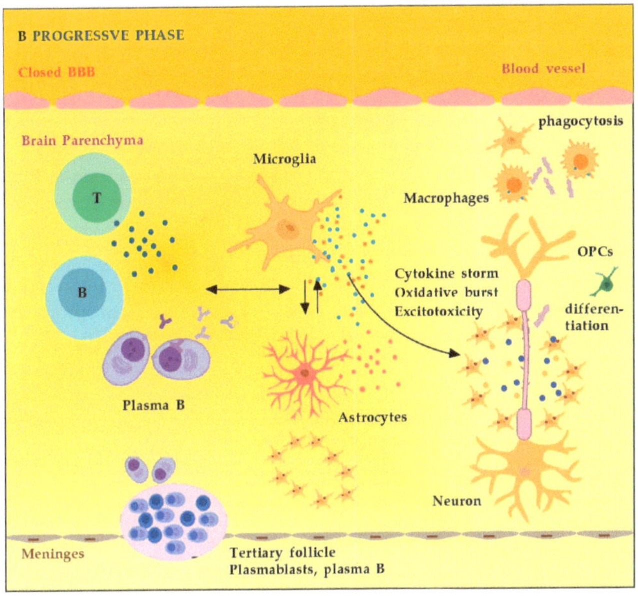

Figure 2. (**A**) The role of peripheral immune cells in MS. Adapted from [18] and modified. (**B**) The role of peripheral immune cells in MS. Adapted from [18] and modified. [dots: in blue and purple (cytokines and cytotoxic products from adjacent cells); in brown (reactive oxygen species)].

3.2.2. The Role of the Innate Resident CNS Cells

The main innate resident CNS cells of relevance to the localized inflammatory response are microglia and astrocytes. They produce cytokines (TNF-α, IL-6) and release ROS in situ, causing myelin damage [28].

Microglia are activated by pathogen-associated molecular pattern molecules (PAMPs) and/or damage-associated molecular pattern molecules (DAMPs) [29]. The classical (M1) microglia activation produces pro-inflammatory cytokines and chemokines, such as tumor necrosis factor-alpha (TNF-α), interleukin (IL)-6, IL-1β, IL-12, and CC chemokine ligand 2 (CCL2), and induce inflammation and neurotoxicity) [30]. The alternative (M2) microglia activation secretes certain growth factors (GFs) and neurotrophic factors (NTFs) and promotes the survival of neurons [31]. The switch from M1 to M2 phenotype may occur via inhibition of nuclear factor kappa-light-chain-enhancer of activated B cells (NF-κB), mitogen-activated protein kinase (MAPK), activator protein 1 (AP-1), and signal transducer and activator of transcription (STAT) transcription factors, and activation of the peroxisome proliferator–activated receptor gamma (PPARγ) pathway [31–36] (Figure 3).

Microglia activation contributes to MS disregulation through antigen presentation, secretion of pro-inflammatory cytokines, and phagocytic processes [37,38]. Although microglia are primed into a pro-inflammatory phenotype, their phagocytic capacities are diminished. Myelin debris are not completely cleared, OPCs are insufficiently recruited and fail to differentiate. Overall, microglial activation in the CNS is heterogeneous and cannot be classified only into two different subtypes: classical (M1) or alternative (M2) [39]. Although M1 microglia promote inflammation and M2 microglia have an anti-inflammatory phenotype, there appears to be a continuum of phenotypes between M1 and M2 that can switch from one to another [40]. Modulation microglia M1/M2 polarization and shifting from M1 to M2 phenotype have been proposed as promising therapeutic strategies in neurodegenerative CNS disorders [41].

Astrocytes may play a role in inhibiting remyelination and axonal regeneration through reactive astrogliosis, glial scar formation, and the secretion of inhibitory molecules which suppress axonal growth [42]. TNF-α-mediated glutamate release from astrocytes leads to excitotoxicity, causing axonal damage. The ferrous iron (Fe^{2+}) released from the myelin is oxidized to produce ROS leading to a major oxidative burst, causing mitochondrial dysfunction, mitochondrial DNA damage, energy failure, and axonal loss [18].

Activated astrocytes show a Janus-faced nature. The A1 astrocytes secrete interleukin (IL)-1β, TNF-α, and C3 components to propagate the neuroinflammatory response. Additionally, they also secrete D-serine and nitric oxide (NO), which may contribute to excitotoxicity with subsequent neuronal and oligodendrocyte death. The alternative A2 astrocytes, however, may secrete anti-inflammatory compounds, such as neurotrophic factors (NTFs, including NGF), IL-10, IL-6, and TGF-β, and promote the neuroprotective and neuroregenerative functions [41,43].

Astrocytes may stop the T-cell response by inducing apoptosis as well [44]. Until recently, astrocytes' formation of the glial scar was considered a harmful process that impedes the regeneration and remyelination of axons. Seen from a different perspective, however, depending on the severity of the injury, the scarring process may also serve to isolate the inflamed area, provide structural support, and restrict damage [42]. Likewise, activated microglia can also promote remyelination by clearing myelin debris from the local environment and by secreting anti-inflammatory cytokines, such as transforming growth factor-beta 1 (TGF-ß1) and certain neurotrophic factors, such as BDNF, that can induce the proliferation of OLs (Figure 3) [45,46].

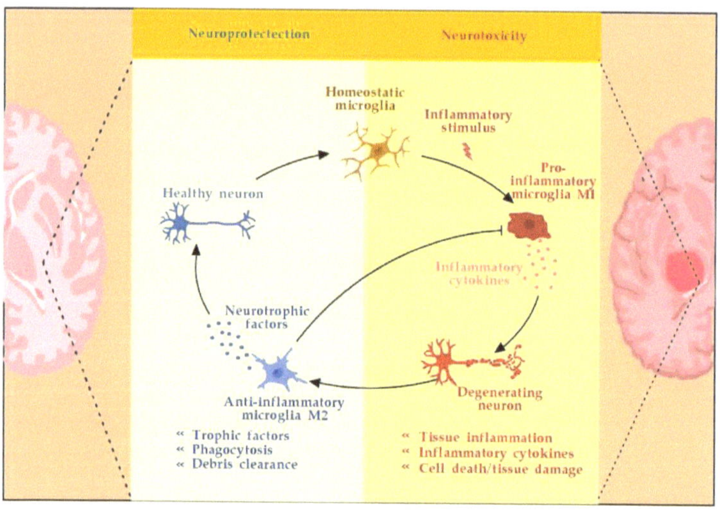

Figure 3. Microglia activation and resolution of inflammation. Adapted from [46] and modified.

4. The Role of Autoantibodies

B cells and their evolving plasma cells, along with the plasma cells producing autoantibodies and complement, have been found in MS lesions [47], indicating their implication in demyelination. Further evidence for antibody-mediated mechanisms in MS comes from the presence of ectopic lymphoid follicles in the CNS of MS patients [48], particularly those with progressive disease. The remarkable success of B-cells depleting therapies suggests that plasmablasts and plasma cells-producing autoantibodies may promote deterioration of the disease. However, the ability of plasma cells and their autoantibodies to significantly affect the course of MS is still a matter of debate [49].

Until recently, the available clinical and experimental evidence suggested that no specific antibodies had been identified in MS [50]. Pathological studies have shown IgG and complement deposition in brain lesions in some MS cases (defined as type II lesions), suggesting the contribution of humoral immunity and autoantibodies to the pathogenesis [51]. In confirmation of these data, some authors reported a subset of patients with type II MS lesions that had autoantibody-induced demyelinating responses [52,53]. Experimental research revealed that MS myelin-specific IgG1 monoclonal recombinant antibodies initiate complement-dependent cytotoxicity to OLs (oligodendrocyte loss) and induce rapid demyelination. The research gives compelling evidence of antibody/complement contribution to the type II MS lesions given the deposition of IgG and activated complement in EAE model. Importantly, antibody-induced demyelination was accompanied by significant activation of microglia [54]. In a human study, serum antibodies against the cytoplasm of OLs were detected in a relatively small proportion of MS patients with primary or secondary progressive disease. Compared to anti-oligodendrocyte autoantibody-negative MS patients, anti-oligodendrocyte antibody-positive MS patients were significantly older at the time of serum sampling, showing significantly greater impairment (significantly higher Kurtzke EDSS scores) and a higher frequency of mental disorders [55]. Another human study demonstrates that myelin obtained post mortem from MS brain donors is bound by IgG antibodies. In addition, IgG immune complexes strongly potentiate the activation of primary human microglia, leading to increased production of key pro-inflammatory cytokines, such as TNF and IL-1b. Thus, IgG immune complexes and activated human microglia may play an increasing role in MS-related inflammation and demyelinating lesion formation [56]. Most recent experimental research revealed that MS plasma IgG antibodies form large aggregates (>100 nm) that generate complement-dependent apoptosis in neurons and astrocytes. These findings provide a direct link between IgG antibodies and neuron death [57]. In real-world clinical practice, with the development of a novel nanomembrane-based TPE technology (with membrane pores 30–50 nm diameter [58]), by removing these pathological antibodies and immune complexes, we could modulate not only the demyelination (oligodendrocyte loss) and microglial activation but the neuronal and astrocyte apoptosis as well [54–57]. This modulation could have a significant impact on the levels of synthesized NGF by OLs, astrocytes, and neurons, which will be discussed.

In the early stage of MS of inflammatory demyelination, increased levels of monosialoganglioside 1 (GM1), the main myelin ganglioside, were found [59]. In addition, anti-ganglioside antibodies were observed that could either contribute to axonal degeneration or appear as a consequence of axonal damage. Whatever is true does not change their potential to cause BBB disruption [60] and inhibition of axonal regeneration [61]. Given the fact that the deleterious effect of anti-ganglioside IgM antibodies on BBB leakage is concentration-dependent but complement-independent [62], the plasma removal of these primary or secondary autoantibodies would also be pathogenetically reasonable.

In general, we could outline the pathogenicity of circulating autoantibodies associated with MS by several different possible mechanisms of actions and interactions (Figure 4). For example, during the early inflammatory phase due to increased BBB permeability induced by encephalitogenic T cells, circulating antibodies can reach the brain and become pathogenic. In addition, these antibodies themselves could induce vascular damage and inflammatory lesions of the CNS by complement-dependent or antibody-dependent cellular cytotoxicity mediated through Fc receptors on microglia and macrophages. Moreover, autoreactive B cells could infiltrate the brain and induce high levels of pathogenic autoantibodies in the cerebrospinal fluid (CSF). In the brain parenchyma, autoantibodies bound to the surface of target cells could cause their direct damage or functional alteration, which in turn leads to demyelination. Finally, autoantibodies may also promote demyelination indirectly by activating autoreactive T cells or microglia and macrophages [7]. By removing the pathogenic antibodies from the circulation and CNS when BBB permeability is available, we can modulate all described mechanisms and pathological consequences of antibodies' actions and interactions.

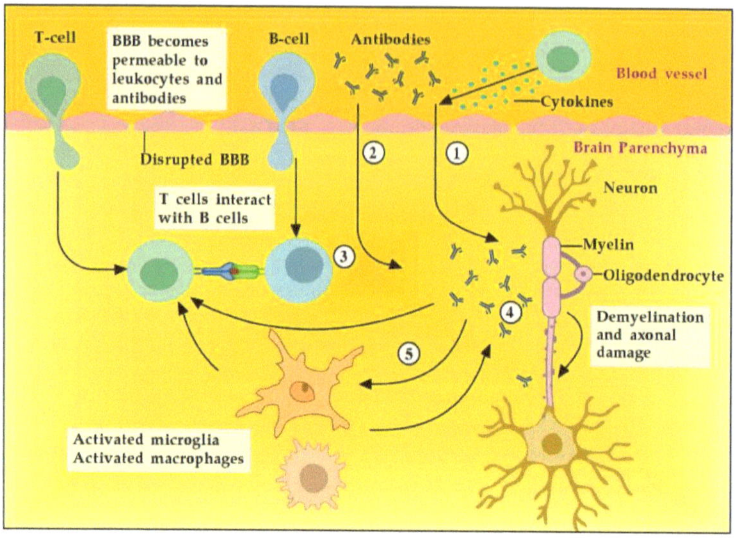

Figure 4. Potential mechanisms of antibody pathogenicity in multiple sclerosis. Adapted from [7] and modified. [activated T cells ① and circulating antibodies ② damage BBB and increase its permeability; activated B cells ③ add to the antibodies production in brain parenchyma; antibodies induce direct damage ④ or promote demyelination indirectly via activation of microglia and macrophages ⑤].

5. The Role of NGF

NGF is the member of the neurotrophin family which has been described in 1952 by Levi-Montalcini [63]. The neurotrophin family also includes neurotrophin-4 (NT4), BDNF, and neurotrophin-3 (NT-3) [64]. NGF activates downstream signaling cascades by binding to two types of membrane receptors, TrkA and p75NTR [65]. TrkA is considered a high-affinity receptor that selectively binds the NGF, thus conveying pro-survival signals [66]. p75NTR belongs to the tumor necrosis factor receptor family (TNFR) binding to all mature neurotrophins with the same affinity, while being considered a high-affinity receptor for the immature isoforms of the neurotrophins, the so-called pro-neurotrophins [67]. Depending on the NGF-specific receptors (high-affinity TrkA and low-affinity p75NTR), signaling pathways for neuronal differentiation, maturation and survival, axonal and dendrite development, or apoptosis can be triggered (Figure 5). The p75NTR forms complexes with various receptors, thus mediating a great number of different and sometimes opposing functions, the latter depending on the cellular and environmental context [68]. When TrkA and p75NTR are co-expressed, they constitute a two-receptor heterotetrameric system that binds to NGF and activates various signaling pathways [69,70].

In the context of demyelinating damage that accompanies MS development, it is essential to emphasize the role of neurotrophins (including NGF) in the activation of the principal signaling pathways driving OLs differentiation, myelination, and corresponding remyelination after injury, namely, Erk1/2-MAPK (Figure 5) [71]. The mitogen-activated protein kinase (MAPK) pathway by extracellular signal-related kinases 1 and 2 (Erk1 and Erk2) is reported to regulate oligodendroglial development, proliferation, apoptosis, differentiation, and myelination [72,73]. The Erk1/2-MAPK pathway is activated by platelet-derived growth factor (PDGF) and neurotrophins (NGF, NT3, and BDNF). This triggers a cascade of processes involving phosphorylation of MAP3K, MEK1, and MEK2, as well asErk1 and Erk2, which are finally translocated to the cellular nucleus [74,75]. Once there, they can regulate the expression of the OLs transcription factor myelin regulatory factor (MYRF), which promotes remyelination in MS [76].

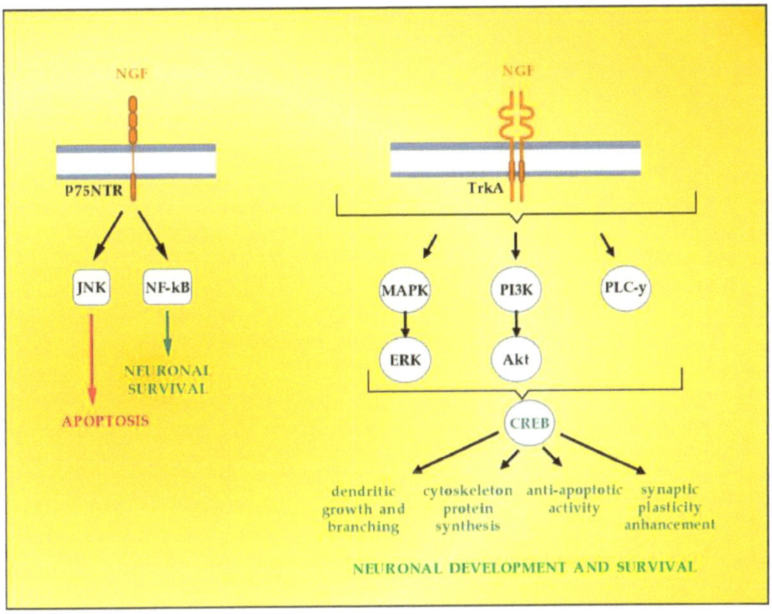

Figure 5. Signaling pathways activated by NGF. Adapted from [41] and modified.

NGF is a neurotrophin that is largely expressed in the CNS in neurons, OLs, and astrocytes as well as in the periphery [77,78]. NGF and its receptors are expressed by almost all different cell types, including T cells, B cells, macrophages, neutrophilic and basophilic granulocytes, mast cells, etc. (Table 1) [79,80]. NGF could affect B cells (proliferation, immunoglobulin production, and cell proliferation), T cells (survival and expression of cytokine receptors) and plays a special role in macrophage antigen presentation and migration into inflamed regions and lesions [81,82]. What is more, NGF activates chemotaxis [83–86], stimulates the phagocytosis of neutrophils [87] and macrophages [84,85], increases the cytotoxic activity of eosinophils [88], and stimulates the degranulation of mast cells [89,90].

Table 1. Expression of NGF and its receptors in the human immune system.

	Cellular Source	Target Receptor	Target Cell
β-NGF (mature)	mast cells, monocytes, macrophages, eosinophils, granulocytes, basophiles, T cells, B cells	TrkA	T cells, macrophages
		p75NTR and TrkA	B cells, mast cells

In the CNS, NGF specifically provides trophic support to cholinergic neurons of the basal forebrain that express TrkA, which makes it particularly interesting for Alzheimer's disease (AD) [91–95]. NGF and its receptors, TrkA and p75, are reported to play a bidirectional role between the immune and nervous systems. NGF plays a dual role both in anti- and pro-inflammatory responses [96]. At the site of inflammation, pro-inflammatory cytokines (such as IL-1β and IL-6) induce overexpression of NGF [97]. p75NTR, in the absence of the TrkA co-receptor, can affect the migration of B cells via BBB, where it has been described to play a crucial role, as well as limit the production of autoantibodies from B cells. By this mechanism, NGF performs neuroprotection in the context of protective autoimmunity, where the organism develops specific mechanisms to cope with CNS damage by restricting and controlling degeneration and/or promoting regeneration [98,99]; and vice versa, NGF using TrkA could upregulate axonal expression of LINGO-1 (a membrane-bound protein, part of the Nogo-A signaling pathway and a myelin-associated inhibitor) and may also negatively affect the process of axonal myelination [100,101]. However, the deletion of Nogo-A signaling (using Nogo-A knockouts animal model) fails to maintain regeneration of axons after spinal cord injury. Hence, the Nogo-A/LINGO1 signaling pathway may not play an important role in the failure of regeneration but instead could participate in an accessory function [102]. The latest research corroborates the regenerative ability of NGF using adipose mesenchymal stem-cell-derived NGF. After injecting into the animals with EAE, the artificial NGF stimulates axon regeneration and also decreases neurogliosis [103]. Moreover, another recent study using an in vitro model of mixed neural stem-cell-derived OPCs revealed that in the mixed culture, astrocytes are the major producer of NGF, and OPCs express both TrkA and p75NTR. NGF treatment increases the percentage of mature OLs, whereas NGF blocking by neutralizing antibodies impairs OPC differentiation. This report clearly demonstrates that NGF is involved in OPC differentiation, maturation, and protection, which also suggests possible implications in the treatment of demyelinating lesions and related diseases [104].

In the course of neuro-inflammation, almost all resident CNS cells overexpress NGF [105]. In addition, NGF in the blood could cross the BBB and reach glial cells, when BBB becomes permeable under pathological conditions, such as, for example, MS [106]. It should be pointed out that NGF levels affect glial physiology. As reported in in vivo mouse model [107], the reduction of NGF leads to A1 activation of astrocytes and neurotoxicity. On the contrary, as previously reported [108], the elevation of NGF steers microglia toward an anti-inflammatory phenotype, thus leading to neuroprotection. In addition, previous research observed the significant effects of intracranial administration of NGF on cytokine expression, which were specific for the CNS parenchyma and were not found in the periphery [109]. As far as MS is concerned, during acute attacks, patients show elevated levels of NGF in the CSF compared with healthy individuals, which can be regarded as an attempt to protect the CNS tissue against inflammation [110]. All these findings suggest the relevance of NGF-based therapeutic approaches in cases of inflammatory and neurodegenerative disorders [107].

The role of NGF in modulating the activity of a number of cellular and tissue structures during CNS inflammation and injury is presented in Table 2.

Table 2. NGF mechanisms of action during CNS inflammation and injury.

Target	Effect
Immune system	Modulation of immune system via enhanced sympathetic innervation of lymph nodes with indirect effect decreasing CD4+ and CD8+ proliferation
BBB	Maintenance of BBB integrity
Lymphocytes	Switch to the anti-inflammatory phenotype by avoiding cytotoxicity and inducing immunosuppressive cytokines (IL-10, TGF-β)
Macrophages/ microglia	Decrease in antigen presentation by macrophage/microglia by reducing the expression of major histocompatibility complex (MHC) molecules; Shift from pro-inflammatory M1 to anti-inflammatory M2 phenotype
Astrocytes	Inactivation of toxic astrocytes mediators; Attenuation of astrogliosis, shift from pro-inflammatory A1 to anti-inflammatory A2 phenotype
OLs	Promotion of proliferation, migration, maturation, and survival of OPCs
Neurons	Promotion of axonal survival during inflammation; Upregulation of axonal LINGO1 with inhibition of axonal receptivity to oligodendrocyte myelination

Recently, it has been shown that TNF-α not only induces NGF over-expression but modulates the NGF signaling pathways as well. The cross talk between these two is possible due to the fact that p75NTR belongs to the tumor necrosis factor receptor family

(TNFR). TNF-α downregulates the mRNA and protein levels of TrkA and also increases p75 mRNA expression [110]. This could shift the role of NGF signaling from neuroprotective to neurotoxic, implying that a specific binding of a certain receptor is of significant importance, especially during inflammation [110]. In turn, NGF can modulate the TNF-α signaling pathways by downregulating TNFR1-mediated apoptosis and promoting preferential signaling through TNFR2, which leads to protection and proliferation. What is more, NGF also induces production of BDNF [22], another CNS neurotrophin and well-established activator of re-myelination in MS [101].

Finally, NGF antibodies were observed to exacerbate neuropathological signs of EAE [111]. This implies not only the significance of NGF in reducing the extent of EAE lesions [112] but also opens up a new possibility to enhance the NGF beneficial anti-inflammatory potential in MS patients by removing these antibodies by means of TPE [113].

6. The Role of S1P

Sphingolipids are functionally active participants in a wide range of extracellular and intracellular processes [114,115]. The balance between sphingosine and sphingosine-1-phosphate (S1P), both being metabolites of the precursor ceramide, and their subsequent phosphorylation by enzymes called kinases were shown to be important in the determination of whether a cell is destined for cell death/apoptosis or proliferation [116]. Although S1P is essential for normal CNS development and maturation [117] and it also may regulate synaptic function [118], it can also have cytotoxic effect at higher concentrations, such as when there is a genetically determined deficiency in its degradative enzymes [119]. S1P also regulates calcium metabolism [120] and may promote presynaptic calcium overload and eventually cell death [121]. Of note, S1P is implicated in both upstream and downstream production of cytokines, and increased interstitial levels of S1P at the inflammatory sites induce the expression of pro-inflammatory cytokines [122]. As described above, free interstitial S1P increases at inflammation sites, where, unlike its plasma anti-inflammatory effects, this sphingolipid is involved in the propagation of inflammation [122].

A distinguishing characteristic of the members of the sphingolipid family is their participation in pro- or anti-proliferative pathways of cell regulation [114]. Especially, S1P is well known for its wide functional activity, influencing processes such as cellular migration, adhesion, differentiation, and survival, among others. It is also an active participant in the genesis of various pathological processes and diseases, involving inflammation, oxidative stress, neurodegenerative pathologies such as MS, etc. [123]. MS is an autoimmune inflammatory neurodegenerative disease, which is characterized by disturbances in the sphingolipid metabolism in the CNS [123]. The levels of S1P are reported to be elevated in the cerebrospinal fluid of MS patients, and this elevation shows specific correlations with the clinical severity of the disease (e.g., Kurtzke EDSS score) [124]. The high concentrations of S1P occurring in cerebrospinal fluid [125] from MS patients support the presumption that the bioactivity of S1P is pro-inflammatory rather than protective [123]. In addition, S1P affects the integrity of the BBB, which is generally damaged in patients with MS [123].

The bioactive lipid, S1P, is generated by phosphorylation of sphingosine, catalyzed by two isoforms of sphingosine kinase (SK1 and SK2). S1P can also be reversibly dephosphorylated by S1P phosphatase to produce sphingosine, the levels of which are generally controlled by flux through de novo ceramide synthesis and sphingosine catabolic pathways [126]. There are numerous studies on the sphingomyelin (SM)–S1P pathway in order to reveal whether SM serves as a major source of S1P through the activities of sphingolipid metabolizing enzymes [127]. The obtained results showed upregulation of certain sphingolipid catabolizing enzymes, implying that SM could serve as a possible source of S1P (Figure 6).

A vast number of the biological effects of S1P are mediated by a family of G-protein-coupled S1P receptors S1P1–S1P5. The complex expression patterns and transmembrane and intracellular signaling pathways of each receptor form the molecular basis for the diversity of S1P functions [122].

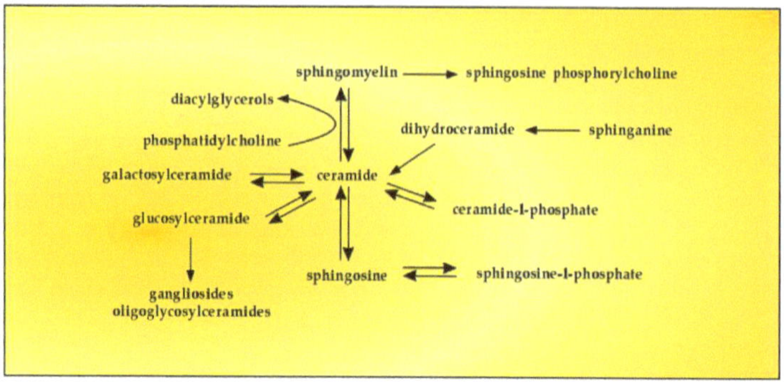

Figure 6. The SM–S1P pathway.

S1P receptors are widely expressed in cells of the CNS [128], including neurons, astrocytes, microglia, and OLs, all of them having potential roles in the pathogenesis of MS. S1P1 upregulates Th17 polarization and increasing neuro-inflammation, which are key factors in MS pathogenesis [129]. During inflammation, an S1PR-1-dependent upregulation of microglia is observed which additionally increases the inflammatory process [130]. The blocking of S1P1 decreases activated microglial production of pro-inflammatory cytokines (TNF-α, IL-1β, and IL-6) and increases production of BDNF and glial-cell-derived neurotrophic factor, the latter being neuroprotective [131]. In addition, S1PR-1 blockade is a potentially important pharmacological target to reduce astrogliosis and promote re-myelination in MS patients [132]. A role of S1P1 in astrocytes has been shown in the disease progression [133]. Both S1PR-1 and S1PR-3 are upregulated by pro-inflammatory astrocytes and are associated with higher production of glial acidic fibrillary protein [134]. The potential of S1P2 to destabilize adherent junctions, promote inflammation, and modulate the infiltration of leukocytes may increase the disease severity [133]. As far as S1P3 signaling in MS is concerned, its actual sequelae regarding detrimental effects (e.g., astrogliosis) and beneficial effects (e.g., remyelination) could not be determined [135]. Clearer evidence for the pro-inflammatory contribution of S1P3 was reported later [136].

Red blood cells (RBCs) and endothelial cells (ECs) are major sources for the production of plasma S1P. About 50–60% of the circulating S1P is bound to apolipoprotein M (ApoM)/high-density lipoprotein (HDL), and 30–40% is bound to albumin. Platelets may also participate in the production of plasma S1P, especially upon platelet activation, which significantly enhances S1P release [137]. Experience from the COVID-19 pandemic implies that during severe inflammation the decrease in S1P is closely connected to the number of RBCs, the major source of plasma S1P, and to ApoM/HDL and albumin, the major transporters of S1P in blood [138].

Alterations in blood flow modulate endothelial S1P secretion and receptor S1P1 expression. In static state, there is a decrease in S1P production and secretion of endothelial S1P. In addition, S1P1 transcription is less active, which leads to lower S1P1 activity. On the contrary, in active state, shear stress substantially upregulates S1P1 expression, which induces an increase in endothelial S1P levels and enhanced S1P1 signaling. S1P enzymatic degradation in tissues is a key factor in the formation of circulatory S1P gradient across the endothelial barrier, which keeps S1P levels at ~1 μM in the blood, at ~0.1 μM in the lymph, and at <1 nM in the interstitial fluids [137].

The above determinants of circulatory S1P gradient along with the S1P plasma levels could be modulated during TPE, which will be discussed later.

7. The Role of TPE

TPE is an invasive therapeutic method that involves extracorporeal blood removal, as well as the return or exchange of blood plasma or components. It usually removes a large volume of plasma (1 to 1.5 of patient's total plasma volume (TPV) per treatment) with adequate volume replacement using colloid solutions (e.g., albumin and/or fresh frozen plasma (FFP)) or a combination of crystalloid/colloid solutions [139]. TPE is applied to remove pathogenic substances with high molecular weight (>150 kDA) including autoantibodies, immune complexes, pro-inflammatory mediators, lipids, and many others from the intravascular space, which ensures its rapid onset of action [139,140]. However, the mechanism of action of TPE in immune-mediated inflammatory and neurodegenerative disorders involves more than the simple removal of large pathogenic molecules. For example, the application of TPE may also modulate cellular immunological response by altering the ratio between T-helper type-1 (Th-1) and type-2 (Th-2) cells in peripheral blood. Th-2 cells maintain the humoral immune response by facilitating B-cell autoantibody production and play an essential role in neurodegenerative autoimmune disorders. By shifting the balance between peripheral T cells from Th-2 predominance to Th-1 predominance, TPE has a modulatory effect on the pathogenic immune response and may play a therapeutic role within and beyond the time of TPE application [141].

The contemporary status of TPE in autoimmune neurological diseases in Japan suggests that it can be considered as an efficient therapy for autoimmune neurological diseases such as MS, myasthenia gravis (MG), neuromyelitis optica spectrum disorders (NMOSD), chronic inflammatory demyelinating polyneuropathy (CIDP), and Guillain–Barré syndrome (GBS), among others, with a low frequency of adverse effects [142]. Our data corroborate these findings in the mentioned neurological disorders after the use of nanomembrane-based TPE [58]. This innovative approach involves passing the patient's blood through several nanomembranes, aiming to filter certain large molecules [113,143–148]. The nanomembrane-based technology involves the use of the "Hemophenix" apparatus (Figure 7) with the ROSA nanomembrane ("Trackpore Technology", Moscow, Russia) (Figure 8). The nanomembrane has pores with a diameter of 30–50 nm, and it can filter molecules with molecular weights less than 40 kDa. The device has a filling volume of up to 70 mL and also possesses the advantage of a single-needle access to a peripheral vein [149].

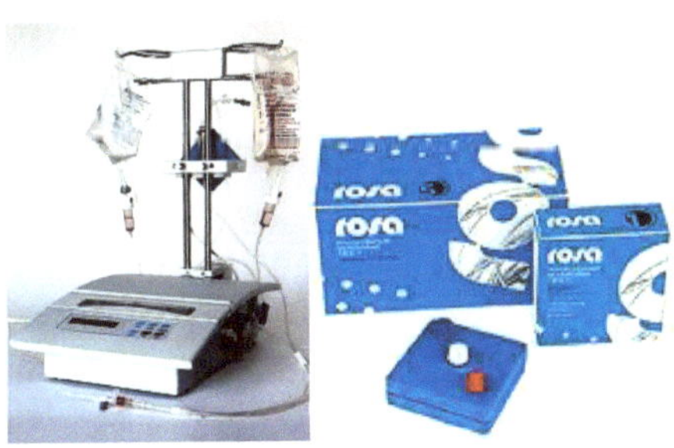

Figure 7. Hemophenix apparatus with ROSA nanomembrane [58].

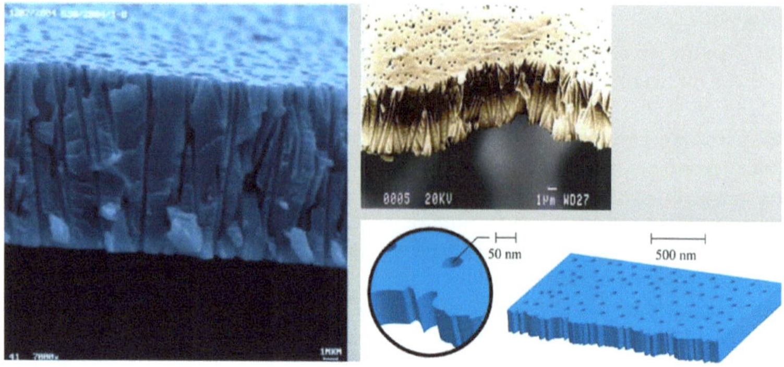

Figure 8. Electron microscopic profile of the track membrane ROSA [58].

The most frequently used replacement fluid in nanomembrane-based TPE is saline (NaCl 0.9), which has low cost and no adverse effects, even when 25% (approximately 700–750 mL plasma) of the circulating plasma is removed [144]. Our practice of saline replacement in the removal of 700–750 mL of plasma is in agreement with the so-called low-volume plasma exchange (LVPE), which ranges from 350 mL to 2 l plasma volume removal per each separate procedure. The LVPE approach is preferred in chronic conditions, in which the separation of smaller volumes of plasma would be justified for long periods of time [150]. The relevance of minimizing the adverse events of colloid replacement by lowering plasma volume exchanged per treatment (0.5–0.7 of TPV) is supported by the German practice in the field of LVPE as well [151,152]. The reported data suggest that effectiveness may be provided with volumes below the currently recommended volumes (1 to 1.5 of TPV) [151,153]. According to the Spanish practice, the LVPE approach suggests good effectiveness in neuro-immunological disorders (GBS, NMOSD, MG, MS). However, more profound studies are needed to confirm LVPE as a better alternative to the classical TPE [150]. Nevertheless, our experience in LVPE adds new insights concerning the effectiveness of the low-volume approach after implementing an innovative nanomembrane-based technology (Figure 9).

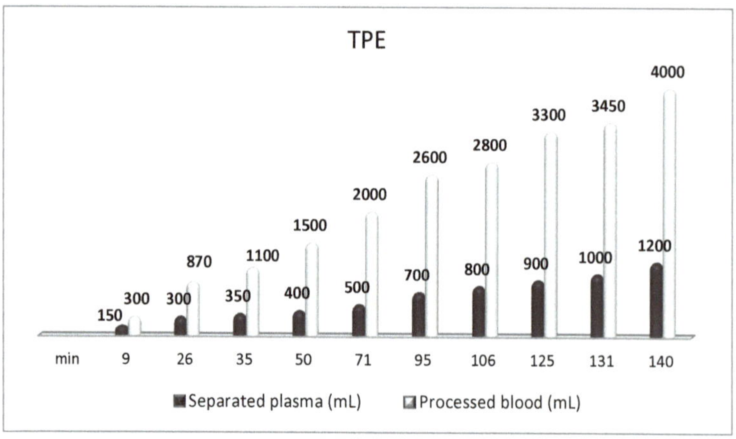

Figure 9. Amount of processed blood and separated plasma (LVPE) during a TPE procedure in a patient with MS.

TPE is presumed to affect NGF and S1P plasma levels in many different ways. In classical filtration TPE (1–1.5 of TPV), membrane pores might be blocked by red blood cells, and hemolysis may occur depending on the hematocrit and the blood flow rate or blood shear rate [154]. In addition, the shear flow and shear stress are factors that affect the leukocyte-material-induced activation [155]. Thus, strict control of the transmembrane pressure is required [154] in order to avoid these TPE-associated adverse effects. In LVPE (0.5–0.7 of TPV), the ratio surface area/plasma volume is more favorable in terms of minimizing hemolysis and leukocytes' activation [156]. This is likely to affect the plasma levels of NGF and S1P. In our clinical settings, the changes in hemoglobin (a major source of S1P synthesis [135]), albumin, and ApoM/HDL (major carriers of circulating S1P [137]), after administering albumin/FFP replacement fluids (infusion of albumin/FFP stimulate the release of S1P from erythrocytes and platelets [157]), activated leukocytes (source of growth factors [158]) and are all balanced by the use of nanomembrane-based LVPE. Beyond these considerations, the most plausible explanation for the observed elevation of NGF plasma levels (Figures 10 and 11) and reduced S1P plasma levels (Figures 12 and 13) in our cases of MS patients could be due to the removal of autoantibodies (Figures 14–16) against NGF-producing cells and NGF itself (discussed above) as well as direct loss of S1P with discarded plasma [159]. The reduction of blood S1P after TPE leads to the inability to maintain the circulatory S1P levels and to the accumulation of mature T cells in lymphoid organs [160]. This may have the same clinical implications for MS patients as the administration of S1P1 receptor modulator fingolimod, causing lymphocyte sequestration in peripheral lymphoid organs and thus preventing autoreactive immune cells' infiltration into the CNS [161]. The increased NGF plasma levels after TPE application could either contribute to or occur as a consequence of increased NGF levels in the CNS (given NGF's ability to cross the permeable BBB according to its gradient [106]). In both cases, they should be considered as a favorable anti-inflammatory response as a result of the reduced pro-inflammatory load related to discarded plasma. The augmented NGF in CNS could steer glia toward an anti-inflammatory phenotype and neuroprotection [108]. Likewise, the removal of circulatory pathogenic factors (autoantibodies, immune complexes, cytokines, etc.) from peripheral and CNS compartments could alleviate their damaging effect on target cells (neurons, OLs) and thus promote neuroprotection. As for the possible interaction between NGF and S1P (NGF stimulates Sphk1 activity via TrkA receptors and increases intracellular S1P [162,163]), the observed increased NGF plasma levels are apparently not sufficient to promote enough synthesis of S1P in order to compensate the lowering effect of TPE on S1P plasma levels.

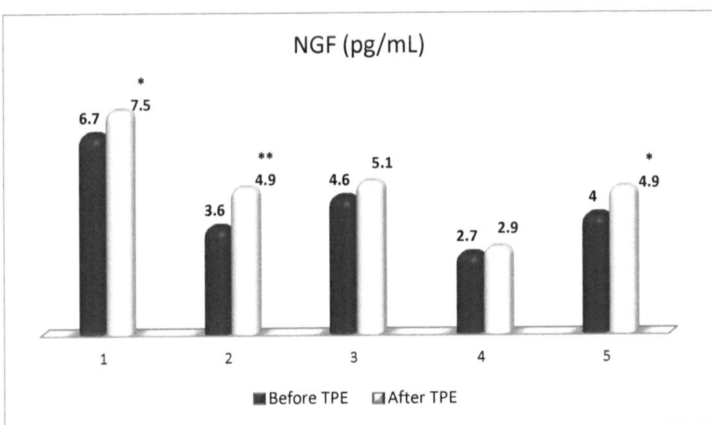

Figure 10. Changes in the level of NGF before and after a TPE procedure in patients (1, 2, 3, 4, 5) with acute exacerbations of relapsing–remitting MS (* $p < 0.05$; ** $p < 0.01$).

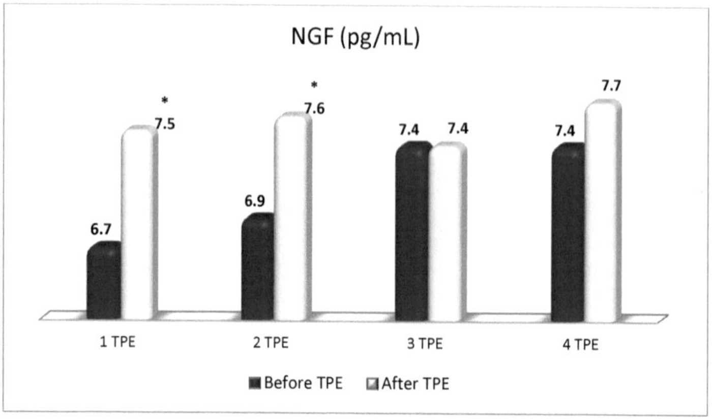

Figure 11. Changes in the level of NGF before and after the course of TPE procedures (1, 2, 3, 4) in a patient with acute exacerbations of relapsing–remitting MS (* $p < 0.05$).

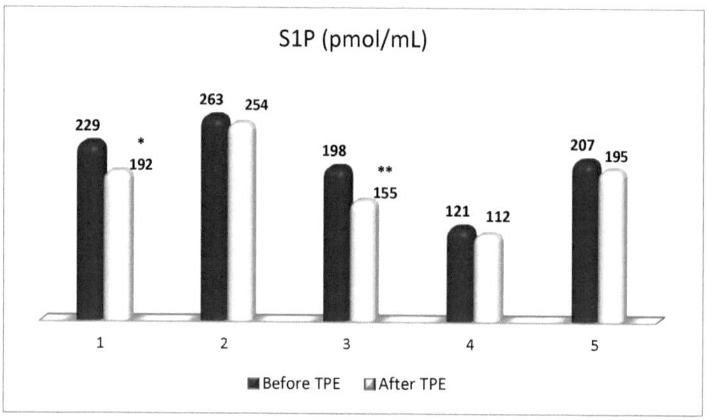

Figure 12. Changes in the level of S1P before and after a TPE procedure in patients (1, 2, 3, 4, 5) with acute exacerbations of relapsing–remitting MS (* $p < 0.05$; ** $p < 0.01$).

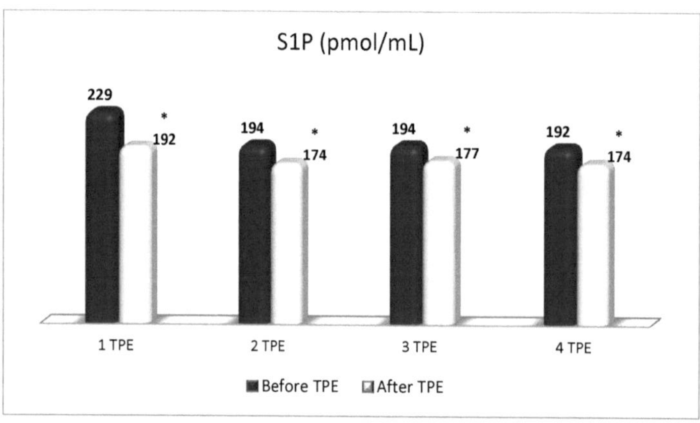

Figure 13. Changes in the level of S1P before and after the course of TPE procedures (1, 2, 3, 4) in a patient with acute exacerbations of relapsing–remitting MS (* $p < 0.05$).

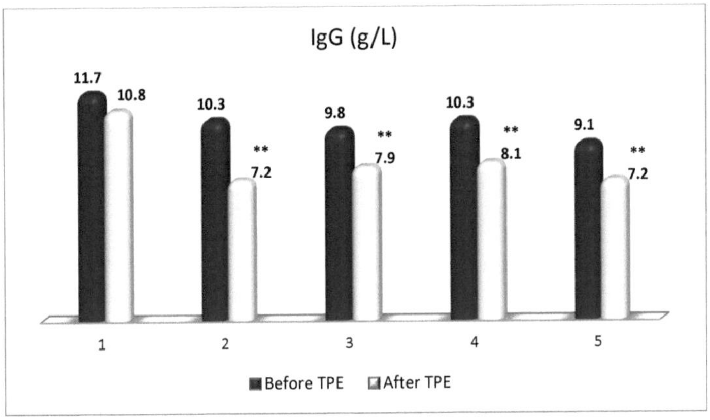

Figure 14. Changes in the level of IgG before and after a TPE procedure in patients (1, 2, 3, 4, 5) with acute exacerbations of relapsing–remitting MS (** $p < 0.01$).

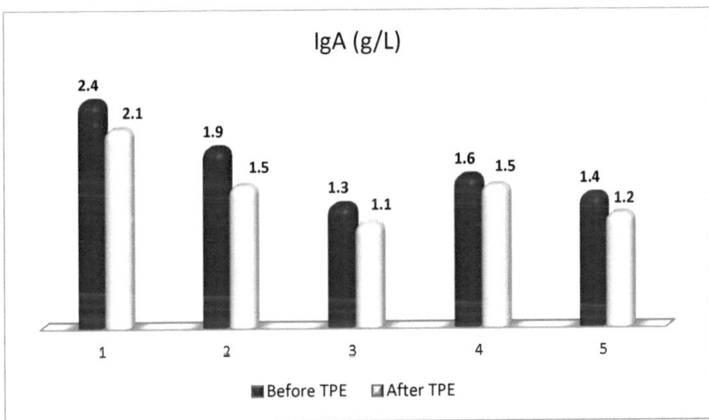

Figure 15. Changes in the level of IgA before and after a TPE procedure in patients (1, 2, 3, 4, 5) with acute exacerbations of relapsing–remitting MS ($p > 0.05$, there is a trend towards reduction).

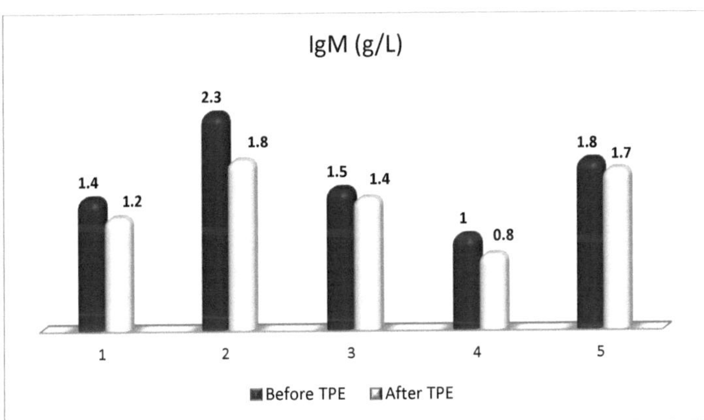

Figure 16. Changes in the level of IgM before and after a TPE procedure in patients (1, 2, 3, 4, 5) with acute exacerbations of relapsing–remitting MS ($p > 0.05$, there is a trend towards reduction).

Hence, the clinical rationale for TPE is that there is a permeable BBB in acute demyelinating attacks, and the pathogenic substances can pass through it in both directions. The removal of plasma antibodies and immune complexes by TPE may facilitate their efflux and clearance from the CNS compartment, especially in MS patients with a highly active disease (involving the progressive forms of MS) [164]. The purpose of a relapse treatment is to accelerate functional recovery after inflammatory demyelination, alleviate the severity of the relapse, and decrease the development of persistent neurologic deficit [165]. If patients are unresponsive to initial corticosteroid treatment, which occurs in 20–25% of all cases, after an interval of 10–14 days a second corticosteroid pulse therapy in combination with TPE is recommended. TPE in steroid-refractory acute attacks/relapses is recommended as an adjunctive treatment by the American Academy of Neurology (AAN) (Level B recommendation) [166] and as a second-line treatment by the American Society for Apheresis (ASFA) (Category II; Grade 1B: strong recommendation, moderate quality evidence) [148]. In this acute clinical setting, a course of 5–7 TPE procedures over two weeks has a response rate of more than 50% [141]. In contrast to the ASFA recommendations, the AAN evidence-based guideline does not recommend TPE for chronic PP or SP forms of MS (Level A recommendation) [166]. It is noteworthy that a recent retrospective study revealed a 50% response rate for the PP/SP subgroup of patients with MS, treated with TPE/IA (both IA and TPE were equally effective) [167]. This observation implies that TPE could also be considered as escalation therapy in progressive MS [165]. In addition, another current retrospective study suggests that the escalation towards TPE should be as early as possible. It is important to point out that the delay between the onset of relapse and the initiation of TPE is crucial for the clinical response to TPE. A 7-day delay was reported to reduce the probability of TPE response by more than 30%. A delay of 14 or 21 days (routine clinical practice) results in a twofold to threefold reduction in the chance of clinically meaningful improvement [168]. All this points to a therapeutic window corresponding to the pathologically permeable BBB during and immediately after the acute demyelinating attack, which, if not used in proper time, reduces the chances of TRE for partial or complete resolution of the active MRI lesions in the great majority of treated patients [169]. This is usually accompanied by a significant improvement in the EDSS scores in post-TPE patients [170].

In addition, we carried out a second-line nanomembrane-based TPE in steroid-refractory MS in 15 patients with RR form of MS [146,147,149,171] and in one patient with progressive MS [149]. Our short-term therapeutic algorithm included 4 sessions of nanomembrane-based TPE with LVPE mode, 0.8 TPV exchange (Figure 6—our MS with LVPE, in TPE file), performed every other day, followed by 5th TPE after 1 month, 6th TPE 3 months later, and 7th TPE 6 months later [171,172]. After the application of a cycle of 4 TPE, usually the symptoms of ocular and vestibular motor function, of visual acuity, of walking without assistance, etc., as well as those of acute neurological deficit (Kurtzke's EDSS) were improved significantly. The latest are in line with the EDSS improvements reported by other authors [170]. A significant reduction of the markers of oxidative stress (published previously) was observed as well [58].

TPE is an efficacious and safe method for the treatment of neurological disorders [58,173]. Nevertheless, its use for acute MS relapses is still modest according to recent UK clinical practice data [173]. Our nanomembrane-based experience suggests a new opportunity in technical terms and is another argument for TPE's extended use in the field. However, it should be interpreted with caution and should be placed in the context of local specificities regarding study population, experience, availability, and insurance coverage [58,149].

Our observations on the plasma levels of immunoglobulins, NGF, and S1P present for the first time insight into the multifaceted role of TPE in the treatment of MS acute demyelinating attacks. Further research is necessary to determine their possible role as reliable biomarkers for appropriate TPE protocols.

8. Summary of Achieving Neuroprotection in MS

In summary, achieving neuroprotection in MS is a multifaceted task requiring drugs or a combination of drugs, with different mechanisms of action, aimed at promoting axonal function (1), glial regulation (2), BBB myelin integrity (3), and restoration of myelin-protective functions (4) (Figure 17). TPE, without being considered as an alternative to the available disease-modifying drugs or new drug formulations in development, may selectively help to advance neuroprotection in all four directions. As described above, TPE could modulate the CNS microenvironment by reducing oxidative stress (less excitotoxicity), by removing the pathological antibodies and immune complexes (less OLs loss, less microglial activation, less neuronal and astrocyte apoptosis, less BBB disruption, etc.), by increasing NGF (shifting TNF-α signaling from TNFR1-mediated apoptosis to TNFR2-mediated protection and survival, steering glia toward an anti-inflammatory phenotype with less secretion of inhibitory molecules, promoting via Erk1/2-MAPK signaling pathway OLs differentiation, myelination, and remyelination, etc.), and by decreasing S1P (leading to the inability to maintain the circulatory S1P gradient and to accumulation of mature T cells in lymphoid organs, decreasing the expression of pro-inflammatory cytokines in inflammatory sites, minimizing S1P promotion of presynaptic calcium overload and cell death, etc.) [54–58,71,108,160,174].

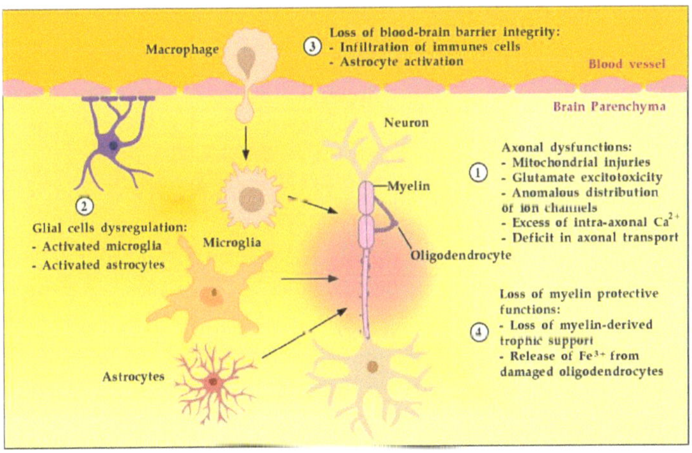

Figure 17. Main targets to achieve neuroprotection in MS. Adapted from [175] and modified.

9. Limitations and Future Directions

The main drawback of TPE is that this is an unspecific blood purification technique for removing plasma without special processing for removing only pathological factors and then replacing the separated plasma with fluids. As a result, some beneficial components, such as antibodies or cytokines with remyelinating features, are eliminated during the procedure as well [10]. Another drawback is that direct evidence for the pathogenic role of serum antibodies in MS is complicated by the marked heterogeneity of the disease and the variability of experimental procedures [7]. In addition, lessons learned from failed phase II–III trials of antibody therapies in MS that were discontinued for various reasons or withdrawn from the market taught us that there is a risk that agents that show promise in preclinical work may not translate into beneficial effects in humans [8,176]. A well-known approach from real clinical practice is to look for evidence of pathogenicity through the effect of the treatment administered. Following best practices in the field, lowering antibody levels alleviates the disease. Therapies that reduce inflammation and the immune response relieve MS symptoms and treat relapses, including prednisone, methylprednisone, apheresis, and ocrelizumab [177]. Regardless of the considered limitations, during acute demyelinating attacks with fulminant lesions and a predominant pro-inflammatory response, the positive effect of TPE administration [7] far outweighs the disadvantages of this therapeutic approach.

At present, we can search for evidence of the effectiveness of TPE based on the relief of MS symptoms from the reduction of pathological substances [177] or after evaluating the percentage of patients who achieved confirmed improvement in disability using the Kurtzke EDSS [176]. From a personalized medicine perspective, a new step in evaluating the effectiveness of new TPE technologies (including the nanomembrane-based one in particular) could be through the use of markers of axonal damage such as the level of neurofilaments in the serum before and after apheresis for acute demyelinating MS attacks [178]. Further research is needed to determine which patients benefit most from this advanced TPE treatment.

10. Conclusions

In conclusion, given the accelerated discovery of novel characteristic autoantibodies, in the near future, it would be expected to see an increase in the number of clinical TPE applications in the field [179,180]. Altered plasma levels of the reviewed molecular compounds in response to TPE treatment of acute MS attacks reflect a successful reduction of the pro-inflammatory burden at the expense of an increase in anti-inflammatory potential in the circulatory and CNS compartments. Plasmapheresis for MS in the twenty-first century should be taken by MS patients.

Author Contributions: All authors made substantial contributions to the conceptualization, methodology, data acquisition and interpretation, and drafting the manuscript. All authors have read and agreed to the published version of the manuscript.

Funding: This research was financially supported by the Bulgarian Ministry of Education and Science: Contract DO1-154/28/08/2018/ Scientific Infrastructure in Cell Technologies in Biomedicine (SICTB); agreement DO1-178/2022.

Data Availability Statement: All data are available under request to corresponding author Dimitar Tonev (dgtsofia@abv.bg).

Conflicts of Interest: The authors declare no conflict of interest.

References

1. Zahoor, I.; Rui, B.; Khan, J.; Datta, I.; Giri, S. An emerging potential of metabolomics in multiple sclerosis: A comprehensive overview. *Cell. Mol. Life Sci.* **2021**, *78*, 3181–3203. [CrossRef]
2. Lassmann, H. Pathogenic mechanisms associated with different clinical courses of multiple sclerosis. *Front. Immunol.* **2018**, *9*, 3116. [CrossRef]
3. Sandi, D.; Kokas, Z.; Biernacki, T.; Bencsik, K.; Klivényi, P.; Vécsei, L. Proteomics in Multiple Sclerosis: The Perspective of the Clinician. *Int. J. Mol. Sci.* **2022**, *23*, 5162. [CrossRef]
4. Vyshkina, T.; Kalman, B. Autoantibodies and neurodegeneration in multiple sclerosis. *Lab. Investig.* **2008**, *88*, 796–807. [CrossRef]
5. Li, Y.; Noto, D.; Hoshino, Y.; Mizuno, M.; Yoshikawa, S.; Miyake, S. Immunoglobulin directly enhances differentiation of oli-godendrocyte-precursor cells and remyelination. *Sci. Rep.* **2023**, *13*, 9394. [CrossRef]
6. Muñoz, U.; Sebal, C.; Escudero, E.; Esiri, M.; Tzartos, J.; Sloan, C.; Sadaba, M.C. Main Role of Antibodies in Demyelination and Axonal Damage in Multiple Sclerosis. *Cell. Mol. Neurobiol.* **2022**, *42*, 1809–1827. [CrossRef]
7. Höftberger, R.; Lassmann, H.; Berger, T.; Reindl, M. Pathogenic autoantibodies in multiple sclerosis—From a simple idea to a complex concept. *Nat. Rev. Neurol.* **2022**, *18*, 681–688. [CrossRef]
8. Cunniffe, N.; Coles, A. Promoting remyelination in multiple sclerosis. *J. Neurol.* **2021**, *268*, 30–44. [CrossRef]
9. Davies, A.J.; Fehmi, J.; Senel, M.; Tumani, H.; Dorst, J.; Rinaldi, S. Immunoadsorption and Plasma Exchange in Seropositive and Seronegative Immune-Mediated Neuropathies. *J. Clin. Med.* **2020**, *9*, 2025. [CrossRef]
10. Farrokhi, M. Plasmapheresis for Multiple Sclerosis in the Twenty-First Century: Take It or Leave It? *J. Rev. Med. Sci.* **2021**, *1*, e1.
11. Lublin, F.D.; Reingold, S.C.; Cohen, J.A.; Cutter, G.R.; Sørensen, P.S.; Thompson, A.J.; Wolinsky, J.S.; Balcer, L.J.; Banwell, B.; Barkhof, F.; et al. Defining the clinical course of multiple sclerosis: The 2013 revisions. *Neurology* **2014**, *83*, 278–286. [CrossRef] [PubMed]
12. Lassmann, H.; Brück, W.; Lucchinetti, C.F. The Immunopathology of Multiple Sclerosis: An Overview. *Brain Pathol.* **2007**, *17*, 210–218. [CrossRef] [PubMed]
13. Dendrou, C.A.; Fugger, L.; Friese, M.A. Immunopathology of multiple sclerosis. *Nat. Rev. Immunol.* **2015**, *15*, 545–558. [CrossRef]

14. Danikowski, K.M.; Jayaraman, S.; Prabhakar, B.S. Regulatory T cells in multiple sclerosis and myasthenia gravis. *J. Neuroinflammation* **2017**, *14*, 117. [CrossRef]
15. Haase, S.; Linker, R.A. Inflammation in multiple sclerosis. *Ther. Adv. Neurol. Disord.* **2021**, *14*, 17562864211007687. [CrossRef]
16. Bordet, R.; Camu, W.; De Seze, J.; Laplaud, D.-A.; Ouallet, J.-C.; Thouvenot, E. Mechanism of action of s1p receptor modulators in multiple sclerosis: The double requirement. *Rev. Neurol.* **2020**, *176*, 100–112. [CrossRef]
17. Stadelmann, C.; Wegner, C.; Bruck, W. Inflammation, demyelination, and degeneration—Recent insights from MS pathology. *Biochim. Biophys. Acta* **2011**, *1812*, 275–282. [CrossRef] [PubMed]
18. Perdaens, O.; van Pesch, V. Molecular Mechanisms of Immunosenescene and Inflammaging: Relevance to the Immunopathogenesis and Treatment of Multiple Sclerosis. *Front. Neurol.* **2022**, *12*, 811518. [CrossRef]
19. Martino, G.; Adorini, L.; Rieckmann, P.; Hillert, J.; Kallmann, B.; Comi, G.; Filippi, M. Inflammation in multiple sclerosis: The good, the bad, and the complex. *Lancet Neurol.* **2002**, *1*, 499–509. [CrossRef]
20. Billiau, A.; Heremans, H.; Vandekerckhove, F.; Dijkmans, R.; Sobis, H.; Meulepas, E.; Carton, H. Enhancement of experimental allergic encephalomyelitis in mice by antibodies against IFN-gamma. *J. Immunol.* **1988**, *140*, 1506–1510. [CrossRef]
21. Arnett, H.A.; Mason, J.; Marino, M.; Suzuki, K.; Matsushima, G.K.; Ting, J.P. TNF alpha promotes proliferation of oligoden-drocyte progenitors and remyelination. *Nat. Neurosci.* **2001**, *4*, 1116–1122. [CrossRef] [PubMed]
22. Acosta, M.; Cortes, C.; MacPhee, H.; Namaka, M.P. Exploring the role of nerve growth factor in multiple sclerosis: Implications in myelin repair. *CNS Neurol. Disord.—Drug Targets* **2013**, *12*, 1242–1256. [CrossRef] [PubMed]
23. Liu, J.; Marino, M.W.; Wong, G.; Grail, D.; Dunn, A.; Bettadapura, J.; Slavin, A.J.; Old, L.; Bernard, C.C. TNF is a potent an-ti-inflammatory cytokine in autoimmune-mediated demyelination. *Nat. Med.* **1998**, *4*, 78–83. [CrossRef]
24. Wang, K.; Song, F.; Fernandez-Escobar, A.; Luo, G.; Wang, J.-H.; Sun, Y. The Properties of Cytokines in Multiple Sclerosis: Pros and Cons. *Am. J. Med. Sci.* **2018**, *356*, 552–560. [CrossRef] [PubMed]
25. Hulshof, S.; Montagne, L.; De Groot, C.J.; Van Der Valk, P. Cellular localization and expression patterns of interleukin-10, interleukin-4, and their receptors in multiple sclerosis lesions. *Glia* **2002**, *38*, 24–35. [CrossRef]
26. Kerschensteiner, M.; Gallmeier, E.; Behrens, L.; Leal, V.V.; Misgeld, T.; Klinkert, W.E.; Kolbeck, R.; Hoppe, E.; Oropeza-Wekerle, R.L.; Bartke, I.; et al. Activated human T cells, B cells, and monocytes produce brain-derived neurotrophic factor in vitro and in inflammatory brain lesions: A neuroprotective role of inflammation? *J. Exp. Med.* **1999**, *189*, 865–870. [CrossRef] [PubMed]
27. Kappos, L.; Hartung, H.-P.; Freedman, M.S.; Boyko, A.; Radü, E.W.; Mikol, D.D.; Lamarine, M.; Hyvert, Y.; Freudensprung, U.; Plitz, T.; et al. Atacicept in multiple sclerosis (ATAMS): A randomised, placebo-controlled, double-blind, phase 2 trial. *Lancet Neurol.* **2014**, *13*, 353–363. [CrossRef]
28. Nociti, V.; Romozzi, M. The Role of BDNF in Multiple Sclerosis Neuroinflammation. *Int. J. Mol. Sci.* **2023**, *24*, 8447. [CrossRef]
29. Rodríguez, A.M.; Rodríguez, J.; Giambartolomei, G.H. Microglia at the Crossroads of Pathogen-Induced Neuroinflammation. *ASN Neuro* **2022**, *14*, 175909142211045. [CrossRef]
30. Colonna, M.; Butovsky, O. Microglia Function in the Central Nervous System During Health and Neurodegeneration. *Annu. Rev. Immunol.* **2017**, *35*, 441–468. [CrossRef]
31. Guo, S.; Wang, H.; Yin, Y. Microglia Polarization From M1 to M2 in Neurodegenerative Diseases. *Front. Aging Neurosci.* **2022**, *14*, 815347. [CrossRef] [PubMed]
32. Liu, X.; Ma, J.; Ding, G.; Gong, Q.; Wang, Y.; Yu, H.; Cheng, X. Microglia Polarization from M1 toward M2 Phenotype Is Promoted by *Astragalus Polysaccharides* Mediated through Inhibition of MiR-155 in Experimental Autoimmune Encephalo-myelitis. *Oxidative Med. Cell. Longev.* **2021**, *2021*, 5753452. [CrossRef] [PubMed]
33. Qie, S.; Ran, Y.; Lu, X.; Su, W.; Li, W.; Xi, J.; Gong, W.; Liu, Z. Candesartan Modulates Microglia Activation and Polarization via NF-KB Signaling Pathway. *Int. J. Immunopathol. Pharmacol.* **2020**, *34*, 205873842097490. [CrossRef] [PubMed]
34. Zhang, B.; Wei, Y.-Z.; Wang, G.-Q.; Li, D.-D.; Shi, J.-S.; Zhang, F. Targeting MAPK Pathways by Naringenin Modulates Mi-croglia M1/M2 Polarization in Lipopolysaccharide-Stimulated Cultures. *Front. Cell Neurosci.* **2019**, *12*, 531. [CrossRef] [PubMed]
35. Ding, Y.; Kang, J.; Liu, S.; Xu, Y.; Shao, B. The Protective Effects of Peroxisome Proliferator-Activated Receptor Gamma in Cerebral Ischemia-Reperfusion Injury. *Front. Neurol.* **2020**, *11*, 588516. [CrossRef] [PubMed]
36. Guerrero, B.L.; Sicotte, N.L. Microglia in Multiple Sclerosis: Friend or Foe? *Front. Immunol.* **2020**, *11*, 374. [CrossRef]
37. Gandhi, R.; Laroni, A.; Weiner, H.L. Role of the innate immune system in the pathogenesis of multiple sclerosis. *J. Neuroimmunol.* **2010**, *221*, 7–14. [CrossRef]
38. Luo, C.; Jian, C.; Liao, Y.; Huang, Q.; Wu, Y.; Liu, X.; Zou, D.; Wu, Y. The role of microglia in multiple sclerosis. *Neuropsychiatr. Dis. Treat.* **2017**, *13*, 1661–1667. [CrossRef]
39. Tang, Y.; Le, W. Differential Roles of M1 and M2 Microglia in Neurodegenerative Diseases. *Mol. Neurobiol.* **2016**, *53*, 1181–1194. [CrossRef]
40. Cherry, J.D.; Olschowka, J.A.; O'Banion, M.K. Neuroinflammation and M2 microglia: The good, the bad, and the inflamed. *J. Neuroinflamm.* **2014**, *11*, 98. [CrossRef]
41. Palasz, E.; Wilkaniec, A.; Stanaszek, L.; Andrzejewska, A.; Adamczyk, A. Glia-Neurotrophic Factor Relationships: Possible Role in Pathobiology of Neuroinflammation-Related Brain Disorders. *Int. J. Mol. Sci.* **2023**, *24*, 6321. [CrossRef] [PubMed]
42. Sofroniew, M.V.; Vinters, H.V. Astrocytes: Biology and pathology. *Acta Neuropathol.* **2010**, *119*, 7–35. [CrossRef] [PubMed]
43. Ponath, G.; Park, C.; Pitt, D. The Role of Astrocytes in Multiple Sclerosis. *Front. Immunol.* **2018**, *9*, 217. [CrossRef]
44. Correale, J.; Farez, M.F. The Role of Astrocytes in Multiple Sclerosis Progression. *Front. Neurol.* **2015**, *6*, 180. [CrossRef] [PubMed]

45. Voss, E.V.; Škuljec, J.; Gudi, V.; Skripuletz, T.; Pul, R.; Trebst, C.; Stangel, M. Characterisation of microglia during de- and remyelination: Can they create a repair promoting environment? *Neurobiol. Dis.* **2012**, *45*, 519–528. [CrossRef] [PubMed]
46. Hao, Z.; Liu, K.; Zhou, L.; Chen, P. Precious but convenient means of prevention and treatment: Physiological molecular mechanisms of interaction between exercise and motor factors and Alzheimer's disease. *Front. Physiol.* **2023**, *14*, 1193031. [CrossRef]
47. Archelos, J.J.; Storch, M.K.; Hartung, H.P. The role of B cells and autoantibodies in multiple sclerosis. *Ann. Neurol.* **2000**, *47*, 694–706. [CrossRef]
48. Serafini, B.; Rosicarelli, B.; Magliozzi, R.; Stigliano, E.; Aloisi, F. Detection of ectopic b-cell follicles with germinal centers in the meninges of patients with secondary progressive multiple sclerosis. *Brain Pathol.* **2004**, *14*, 164–174. [CrossRef]
49. Castillo-Trivino, T.; Braithwaite, D.; Bacchetti, P.; Waubant, E. Rituximab in relapsing and progressive forms of multiple sclerosis: A systematic review. *PLoS ONE* **2013**, *8*, e66308. [CrossRef]
50. Nourbakhsh, B.; Mowry, E.M. Multiple Sclerosis Risk Factors and Pathogenesis. *Contin. Lifelong Learn. Neurol.* **2019**, *25*, 596–610. [CrossRef]
51. Lassmann, H. Multiple sclerosis pathology. *Cold Spring Harb. Perspect. Med.* **2018**, *8*, a028936. [CrossRef] [PubMed]
52. Elliott, C.; Lindner, M.; Arthur, A.; Brennan, K.; Jarius, S.; Hussey, J.; Chan, A.; Stroet, A.; Olsson, T.; Willison, H.; et al. Functional identification of pathogenic autoantibody responses in patients with multiple sclerosis. *Brain* **2012**, *135*, 1819–1833. [CrossRef]
53. Pröbstel, A.-K.; Sanderson, N.S.R.; Derfuss, T. B Cells and autoantibodies in multiple sclerosis. *Int. J. Mol. Sci.* **2015**, *16*, 16576–16592. [CrossRef] [PubMed]
54. Liu, Y.; Given, K.S.; Harlow, D.E.; Matschulat, A.M.; Macklin, W.B.; Bennett, J.L.; Owens, G.P. Myelin-specific multiple sclerosis antibodies cause complement-dependent oligodendrocyte loss and demyelination. *Acta Neuropathol. Commun.* **2017**, *5*, 25. [CrossRef]
55. Miyachi, Y.; Fujii, T.; Yamasaki, R.; Tsuchimoto, D.; Iinuma, K.; Sakoda, A.; Fukumoto, S.; Matsushita, T.; Masaki, K.; Isobe, N.; et al. Serum Anti-oligodendrocyte Autoantibodies in Patients With Multiple Sclerosis Detected by a Tissue-Based Immunofluores-cence Assay. *Front. Neurol.* **2021**, *12*, 681980. [CrossRef] [PubMed]
56. van der Poel, M.; Hoepel, W.; Hamann, J.; Huitinga, I.; Dunnen, J.D. IgG Immune Complexes Break Immune Tolerance of Human Microglia. *J. Immunol.* **2020**, *205*, 2511–2518. [CrossRef]
57. Zhou, W.; Graner, M.; Paucek, P.; Beseler, C.; Boisen, M.; Bubak, A.; Asturias, F.; George, W.; Graner, A.; Ormond, D.; et al. Multiple sclerosis plasma IgG aggregates induce complement-dependent neuronal apoptosis. *Cell Death Dis.* **2023**, *14*, 254. [CrossRef] [PubMed]
58. Tonev, D.G.; Momchilova, A.B. Therapeutic Plasma Exchange in Certain Immune-Mediated Neurological Disorders: Focus on a Novel Nanomembrane-Based Technology. *Biomedicines* **2023**, *11*, 328. [CrossRef] [PubMed]
59. Zaprianova, E.; Deleva, D.; Ilinov, P.; Sultanov, E.; Filchev, A.; Christova, L.; Sultanov, B. Serum ganglioside patterns in multiple sclerosis. *Neurochem. Res.* **2001**, *26*, 95–100. [CrossRef]
60. Kanda, T.; Iwasaki, T.; Yamawaki, M.; Tai, T.; Mizusawa, H. Anti-GM1 antibody facilitates leakage in an in vitro blood-nerve barrier model. *Neurology* **2000**, *55*, 585–587. [CrossRef]
61. Lehmann, H.C.; Lopez, P.H.H.; Zhang, G.; Ngyuen, T.; Zhang, J.; Kieseier, B.C.; Mori, S.; Sheikh, K.A. Passive immunization with anti-ganglioside antibodies directly inhibits axon regeneration in an animal model. *J. Neurosci.* **2007**, *27*, 27–34. [CrossRef]
62. Ravindranath, M.H.; Muthugounder, S.; Saravanan, T.S.; Presser, N.; Morton, D.L. Human antiganglioside autoantibodies: Validation of ELISA. *Ann. N. Y. Acad. Sci.* **2005**, *1050*, 229–242. [CrossRef] [PubMed]
63. Levi-Montalcini, R.; Skaper, S.D.; Dal Toso, R.; Petrelli, L.; Leon, A. Nerve growth factor: From neurotrophin to neurokine. *Trends Neurosci.* **1996**, *19*, 514–520. [CrossRef]
64. Bibel, M.; Barde, Y.-A. Neurotrophins: Key regulators of cell fate and cell shape in the vertebrate nervous system. *Genes Dev.* **2000**, *14*, 2919–2937. [CrossRef] [PubMed]
65. Barbacid, M. Neurotrophic factors and their receptors. *Curr. Opin. Cell Biol.* **1995**, *7*, 148–155. [CrossRef] [PubMed]
66. Patapoutian, A.; Reichardt, L.F. Trk receptors: Mediators of neurotrophin action. *Curr. Opin. Neurobiol.* **2001**, *11*, 272–280. [CrossRef]
67. Chao, M.V. The p75 neurotrophin receptor. *J. Neurobiol.* **1994**, *25*, 1373–1385. [CrossRef]
68. Barker, P.A. p75NTR is positively promiscuous: Novel partners and new insights. *Neuron* **2004**, *42*, 529–533. [CrossRef]
69. Chao, M.V. Neurotrophins and their receptors: A convergence point for many signalling pathways. *Nat. Rev. Neurosci.* **2003**, *4*, 299–309. [CrossRef]
70. Chao, M.V.; Hempstead, B.L. p75 and Trk: A two-receptor system. *Trends Neurosci.* **1995**, *18*, 321–326. [CrossRef]
71. Alcover-Sanchez, B.; Garcia-Martin, G.; Wandosell, F.; Cubelos, B. R-Ras GTPases Signaling Role in Myelin Neurodegenerative Diseases. *Int. J. Mol. Sci.* **2020**, *21*, 5911. [CrossRef]
72. Gaesser, J.M.; Fyffe-Maricich, S.L. Intracellular signaling pathway regulation of myelination and remyelination in the CNS. *Exp. Neurol.* **2016**, *283*, 501–511. [CrossRef] [PubMed]
73. Gonsalvez, D.; Ferner, A.H.; Peckham, H.; Murray, S.S.; Xiao, J. The roles of extracellular related-kinases 1 and 2 signaling in CNS myelination. *Neuropharmacology* **2016**, *110*, 586–593. [CrossRef] [PubMed]

74. Ishii, A.; Fyffe-Maricich, S.L.; Furusho, M.; Miller, R.H.; Bansal, R. ERK1/ERK2 MAPK signaling is required to increase myelin thickness independent of oligodendrocyte differentiation and initiation of myelination. *J. Neurosci.* **2012**, *32*, 8855–8864. [CrossRef] [PubMed]
75. Ishii, A.; Furusho, M.; Dupree, J.L.; Bansal, R. Role of ERK1/2 MAPK signaling in the maintenance of myelin and axonal in-tegrity in the adult CNS. *J. Neurosci.* **2014**, *34*, 16031–16045. [CrossRef]
76. Duncan, G.J.; Plemel, J.R.; Assinck, P.; Manesh, S.B.; Muir, F.G.W.; Hirata, R.; Berson, M.; Liu, J.; Wegner, M.; Emery, B.; et al. Myelin regulatory factor drives remyelination in multiple sclerosis. *Acta Neuropathol.* **2017**, *134*, 403–422. [CrossRef]
77. Niewiadomska, G.; Mietelska-Porowska, A.; Mazurkiewicz, M. The Cholinergic System, Nerve Growth Factor and the Cyto-skeleton. *Behav. Brain Res.* **2011**, *221*, 515–526. [CrossRef]
78. Du, Y.; Dreyfus, C.F. Oligodendrocytes as Providers of Growth Factors. *J. Neurosci. Res.* **2002**, *68*, 647–654. [CrossRef]
79. Bracci-Laudiero, L.; Bonini, S.; Manni, L.; Aloe, L. The expanding role of nerve growth factor: From neurotrophic activity to immunologic diseases. *Allergy* **1997**, *52*, 883–894. [CrossRef]
80. Kalinowska-Lyszczarz, A.; Losy, J. The role of neurotrophins in multiple sclerosis-pathological and clinical implications. *Int. J. Mol. Sci.* **2012**, *13*, 13713–13725. [CrossRef]
81. Linker, R.; Gold, R.; Luhder, F. Function of neurotrophic factors beyond the nervous system: Infammation and autoimmune demyelination. *Crit. Rev. Immunol.* **2009**, *29*, 43–68. [CrossRef] [PubMed]
82. Hohlfeld, R. Neurotrophic cross-talk between the nervous and immune systems: Relevance for repair strategies in multiple sclerosis? *J. Neurol. Sci.* **2008**, *265*, 93–96. [CrossRef] [PubMed]
83. Sawada, J.; Itakura, A.; Tanaka, A.; Furusaka, T.; Matsuda, H. Nerve growth factor functions as a chemoattractant for mast cells through both mitogen-activated protein kinase and phosphatidylinositol 3-kinase signaling pathways. *Blood* **2000**, *95*, 2052–2058. [CrossRef] [PubMed]
84. Samah, B.; Porcheray, F.; Gras, G. Neurotrophins modulate monocyte chemotaxis without affecting macrophage function. *Clin. Exp. Immunol.* **2008**, *151*, 476–486. [CrossRef] [PubMed]
85. Susaki, Y.; Shimizu, S.; Katakura, K.; Watanabe, N.; Kawamoto, K.; Matsumoto, M.; Tsudzuki, M.; Furusaka, T.; Kitamura, Y.; Matsuda, H. Functional properties of murine macrophages promoted by nerve growth factor. *Blood* **1996**, *88*, 4630–4637. [CrossRef]
86. Beigelman, A.; Levy, J.; Hadad, N.; Pinsk, V.; Haim, A.; Fruchtman, Y.; Levy, R. Abnormal neutrophil chemotactic activity in children with congenital insensitivity to pain with anhidrosis (CIPA): The role of nerve growth factor. *Clin. Immunol.* **2009**, *130*, 365–372. [CrossRef]
87. Kannan, Y.; Ushio, H.; Koyama, H.; Okada, M.; Oikawa, M.; Yoshihara, T.; Kaneko, M.; Matsuda, H. Nerve growth factor enhances survival, phagocytosis, and superoxide production of murine neutrophils. *Blood* **1991**, *77*, 1320–1325. [CrossRef]
88. Hamada, A.; Watanabe, N.; Ohtomo, H.; Matsuda, H. Nerve growth factor enhances survival and cytotoxic activity of human eosinophils. *Br. J. Haematol.* **1996**, *93*, 299–302. [CrossRef]
89. Mazurek, N.; Weskamp, G.; Erne, P.; Otten, U. Nerve growth factor induces mast cell degranulation without changing intra-cellular calcium levels. *FEBS Lett.* **1986**, *198*, 315–320. [CrossRef]
90. Kawamoto, K.; Okada, T.; Kannan, Y.; Ushio, H.; Matsumoto, M.; Matsuda, H. Nerve growth factor prevents apoptosis of rat peritoneal mast cells through the Trk proto-oncogene receptor. *Blood* **1995**, *86*, 4638–4644. [CrossRef]
91. Tuszynski, M.H.; Thal, L.; Pay, M.; Salmon, D.P.; U, H.S.; Bakay, R.; Patel, P.; Blesch, A.; Vahlsing, H.L.; Ho, G.; et al. A phase 1 clinical trial of nerve growth factor gene therapy for Alzheimer disease. *Nat. Med.* **2005**, *11*, 551–555. [CrossRef] [PubMed]
92. Hadaczek, P.; Eberling, J.L.; Pivirotto, P.; Bringas, J.; Forsayeth, J.; Bankiewicz, K.S. Eight years of clinical improvement in mptp-lesioned primates after gene therapy with AAV2-hAADC. *Mol. Ther.* **2010**, *18*, 1458–1461. [CrossRef]
93. Tuszynski, M.H.; Yang, J.H.; Barba, D.; Hoi-Sang, U.; Bakay, R.A.E.; Pay, M.M.; Masliah, E.; Conner, J.M.; Kobalka, P.; Roy, S.; et al. Nerve growth factor gene therapy activation of neuronal responses in Alzheimer disease. *JAMA Neurol.* **2015**, *72*, 1139–1147. [CrossRef] [PubMed]
94. Tuszynski, M.H. Intraparenchymal NGF infusions rescue degenerating cholinergic neurons. *Cell Transplant.* **2000**, *9*, 629–636. [CrossRef] [PubMed]
95. Jönhagen, M.E.; Nordberg, A.; Amberla, K.; Bäckman, L.; Ebendal, T.; Meyerson, B.; Olson, L.; Seiger, Å.; Shigeta, M.; Theodorsson, E.; et al. Intracerebroventricular infusion of nerve growth factor in three patients with alzheimer's disease. *Dement. Geriatr. Cogn. Disord.* **1998**, *9*, 246–257. [CrossRef]
96. Delivanoglou, N.; Boziki, M.; Theotokis, P.; Kesidou, E.; Touloumi, O.; Dafi, N.; Nousiopoulou, E.; Lagoudaki, R.; Grigoriadis, N.; Charalampopoulos, I.; et al. Spatio-temporal expression profile of NGF and the two-receptor system, TrkA and p75NTR, in experimental autoimmune encephalomyelitis. *J. Neuroinflamm.* **2020**, *17*, 41. [CrossRef]
97. Minnone, G.; De Benedetti, F.; Bracci-Laudiero, L. NGF and its receptors in the regulation of inflammatory response. *Int. J. Mol. Sci.* **2017**, *18*, 1028. [CrossRef]
98. Cohen, I.R.; Schwartz, M. Autoimmune maintenance and neuroprotection of the central nervous system. *J. Neuroimmunol.* **1999**, *100*, 111–114. [CrossRef]
99. Schwartz, M.; Raposo, C. Protective autoimmunity: A unifying model for the immune network involved in CNS repair. *Neuroscientist* **2014**, *20*, 343–358. [CrossRef]

100. Lee, X.; Yang, Z.; Shao, Z.; Rosenberg, S.S.; Levesque, M.; Pepinsky, R.B.; Qiu, M.; Miller, R.H.; Chan, J.R.; Mi, S. NGF regulates the expression of axonal LINGO-1 to inhibit oligodendrocyte differentiation and myelination. *J. Neurosci.* **2007**, *27*, 220–225. [CrossRef]
101. Plemel, J.R.; Liu, W.Q.; Yong, V.W. Remyelination therapies: A new direction and challenge in multiple sclerosis. *Nat. Rev. Drug Discov.* **2017**, *16*, 617–634. [CrossRef] [PubMed]
102. Lee, J.K.; Geoffroy, C.G.; Chan, A.F.; Tolentino, K.E.; Crawford, M.J.; Leal, M.A.; Kang, B.; Zheng, B. Assessing spinal axon regen-eration and sprouting in Nogo-, MAG-, and OMgp-deficient mice. *Neuron* **2010**, *66*, 663–670. [CrossRef] [PubMed]
103. Alatrash, R.; Golubenko, M.; Martynova, E.; Garanina, E.; Mukhamedshina, Y.; Khaiboullina, S.; Rizvanov, A.; Salafutdinov, I.; Arkhipova, S. Genetically Engineered Artificial Microvesicles Carrying Nerve Growth Factor Restrains the Progression of Au-toimmune Encephalomyelitis in an Experimental Mouse Model. *Int. J. Mol. Sci.* **2023**, *24*, 8332. [CrossRef] [PubMed]
104. Baldassarro, V.A.; Cescatti, M.; Rocco, M.L.; Aloe, L.; Lorenzini, L.; Giardino, L.; Calzà, L. Nerve growth factor promotes differ-entiation and protects the oligodendrocyte precursor cells from in vitro hypoxia/ischemia. *Front Neurosci.* **2023**, *17*, 1111170. [CrossRef] [PubMed]
105. Lorenzini, L.; Baldassarro, V.A.; Stanzani, A.; Giardino, L. Nerve Growth Factor: The First Molecule of the Neurotrophin Family. *Adv. Exp. Med. Biol.* **2021**, *1331*, 3–10. [CrossRef] [PubMed]
106. Loy, R.; Taglialatela, G.; Angelucci, L.; Heyer, D.; Perez-Polo, R. Regional CNS uptake of blood-borne nerve growth factor. *J. Neurosci. Res.* **1994**, *39*, 339–346. [CrossRef]
107. Tiberi, A.; Carucci, N.M.; Testa, G.; Rizzi, C.; Pacifico, P.; Borgonovo, G.; Arisi, I.; D'onofrio, M.; Brandi, R.; Gan, W.-B.; et al. Reduced levels of NGF shift astrocytes toward a neurotoxic phenotype. *Front. Cell Dev. Biol.* **2023**, *11*, 1165125. [CrossRef]
108. Rizzi, C.; Tiberi, A.; Giustizieri, M.; Marrone, M.C.; Gobbo, F.; Carucci, N.M.; Meli, G.; Arisi, I.; D'Onofrio, M.; Marinelli, S.; et al. NGF steers microglia toward a neuroprotective phenotype. *Glia* **2018**, *66*, 1395–1416. [CrossRef]
109. Villoslada, P.; Genain, C.P. Role of nerve growth factor and other trophic factors in brain inflammation. *Prog. Brain Res.* **2004**, *146*, 403–414. [CrossRef]
110. Guarnieri, G.; Sarchielli, E.; Comeglio, P.; Herrera-Puerta, E.; Piaceri, I.; Nacmias, B.; Benelli, M.; Kelsey, G.; Maggi, M.; Gallina, P.; et al. Tumor necrosis factor α influences phenotypic plasticity and promotes epigenetic changes in human basal forebrain cholinergic neuroblasts. *Int. J. Mol. Sci.* **2020**, *21*, 6128. [CrossRef]
111. Micera, A.; Properzi, F.; Triaca, V.; Aloe, L. Nerve growth factor antibody exacerbates neuropathological signs of experimental allergic encephalomyelitis in adult Lewis rats. *J. Neuroimmunol.* **2000**, *104*, 116–123. [CrossRef]
112. Villoslada, P.; Hauser, S.L.; Bartke, I.; Unger, J.; Heald, N.; Rosenberg, D.; Cheung, S.W.; Mobley, W.C.; Fisher, S.; Genain, C.P. Human nerve growth factor protects common marmosets against autoimmune encephalomyelitis by switching the balance of t helper cell type 1 and 2 cytokines within the central nervous system. *J. Exp. Med.* **2000**, *191*, 1799–1806. [CrossRef] [PubMed]
113. Kenarov, P.; Petrov, N.; Voinov, V.; Daskalov, M.; Anaya, F.; Russo, G.; Momchilova, A. A new approach using nanomem-brane—Based therapeutic plasmapheresis for treatment of patients with multiple sclerosis. A case report. *J. Pharmacol. Clin. Toxicol.* **2014**, *2*, 1031.
114. Hannun, Y.A. The sphingomyelin cycle and the second messenger function of ceramide. *J. Biol. Chem.* **1994**, *269*, 3125–3128. [CrossRef] [PubMed]
115. Igarashi, Y. Functional roles of sphingosine and sphingosine-1-phosphate in regard to membrane sphingolipid signaling pathways. *J. Biochem.* **1997**, *122*, 1080–1087. [CrossRef]
116. Lucaciu, A.; Brunkhorst, R.; Pfeilschifter, J.M.; Pfeilschifter, W.; Subburayalu, J. The S1P-S1PR Axis in Neurological Disor-ders-Insights into Current and Future Therapeutic Perspectives. *Cells* **2020**, *9*, 1515. [CrossRef]
117. Mizugishi, K.; Yamashita, T.; Olivera, A.; Miller, G.F.; Spiegel, S.; Proia, R.L. Essential Role for Sphingosine Kinases in Neural and Vascular Development. *Mol. Cell. Biol.* **2005**, *25*, 11113–11121. [CrossRef]
118. Riganti, L.; Antonucci, F.; Gabrielli, M.; Prada, I.; Giussani, P.; Viani, P.; Valtorta, F.; Menna, E.; Matteoli, M.; Verderio, C. Sphingosine-1-Phosphate (S1P) Impacts Presynaptic Functions by Regulating Synapsin I Localization in the Presynaptic Com-partment. *J. Neurosci.* **2016**, *36*, 4624–4634. [CrossRef]
119. Moore, A.N.; Kampfl, A.W.; Zhao, X.; Hayes, R.L.; Dash, P.K. Sphingosine-1-phosphate induces apoptosis of cultured hippo-campal neurons that requires protein phosphatases and activator protein-1 complexes. *Neuroscience* **1999**, *94*, 405–415. [CrossRef]
120. Giussani, P.C.; Ferraretto, A.; Gravaghi, C.; Bassi, R.; Tettamanti, G.; Riboni, L.; Viani, P. Sphingosine-1-Phosphate and Cal-cium Signaling in Cerebellar Astrocytes and Differentiated Granule Cells. *Neurochem. Res.* **2006**, *32*, 27–37. [CrossRef]
121. Mitroi, D.N.; Deutschmann, A.U.; Raucamp, M.; Karunakaran, I.; Glebov, K.; Hans, M.; Walter, J.; Saba, J.; Gräler, M.; Ehninger, D.; et al. Sphingosine 1-phosphate lyase ablation disrupts presynaptic architecture and function via an ubiquitin- proteasome mediated mechanism. *Sci. Rep.* **2016**, *6*, 37064. [CrossRef]
122. Obinata, H.; Hla, T. Sphingosine 1-phosphate and inflammation. *Int. Immunol.* **2019**, *31*, 617–625. [CrossRef] [PubMed]
123. Jana, A.; Pahan, K. Sphingolipids in multiple sclerosis. *Neuromolecular Med.* **2010**, *12*, 351–361. [CrossRef] [PubMed]
124. Kułakowska, A.; Żendzian-Piotrowska, M.; Baranowski, M.; Konończuk, T.; Drozdowski, W.; Górski, J.; Bucki, R. Intrathecal increase of sphingosine 1-phosphate at early stage multiple sclerosis. *Neurosci. Lett.* **2010**, *477*, 149–152. [CrossRef]
125. Hopkin, S.J.; Lewis, J.W.; Krautter, F.; Chimen, M.; McGettrick, H.M. Triggering the Resolution of Immune Mediated Inflammatory Diseases: Can Targeting Leukocyte Migration Be the Answer? *Front. Pharmacol.* **2019**, *10*, 184. [CrossRef] [PubMed]

126. Pyne, N.J.; Pyne, S. Sphingosine 1-Phosphate Receptor 1 Signaling in Mammalian Cells. *Molecules* **2017**, *22*, 344. [CrossRef] [PubMed]
127. Momchilova, A.; Pankov, R.; Alexandrov, A.; Markovska, T.; Pankov, S.; Krastev, P.; Staneva, G.; Vassileva, E.; Krastev, N.; Pinkas, A. Sphingolipid Catabolism and Glycerophospholipid Levels Are Altered in Erythrocytes and Plasma from Multiple Sclerosis Patients. *Int. J. Mol. Sci.* **2022**, *23*, 7592. [CrossRef]
128. Bravo, G.; Cedeño, R.R.; Casadevall, M.P.; Ramió-Torrentà, L. Sphingosine-1-Phosphate (S1P) and S1P Signaling Pathway Modulators, from Current Insights to Future Perspectives. *Cells* **2022**, *11*, 2058. [CrossRef]
129. Garris, C.S.; Wu, L.; Acharya, S.; Arac, A.; Blaho, V.A.; Huang, Y.; Moon, B.S.; Axtell, R.C.; Ho, P.P.; Steinberg, G.K.; et al. Defective sphingosine 1-phosphate receptor 1 (S1P1) phosphorylation exacerbates TH17-mediated autoimmune neuroin-flammation. *Nat. Immunol.* **2013**, *14*, 1166–1172. [CrossRef]
130. Assi, E.; Cazzato, D.; De Palma, C.; Perrotta, C.; Clementi, E.; Cervia, D. Sphingolipids and Brain Resident Macrophages in Neuroinflammation: An Emerging Aspect of Nervous System Pathology. *J. Immunol. Res.* **2013**, *2013*, 309302. [CrossRef]
131. Noda, H.; Takeuchi, H.; Mizuno, T.; Suzumura, A. Fingolimod phosphate promotes the neuroprotective effects of microglia. *J. Neuroimmunol.* **2013**, *256*, 13–18. [CrossRef] [PubMed]
132. Cohan, S.; Lucassen, E.; Smoot, K.; Brink, J.; Chen, C. Sphingosine-1-Phosphate: Its Pharmacological Regulation and the Treatment of Multiple Sclerosis: A Review Article. *Biomedicines* **2020**, *8*, 227. [CrossRef] [PubMed]
133. Proia, R.L.; Hla, T. Emerging biology of sphingosine-1-phosphate: Its role in pathogenesis and therapy. *J. Clin. Invest.* **2015**, *125*, 1379–1387. [CrossRef]
134. Grassi, S.; Mauri, L.; Prioni, S.; Cabitta, L.; Sonnino, S.; Prinetti, A.; Giussani, P. Sphingosine 1-Phosphate Receptors and Met-abolic Enzymes as Druggable Targets for Brain Diseases. *Front. Pharmacol.* **2019**, *10*, 807. [CrossRef]
135. Fischer, I.; Alliod, C.; Martinier, N.; Newcombe, J.; Brana, C.; Pouly, S. Sphingosine Kinase 1 and sphingosine 1-Phosphate receptor 3 are functionally upregulated on astrocytes under pro-inflammatory conditions. *PLoS ONE* **2011**, *6*, e23905. [CrossRef]
136. Dusaban, S.S.; Chun, J.; Rosen, H.; Purcell, N.H.; Brown, J.H. Sphingosine 1-phosphate receptor 3 and RhoA signaling mediate inflammatory gene expression in astrocytes. *J. Neuroinflamm.* **2017**, *14*, 111. [CrossRef] [PubMed]
137. Yanagida, K.; Hla, T. Vascular and Immunobiology of the Circulatory Sphingosine 1-Phosphate Gradient. *Annu. Rev. Physiol.* **2017**, *79*, 67–91. [CrossRef]
138. Marfia, G.; Navone, S.; Guarnaccia, L.; Campanella, R.; Mondoni, M.; Locatelli, M.; Barassi, A.; Fontana, L.; Palumbo, F.; Garzia, E.; et al. Decreased serum level of sphingosine-1-phosphate: A novel predictor of clinical severity in COVID-19. *EMBO Mol. Med.* **2021**, *13*, e13424. [CrossRef]
139. Connelly-Smith, L.; Alquist, C.R.; Aqui, N.A.; Hofmann, J.C.; Klingel, R.; Onwuemene, O.A.; Patriquin, C.J.; Pham, H.P.; Sanchez, A.P.; Schneiderman, J.; et al. Guidelines on the Use of Therapeutic Apheresis in Clinical Practice—Evidence-Based Approach from the Writing Committee of the American Society for Apheresis: The Ninth Special Issue. *J. Clin. Apher.* **2023**, *38*, 77–278. [CrossRef]
140. Redant, S.; De Bels, D.; Ismaili, K.; Honoré, P.M. Membrane-based therapeutic plasma exchange in intensive care. *Blood Purif.* **2021**, *50*, 290–297. [CrossRef]
141. Reeves, H.M.; Winters, J.L. The mechanisms of action of plasma exchange. *Br. J. Haematol.* **2014**, *164*, 342–351. [CrossRef] [PubMed]
142. Lin, Y.; Oji, S.; Miyamoto, K.; Narita, T.; Kameyama, M.; Matsuo, H. Real-world application of plasmapheresis for neurological disease: Results from the Japan-Plasmapheresis Outcome and Practice Patterns Study. *Ther. Apher. Dial.* **2023**, *27*, 123–135. [CrossRef] [PubMed]
143. Yamakova, Y.; Ilieva, V.A.; Petkov, R.; Yankov, G. Nanomembrane-Based Therapeutic Plasmapheresis after Non-Invasive Ventilation Failure for Treatment of a Patient with Acute Respiratory Distress Syndrome and Myasthenia Gravis: A Case Re-port. *Blood Purif.* **2019**, *48*, 382–384. [CrossRef] [PubMed]
144. Alexandrov, A.; Vassileva, P.; Momchilova, A.; Tsonchev, Z.; Kirilova, Y.; Ivanova, R.; Sapundzhiev, P.; Petkova, D.; Tzoneva, R.; Daskalov, M.; et al. A new approach using nanomembrane-based therapeutic plasmapheresis for treatment of patients with multiple sclerosis and neuromyelitis optica. *Comptes Rendus L'academie Bulg. Sci.* **2016**, *69*, 373–384.
145. Momchilova, A.; Tsonchev, Z.; Hadzhilazova, M.; Tzoneva, R.; Alexandrov, A.; Nikolakov, D.; Ilieva, V.; Pankov, R. Sphin-golipid Metabolism Is Dysregulated in Erythrocytes from Multiple Sclerosis Patient. *Comptes Rendus L'academie Bulg. Des Sci.* **2020**, *73*, 426–432.
146. Sapundzhiev, P.; Momchilova, A.; Vassileva, P.; Kirilova, Y.; Ivanova, R.; Bozhilova, M.; Orozova, M.; Staneva, G.; Krastev, P.; Pankov, R.; et al. Plasmapheresis Affects Ophthalmological Parameters and Oxidative Stress in Patients with Multiple Sclerosis and Neuromyelitis Optica. *Arch. Biomed. Eng. Biotechnol.* **2021**, *5*, 000617.
147. Tenchov, B.; Koynova, R.; Antonova, B.; Zaharinova, S.; Abarova, S.; Tsonchev, Z.; Komsa-Penkova, R.; Momchilova, A. Blood plasma thermal behavior and protein oxidation as indicators of multiple sclerosis clinical status and plasma exchange therapy progression. *Thermochim. Acta* **2019**, *671*, 193–199. [CrossRef]
148. Tsonchev, Z.; Alexandrov, A.; Momchilova, A.; Pankov, R.; Orozova, M.; Georgieva, R.; Georgiev, S.; Alexandrov, S.; Voinov, V.; Anaya, F.; et al. *Therapeutic Apheresis with Nanotechnology Membrane for Human Diseases*; Bulgarian Academy of Science Prof. Marin Drinov Publishing House: Sofia, Bulgaria, 2020; Volume 2, pp. 1–163.
149. Tonev, D.; Georgieva, R.; Vavrek, E. Our Clinical Experience in the Treatment of Myasthenia Gravis Acute Exacerbations with a Novel Nanomembrane-Based Therapeutic Plasma Exchange Technology. *J. Clin. Med.* **2022**, *11*, 4021. [CrossRef]

150. Escolar, G.; Páez, A.; Cid, J. Conventional Therapeutic Plasma Exchange Versus Low Volume Plasma Exchange in Chronic Pathologies: Potential Benefit in Alzheimer's Disease. *Plasmatology* **2022**, *16*, 26348535221131685. [CrossRef]
151. Klingele, M.; Allmendinger, C.; Thieme, S.; Baerens, L.; Fliser, D.; Jan, B. Therapeutic apheresis within immune-mediated neurological disorders: Dosing and its effectiveness. *Sci. Rep.* **2020**, *10*, 7925. [CrossRef]
152. Dorst, J.; Fillies, F.; Dreyhaupt, J.; Senel, M.; Tumani, H. Safety and Tolerability of Plasma Exchange and Immunoadsorption in Neuroinflammatory Diseases. *J. Clin. Med.* **2020**, *9*, 2874. [CrossRef]
153. Padmanabhan, A.; Connelly-Smith, L.; Aqui, N.; Balogun, R.A.; Klingel, R.; Meyer, E.; Pham, H.P.; Schneiderman, J.; Witt, V.; Wu, Y.; et al. Guidelines on the Use of Therapeutic Apheresis in Clinical Practice—Evidence-Based Approach from the Writing Committee of the American Society for Apheresis: The Eighth Special Issue. *J. Clin. Apher.* **2019**, *34*, 171–354. [CrossRef]
154. Strasser, E. Principles of Therapeutic Apheresis in Neurological Disease. *Transfus. Med. Hemotherapy* **2023**, *50*, 88–97. [CrossRef]
155. Chang, X.; Gorbet, M. The effect of shear on in vitro platelet and leukocyte material-induced activation. *J. Biomater. Appl.* **2013**, *28*, 407–415. [CrossRef]
156. Yeh, J.H.; Chien, P.J.; Hsueh, Y.M.; Shih, C.M.; Chiu, H.C. Changes in the lymphocyte subset after double-filtration plasmapheresis. *Am. J. Clin. Pathol.* **2007**, *128*, 940–944. [CrossRef] [PubMed]
157. Adamson, R.H.; Clark, J.F.; Radeva, M.; Kheirolomoom, A.; Ferrara, K.W.; Curry, F.E. Albumin modulates S1P delivery from red blood cells in perfused microvessels: Mechanism of the protein effect. *Am. J. Physiol. Heart Circ. Physiol.* **2014**, *306*, H1011–H1017. [CrossRef] [PubMed]
158. Hardersen, R.; Enebakk, T.; Christiansen, D.; Ludviksen, J.K.; Mollnes, T.E.; Lappegård, K.T.; Hovland, A. Comparison of cytokine changes in three different lipoprotein apheresis systems in an ex vivo whole blood model. *J. Clin. Apher.* **2020**, *35*, 104–116. [CrossRef] [PubMed]
159. Alexandrov, A.; Momchilova, A.; Orozova, M.; Alexandrov, S.; Krastev, P.; Stanev, G.; Nikolova, B.; Tsonchev, Z. *Therapeutic Apheresis*; Bulgarian Academy of Science Prof. Marin Drinov Publishing House: Sofia, Bulgaria, 2022; pp. 1–120.
160. Dixit, D.; Okuniewska, M.; Schwab, S.R. Secrets and lyase: Control of sphingosine 1-phosphate distribution. *Immunol. Rev.* **2019**, *289*, 173–185. [CrossRef] [PubMed]
161. Brinkmann, V.; Billich, A.; Baumruker, T.; Heining, P.; Schmouder, R.; Francis, G.; Aradhye, S.; Burtin, P. Fingolimod (FTY720): Discovery and development of an oral drug to treat multiple sclerosis. *Nat. Rev. Drug Discov.* **2010**, *9*, 883–897. [CrossRef]
162. Pyne, S.; Rakhit, S.; Conway, A.M.; McKie, A.; Darroch, P.; Tate, R.; Pyne, N. Extracellular actions of sphingosine I-phosphate through endothelial differentiation gene products in mammalian cells: Role in regulating proliferation and apoptosis. *Biochem. Soc. Trans.* **1999**, *27*, 404–409. [CrossRef]
163. Ghasemi, R.; Dargahi, L.; Ahmadiani, A. Integrated sphingosine-1 phosphate signaling in the central nervous system: From physiological equilibrium to pathological damage. *Pharmacol. Res.* **2016**, *104*, 156–164. [CrossRef] [PubMed]
164. Petrou, P.; Ben-Hur, T.; Vaknin-Dembinsky, A.; Abramsky, O.; Karussis, D. Clinical Efficacy of Plasma-Exchange in Patients with Progressive forms of Multiple Sclerosis and NMO-Spectrum Disease. *J. Mult. Scler.* **2016**, *3*, 1–6. [CrossRef]
165. Jacob, S.; Mazibrada, G.; Irani, S.R.; Jacob, A.; Yudina, A. The Role of Plasma Exchange in the Treatment of Refractory Autoimmune Neurological Diseases: A Narrative Review. *J. Neuroimmune Pharmacol.* **2021**, *16*, 806–817. [CrossRef] [PubMed]
166. Cortese, I.; Chaudhry, V.; So, Y.T.; Cantor, F.; Cornblath, D.R.; Rae-Grant, A. Evidence-based guideline update: Plasmapheresis in neurologic disorders: Report of the Therapeutics and Technology Assessment Subcommittee of the American Academy of Neurology. *Neurology* **2011**, *76*, 294–300. [CrossRef]
167. Lipphardt, M.; Mühlhausen, J.; Kitze, B.; Heigl, F.; Mauch, E.; Helms, J.; Müller, G.A.; Koziolek, M.J. Immunoadsorption or plasma exchange in steroid-refractory multiple sclerosis and neuromyelitis optica. *J. Clin. Apher.* **2019**, *34*, 381–391. [CrossRef]
168. Blechinger, S.; Ehler, J.; Bsteh, G.; Winkelmann, A.; Leutmezer, F.; Meister, S.; Santer, A.; Hecker, M.; Berger, T.; Rommer, P.; et al. Therapeutic plasma exchange in steroid-refractory multiple sclerosis relapses. A retrospective two-center study. *Ther. Adv. Neurol. Disord.* **2021**, *14*, 1756286420975642. [CrossRef]
169. Meca-Lallana, J.E.; Hernández-Clares, R.; León-Hernández, A.; Genovés Aleixandre, A.; Cacho Pérez, M.; Martín-Fernández, J.J. Plasma exchange for steroidrefractory relapses in multiple sclerosis: An observational, MRI pilot study. *Clin. Ther.* **2013**, *35*, 474–485. [CrossRef]
170. Bunganic, R.; Blahutova, S.; Revendova, K.; Zapletalova, O.; Hradilek, P.; Hrdlickova, R.; Ganesh, A.; Cermakova, Z.; Bar, M.; Volny, O. Therapeutic plasma exchange in multiple sclerosis patients with an aggressive relapse: An observational analysis in a high-volume center. *Sci. Rep.* **2022**, *12*, 18374. [CrossRef]
171. Kenarov, P.; Momchilova, A.; Anaya, F.; Voynov, V.; Alexandrov, A.; Tsonchev, Z.; Daskalov, M. *Therapeutic Apheresis with Nanotechnology Membrane for Human Diseases*; St. Kliment Ohridski University Press: Sofia, Bulgaria, 2014; Volume 1, pp. 1–155.
172. Kolev, O.I.; Kenarov, P. Vestibular and ocular motor function prior to and after therapeutic apheresis with small plasmafilter in multiple sclerosis. *J. Clin. Apher.* **2016**, *31*, 470–472. [CrossRef]
173. Das, J.; Chauhan, V.D.; Mills, D.; Johal, N.J.; Tan, M.; Matthews, R.; Keh, R.; Lilleker, J.B.; Gosal, D.; Sharaf, N. Therapeutic plasma exchange in neurological dis-orders: Experience from a tertiary neuroscience centre. *Transfus. Apher. Sci.* **2019**, *58*, 102654. [CrossRef]
174. Podbielska, M.; Ariga, T.; Pokryszko-Dragan, A. Sphingolipid Players in Multiple Sclerosis: Their Influence on the Initiation and Course of the Disease. *Int. J. Mol. Sci.* **2022**, *23*, 5330. [CrossRef] [PubMed]

175. Collongues, N.; Becker, G.; Jolivel, V.; Ayme-Dietrich, E.; de Seze, J.; Binamé, F.; Patte-Mensah, C.; Monassier, L.; Mensah-Nyagan, A.G. A Narrative Review on Axonal Neuroprotection in Multiple Sclerosis. *Neurol. Ther.* **2022**, *11*, 981–1042. [CrossRef]
176. Krämer, J.; Wiendl, H. What Have Failed, Interrupted, and Withdrawn Antibody Therapies in Multiple Sclerosis Taught Us? *Neurotherapeutics* **2022**, *19*, 785–807. [CrossRef] [PubMed]
177. Lopez, J.A.; Denkova, M.; Ramanathan, S.; Dale, R.C.; Brilot, F. Pathogenesis of autoimmune demyelination: From multiple scle-rosis to neuromyelitis optica spectrum disorders and myelin oligodendrocyte glycoprotein antibody-associated disease. *Clin. Transl. Immunol.* **2021**, *10*, e1316. [CrossRef] [PubMed]
178. Barizzone, N.; Leone, M.; Pizzino, A.; Kockum, I.; MultipleMS Consortium; Martinelli-Boneschi, F.; D'alfonso, S. A Scoping Review on Body Fluid Biomarkers for Prognosis and Disease Activity in Patients with Multiple Sclerosis. *J. Pers. Med.* **2022**, *12*, 1430. [CrossRef] [PubMed]
179. Fernández-Fournier, M.; Lacruz, L.; Nozal, P.; Chico, J.L.; Barranco, A.T.; Otero-Ortega, L.; Corral, I.; Carrasco, A. The study of neural antibodies in neurology: A practical summary. *Front. Immunol.* **2022**, *13*, 1043723. [CrossRef]
180. David, S.; Russell, L.; Castro, P.; van de Louw, A.; Zafrani, L.; Pirani, T.; Nielsen, N.D.; Mariotte, E.; Ferreyro, B.L.; Kielstein, J.T.; et al. Research priorities for therapeutic plasma exchange in critically ill patients. *Intensiv. Care Med. Exp.* **2023**, *11*, 26. [CrossRef]

current issues in molecular biology

MDPI

Review

The Roles of Caloric Restriction Mimetics in Central Nervous System Demyelination and Remyelination

Despoina Kaffe [1], Stefanos Ioannis Kaplanis [2,3] and Domna Karagogeos [2,3,*]

1 Department of Biology, University of Crete, Vassilika Vouton, 70013 Heraklion, Greece; biolp443@edu.biology.uoc.gr
2 Department of Basic Science, School of Medicine, University of Crete, Vassilika Vouton, 70013 Heraklion, Greece; ioannis_kaplanis@imbb.forth.gr
3 Institute of Molecular Biology & Biotechnology (IMBB), Foundation for Research and Technology-Hellas (FORTH), Vassilika Vouton, 70013 Heraklion, Greece
* Correspondence: karagoge@imbb.forth.gr; Tel.: +30-2810394542

Abstract: The dysfunction of myelinating glial cells, the oligodendrocytes, within the central nervous system (CNS) can result in the disruption of myelin, the lipid-rich multi-layered membrane structure that surrounds most vertebrate axons. This leads to axonal degeneration and motor/cognitive impairments. In response to demyelination in the CNS, the formation of new myelin sheaths occurs through the homeostatic process of remyelination, facilitated by the differentiation of newly formed oligodendrocytes. Apart from oligodendrocytes, the two other main glial cell types of the CNS, microglia and astrocytes, play a pivotal role in remyelination. Following a demyelination insult, microglia can phagocytose myelin debris, thus permitting remyelination, while the developing neuroinflammation in the demyelinated region triggers the activation of astrocytes. Modulating the profile of glial cells can enhance the likelihood of successful remyelination. In this context, recent studies have implicated autophagy as a pivotal pathway in glial cells, playing a significant role in both their maturation and the maintenance of myelin. In this Review, we examine the role of substances capable of modulating the autophagic machinery within the myelinating glial cells of the CNS. Such substances, called caloric restriction mimetics, have been shown to decelerate the aging process by mitigating age-related ailments, with their mechanisms of action intricately linked to the induction of autophagic processes.

Keywords: oligodendrocyte progenitor cells; oligodendrocytes; microglia; astrocytes; caloric restriction; caloric restriction mimetics; demyelination; remyelination; autophagy

1. Introduction

Myelin is a lipid-rich multi-layered membrane structure that surrounds most vertebrate axons. It is characterized by a high lipid-to-protein ratio, containing 75–80% lipids (by dry weight) and 25–30% proteins [1]. A hallmark of myelinated fibers is saltatory conduction, a mechanism that enables the rapid and efficient propagation of action potentials along the axonal length. Beyond its insulating function, myelin also plays an active role in providing metabolic support to axons [2]. In the central nervous system (CNS), myelin is produced by oligodendrocytes (OLs), while in the peripheral nervous system (PNS), it is synthesized by Schwann cells (SCs) [3].

The dysfunction of myelinating glial cells within the CNS can result in the disruption of myelin, a phenomenon that can subsequently lead to axonal demyelination and contribute to eventual axonal degeneration [4]. In response to demyelination in the CNS, the formation of new myelin sheaths occurs through the homeostatic process of remyelination, facilitated by the differentiation of newly formed OLs [5]. It is important to note, however, that remyelination is often inadequate for fully replicating the original myelin ultrastructure [5].

Apart from OLs, microglia and astrocytes, the two other main glial cell types of the CNS, play a pivotal role in remyelination [6–8]. Microglia constitute the resident macrophages within the CNS and display dynamic diversity [9,10]. Following a demyelination insult, they can phagocytose myelin debris, which is vital for recruiting and differentiating oligodendrocyte progenitor cells (OPCs), and they secrete growth factors and chemotactic substances. They also alter the extracellular matrix to support OPCs, aiding remyelination [11–14]. The developing neuroinflammation in the demyelinated region triggers the activation of astrocytes, the third glial population involved in remyelination, in a process known as reactive astrogliosis [15]. Activated astrocytes play a dual role, sometimes favoring or hindering remyelination based on their specific phenotype [16,17]. Astrocytes can directly impact remyelination because they recruit microglia to the lesion site and, thus, modulate the removal of myelin debris, which is essential for the resolution of the inflammatory response and, ultimately, remyelination [18]. Additionally, they modulate the extracellular matrix, affecting OPC proliferation and differentiation [19]. Modulating the expression profile of these glial cell types can enhance the likelihood of successful CNS remyelination.

In addition, recently, studies have implicated autophagy as a pivotal pathway in glial cells, playing a significant role in both their maturation and the maintenance of myelin. A study by Bankston and colleagues reveals that autophagy deficiency hinders OL differentiation both in vitro and in vivo. Specifically, their findings indicate that inhibiting autophagy alters the ultrastructure of myelin, thus underscoring the critical role of autophagy in OLs for proper myelination. Additionally, the observed enrichment of autolysosomes in OL processes suggests a specialized role of autophagy in these cellular processes. Notably, this research group also reports an increase in autophagic flux during oligodendrocyte differentiation in vitro [20]. Two recent consecutive studies have highlighted the essential role of autophagy in OLs not only in myelination but also in maintaining myelin throughout the lifespan of mice. Aber et al. demonstrate that OLs orchestrate the autophagic machinery to turnover myelin sheaths during adulthood, as autophagy deficiency leads to increased myelin deposition, a phenomenon that intensifies over time [21]. Furthermore, Ktena et al. corroborate the hypothesis that autophagy plays a pivotal role in myelin maintenance. The inhibition of autophagy, both genetically and pharmacologically, results in defects in OL maturation in vitro. The ablation of the core autophagic gene atg5 in OLs in vivo in 2.5 month-old mice, following the completion of myelination, leads to an excess of both PLP protein and mRNA levels at the age of 6 months, also implicating the autophagic machinery in PLP mRNA degradation. Moreover, conditional knockout mice in which autophagy is ablated in OLs exhibit myelin decompaction with subsequent axonal degeneration and behavioral deficits at the age of 6 months [22]. Collectively, these recent findings regarding autophagy and its pivotal role in CNS myelination and myelin maintenance have made autophagy an attractive therapeutic target for repairing myelin insults and/or abnormalities.

In the context of this Review, we focused on substances capable of modulating the autophagic machinery within the myelinating glial cells of the CNS. This modulation is achieved through a process akin to caloric restriction (CR), and the substances are named caloric restriction mimetics (CRMs) [23,24]. Dietary or caloric restriction is defined as the deliberate reduction of food consumption while maintaining proper nutrition, irrespective of the selective restriction of specific food groups. After nearly a century of extensive investigation across various model organisms, including *Saccharomyces cerevisiae*, *Drosophila melanogaster*, rodents, and non-human primates, and the analysis of human epidemiological data, CR is presently widely acknowledged for its capacity to enhance the longevity of organisms and decelerate the aging process [25,26]. Furthermore, it is recognized for its ability to mitigate age-related ailments, with its mechanisms of action being intricately linked to the induction of autophagic processes [27].

In the specific context of the CNS myelin, the advantageous effects of CR have been demonstrated. Piccio and colleagues provided compelling evidence illustrating the efficacy of a chronic CR regimen in enhancing the clinical outcomes of both relapsing–remitting and chronic experimental autoimmune encephalomyelitis (EAE) models [23]. These improvements in clinical outcomes were further validated through the observation of reduced severity in CNS pathology among the mice subjected to CR. Furthermore, the beneficial impact of CR on myelin recovery has also been observed in the cuprizone (CPZ) model of demyelination. Studies have shown that CR fosters the remyelination process by significantly increasing the survival rates of OLs. Additionally, it leads to a decrease in both astrogliosis and microgliosis within the corpus callosum (cc) of mice with CPZ-induced demyelination [24]. Nevertheless, owing to the systemic and extensive impacts of CR, unraveling the specific signaling pathways and the exact mechanisms underpinning its favorable effects mediated via autophagy can prove to be a complex endeavor. Over the course of decades of research, several hypotheses have arisen, among which the predominant one suggests that CR primarily acts to preserve cellular homeostasis and overall health [28].

The depletion of nutrients leads to a reduction in intracellular acetyl coenzyme A (AcCoA) levels, concurrent with the deacetylation of cellular proteins. Within this conceptual framework, there are three potential approaches to replicate these effects: (i) decrease cytosolic AcCoA levels by disrupting its biosynthesis; (ii) inhibit acetyltransferases, enzymes responsible for transferring acetyl groups from AcCoA to various molecules; or (iii) promote the activity of deacetylases, which facilitate the removal of acetyl groups from leucine residues [27,29,30]. The impact of CR can be replicated through the use of specific pharmacological agents referred to as CRMs. These agents, including metformin, nicotinamide adenine dinucleotide (NAD+) precursors, and resveratrol, are non-toxic natural compounds, which exhibit the capability to modulate the autophagic flux by triggering pathways similar to those activated during nutrient deprivation [31]. For the reasons mentioned above, we will focus this Review on the roles of metformin, NAD+ precursors, and resveratrol, mainly in demyelinating diseases.

2. Metformin

Metformin is a derivative of the natural guanidines present in the plant *Galega officinalis* and is widely used as a drug for type II diabetes, primarily operating through the inhibition of hepatic gluconeogenesis [32–34]. Beyond its established role in managing type II diabetes, metformin administration seems to exert beneficial effects on diseases, including cancer [35,36], cardiovascular disease [37], and obesity [38], as well as on neurodegeneration [39] and aging [40]. However, the precise underlying mechanisms responsible for these diverse therapeutic benefits remain to be elucidated [41].

Metformin inhibits mitochondrial complex I [42], a crucial component of the electron transport chain, thereby leading to decreased cellular ATP/ADP and ATP/AMP ratios and, thus, adenosine 5′-monophosphate-activated protein kinase (AMPK) activation [43,44]. Importantly, metformin-mediated AMPK activation exerts regulatory effects on cell energy metabolism and the autophagic cascade by reducing the activity of EP300 acetyl-transferase [45] and simultaneously enhancing the activity of sirtuin 1 (SIRT1) protein deacetylase [46]. Furthermore, a recent study has highlighted an additional mode of AMPK activation by metformin, which directly acts on the lysosomal vacuolar-type ATPase (v-ATPase), promoting the formation of the v-ATPase-regulator-AXIN/liver kinase B1 (LKB1)-AMPK complex in the lysosome, ultimately leading to AMPK activation. Interestingly, when the v-ATPase-regulator complex is engaged by AXIN, it inactivates mammalian target of rapamycin complex 1 (mTORC1), demonstrating that metformin's effects extend beyond AMPK activation, also encompassing mTORC1 inactivation [47]. The activation of AMPK together with the inactivation of mTORC1, the two major energy and nutrient sensors of the cell, induce the activation of the autophagic pathway [48].

It has long been reported that metformin exerts neuroprotective effects on several neurodegenerative diseases, such as Alzheimer's disease (AD), Parkinson's disease (PD), and Huntington's disease (HD). Chronic metformin administration was found to ameliorate synaptic malfunctions and cognitive impairment in the amyloid precursor protein (APP)swe/presenilin-1(PS1)DE9 (APP/PS1) mouse model of AD via the inhibition of cyclin-dependent kinase 5 (Cdk5) activity [49]. In the same mouse model of early-onset AD, metformin promoted the phagocytosis of pathological amyloid-β (Aβ) and tau proteins by microglia via the enhancement of the autophagic pathway, thus reducing the abundance of Aβ deposits and severity of neuritic plaque (NP) tau-pathology [50]. Metformin was also found to exert neuroprotective effects on dopaminergic neurodegeneration and alpha-synuclein aggregation in *Caenorhabditis elegans* models of PD [51], while it alleviated motor and neuropsychiatric manifestations in the zQ175 mouse model of HD [52].

Even though most of the current evidence suggests a beneficial effect of metformin on the prevention of AD in humans, its efficacy seems to be controversial. Recently, an observational study has indicated that metformin was associated with slower cognitive decline and reduced risk of dementia in patients with type II diabetes [53]. Furthermore, a randomized, double-blinded, placebo-controlled crossover pilot study demonstrated that metformin is safe and well tolerated by individuals, while being able to penetrate the blood–brain barrier [54]. Interestingly, metformin improved the executive function and tended to ameliorate memory, learning, and attention [54]. However, results from a prospective trial revealed that metformin impaired cognitive performance and that this effect was, at least in part, mediated by metformin-induced vitamin B12 deficiency [55]. This controversy could be attributed to different sample sizes, statistical methods, and drug administration, suggesting that more clinical trials need to be conducted [40].

In line with the multitude of evidence indicating metformin's favorable results in neurodegenerative conditions, many recent studies have diligently scrutinized the potential therapeutic implications of metformin in the context of multiple sclerosis (MS) [56]. MS, a complex and heterogeneous neurodegenerative disorder affecting the CNS, is primarily characterized by profound demyelination, inflammation, and reactive gliosis [57]. Metformin treatment was shown to protect against intense demyelination in the cc of the CPZ-induced demyelination mouse model, when administered with the copper chelator CPZ, by attenuating reactive microgliosis and astrogliosis in the cc (Figures 1 and 2) [58,59].

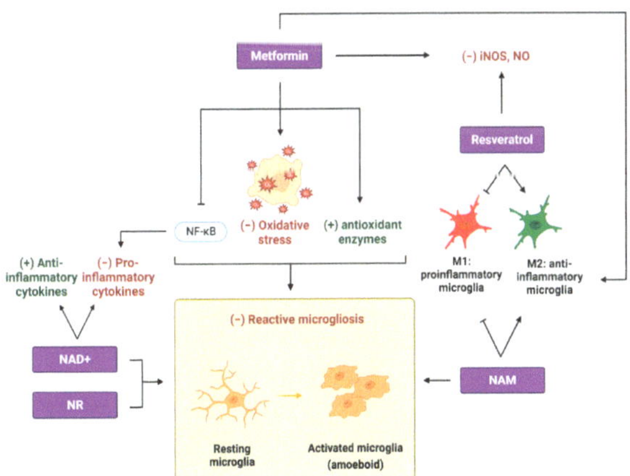

Figure 1. The effects of different caloric restriction mimetics (CRMs) on microglia. Metformin treatment reduces oxidative stress, upregulates antioxidant enzymes, and downregulates NF-κB signaling in microglia, thus attenuating the production of pro-inflammatory cytokines, ultimately leading to reduced microgliosis. Moreover, a similar reduction in reactive microgliosis is observed following treatment with NR, NAD+, and NAM. NAD+ administration results in a decreased expression of pro-inflammatory cytokines and an increased expression of anti-inflammatory ones. In parallel, NAM facilitates the polarization of microglia toward their anti-inflammatory phenotype, an effect that is also evident in response to metformin and resveratrol treatment, which additionally re-

duce iNOS and NO levels. The cumulative impact of these cellular responses contributes to the establishment of a less inflammatory milieu that could support the remyelination process. iNOS: inducible nitric oxide synthase; NF-κB: nuclear factor kappa-light-chain-enhancer of activated B cells; NR: nicotinamide riboside; NAD+: nicotinamide adenine dinucleotide; NAM: nicotinamide; NO: nitric oxide. Created with BioRender.com (accessed on 21 November 2023).

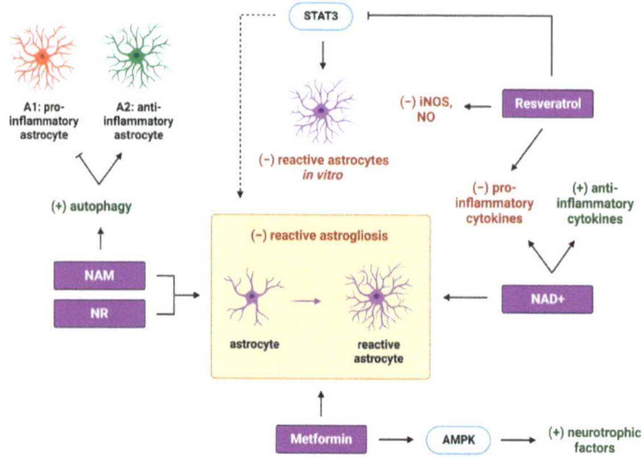

Figure 2. The effects of different CRMs on astrocytes. Resveratrol attenuates the expression of pro-inflammatory cytokines and inflammatory markers, such as iNOS and NO, while it also downregulates STAT3 signaling, leading to reduced proliferation and activation of reactive astrocytes. Given that STAT3 is implicated in the formation of glial scars in response to CNS demyelination, it is possible that resveratrol can reduce reactive astrogliosis in vivo. Furthermore, reduced reactive astrogliosis is observed upon NR, NAD+, NAM, and metformin treatments. NAD+ administration results in a decreased expression of pro-inflammatory cytokines and an increased expression of anti-inflammatory ones. In a similar way, NAM facilitates the polarization of astrocytes toward their anti-inflammatory phenotype, partially through the induction of autophagy. Metformin, in turn, acts through the activation of AMPK and induces the production of neurotrophic factors by astrocytes. This protective, less inflammatory microenvironment can support the process of remyelination in vivo after a demyelination insult. STAT3: signal transducer and activator of transcription 3; AMPK: adenosine 5′-monophosphate-activated protein kinase. Created with BioRender.com (accessed on 21 November 2023).

Largani et al. attributed the beneficial effects of metformin on myelin maintenance and reduced gliosis to its ability to reduce oxidative stress and upregulate antioxidant enzymes. There have been reports suggesting that reactive oxygen species (ROS) can regulate the expression of pro-inflammatory genes in microglia [60] and stimulate astrocytes to secrete inflammatory cytokines [61]. Abdi and his colleagues showed that metformin reduced levels of pro-inflammatory microglia markers through suppressing nuclear factor kappa-light-chain-enhancer of activated B cells (NF-κB) in the CPZ model of MS, an effect that was accompanied by the delayed initiation of gliosis. Moreover, metformin administration was shown to decrease inducible nitric oxide synthase (iNOS) mRNA levels in EAE mice (Figure 1) [62] as well as to protect myelin and promote an anti-inflammatory microglial phenotype that promotes the clearance of myelin debris in a rat spinal cord injury model (Figure 1) [63]. In this case, the effects of metformin were mediated by the induction of autophagy through the activation of AMPK and the inhibition of mTORC1 [63]. These results indicate that metformin can act in favor of a less inflammatory environment under demyelinating conditions, thus enabling the physiological process of remyelination to take over demyelination. In particular, metformin administration during the recovery period significantly promoted the recruitment of intermediate and premature OPCs to the lesion site in favor of the remyelination process in a CPZ-induced demyelination mouse model [64]. In this case, accelerated myelin recovery upon metformin treatment was mediated by AMPK activation and m-TORC inactivation in mature OLs (Figure 3), indicating a possible implication of the autophagic machinery in the recovery process.

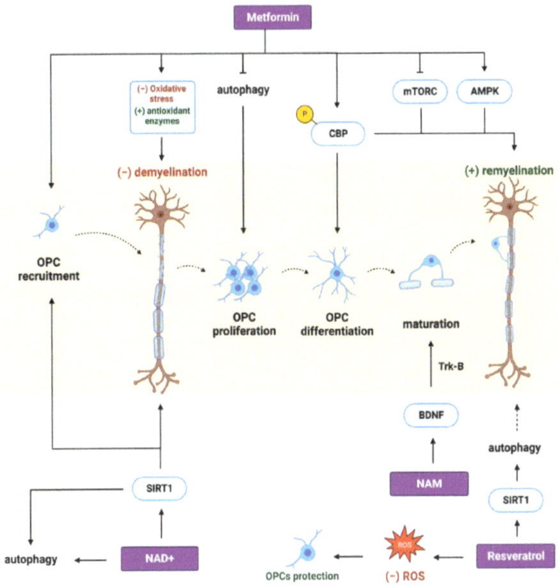

Figure 3. The effects of different CRMs on oligodendrocyte lineage cells and the process of remyelination. Metformin administration promotes the recruitment of OPCs to the lesion site and attenuates demyelination through its ability to reduce oxidative stress and upregulate antioxidant enzymes. Furthermore, metformin promotes OPC proliferation via the blockage of autophagy and enhances OPC differentiation and maturation into myelinating OLs via CBP phosphorylation. The remyelination process is also enhanced by the modulation of AMPK/mTORC pathways in mature OLs. Apart from metformin, NAM and resveratrol can promote the remyelination process. NAM treatment promotes the maturation of OPCs via the BDNF/TrkB pathway. Resveratrol protects OLs by reducing the abundance of ROS while it also induces autophagy through the activation of SIRT1, a mechanism that likely supports remyelination. Finally, direct NAD+ supplementation facilitates the recruitment of OPCs and alleviates demyelination through the activation of the SIRT1 signaling pathway and, probably, through the induction of autophagy. OPCs: oligodendrocyte progenitor cells; OLs: oligodendrocytes; CBP: CREB-binding protein; mTORC: mammalian target of rapamycin complex; BDNF: brain-derived neurotrophic factor; TrkB: tropomyosin receptor kinase B; SIRT1: sirtuin 1. Created with BioRender.com (accessed on 21 November 2023).

Despite the positive impacts of metformin on myelin protection and recovery through the inhibition of mTOR, it has been demonstrated that mTOR signaling regulates the developmental myelination of the CNS [65]. In particular, the ablation of raptor, the defining subunit of mTORC1, in OLs results in impaired OPC differentiation and delayed initiation of myelination in the spinal cords of mutant mice, which are also characterized by the formation of thinner myelin sheaths [65]. Interestingly, mTORC1 signaling driven by phosphoinositide 3-kinase (PI3K)/Akt, rather than ERK1/2, regulates the differentiation of progenitors, whereas both pathways converge at the level of mTORC1 to modulate myelin growth during active myelination [66]. Nevertheless, it has been shown that the prevention of the expression of tuberous sclerosis complex 1 (TSC1), a suppressor of mTOR signaling, resulted unexpectedly in hypomyelination during development [67]. On the other hand, the loss of TSC1 in adult OPCs enhanced remyelination and increased myelin thickness following lysolecithin (LPC)-induced focal demyelination [68], indicating that the deficiency in mTOR suppressors may exert either beneficial or detrimental effects on the differentially regulated processes of developmental myelination and remyelination. Therefore, more research is warranted to elucidate the interactions between AMPK and mTOR upon metformin administration.

Regarding AMPK, it is a cellular energy regulator found in many types of brain cells, including neurons, astrocytes, and microglia, as well as OLs [69]. Metformin treatment accelerates the differentiation of OLs in an AMPK-dependent manner, also requiring active glycolysis and/or oxidative phosphorylation to mediate OL differentiation [70]. The same study demonstrates the potential of metformin to improve myelin recovery from CPZ-induced demyelination by promoting OL differentiation in vivo [70]. Metformin-mediated AMPK activation seems to protect OLs against cytokine toxicity and oxidative stress rescuing their loss in the spinal cords of EAE rats, thus attenuating the clinical impairments of the disease and restoring the CNS integrity [71]. These immunomodulatory activities of AMPK signaling are concomitant with the stimulation of neurotrophic factor production in astrocytes within the CNS, which subsequently provides a myelinogenic environment for OLs (Figure 1) [71]. Furthermore, metformin treatment leads to increased synthesis of neurotrophic factors, like nerve growth factor (NGF), brain-derived neurotrophic factor (BDNF), and ciliary neurotrophic factor (CNTF), while it also induces the expression of mature oligodendrocyte markers and the activation of AMPK in the CPZ-induced demyelination mouse model [72]. Because neurotrophic factors are reported to enhance OPC survival, migration, proliferation, differentiation, and maturation [73], it is suggested that metformin enhances the secretion of these factors during the recovery phase after demyelination, thus affecting the migration and differentiation of oligodendrocyte transcription factor 2 (Olig2)+ cells in favor of remyelination, effects that are mediated by AMPK activation [72].

Apart from its AMPK-mediated effects on remyelination, metformin was also found to act via the phosphorylation of the histone acetyltransferase CREB-binding protein (CBP), ultimately promoting OPC recruitment and differentiation to the lesion site in an LPC-induced focal demyelination mouse model. In particular, in vitro experiments confirmed that CBP Ser436 phosphorylation is required for metformin to promote the differentiation of OPCs into mature OLs. However, it is not responsible for metformin-induced OPC proliferation, an effect that was connected with the ability of metformin to block autophagy at early stages (Figure 3) [74].

When the remyelination process is delayed or fails, demyelinated axons are susceptible to irreversible degeneration, which can eventually lead to neuronal death [75]. The deceleration of remyelination that occurs in aging is marked by the deficient recruitment of OPCs to the site of the injury, coupled with the delayed progression in their differentiation into mature OLs [76]. Reversing the age-related intrinsic deficiencies of OPCs that are associated with their inability to respond to pro-differentiation factors was able to enhance OPC differentiation and remyelination in aged animals [77]. In this study, metformin was found to improve the mitochondrial function of aged OPCs by modulating the AMPK pathway and to restore the CNS remyelination capacity in aged rats, following ethidium bromide-induced focal demyelination in the cerebellar white matter (Figure 4). The authors postulated that metformin's impact on remyelination could also be attributed to its capacity to enhance DNA repair and induce autophagy, both of which are established effects associated with metformin [78,79].

Regarding its functional behavioral effects, metformin treatment improved motor impairment and reduced anxiety in the CPZ-induced demyelination mouse model [64], while it also improved the social interaction of juvenile mice in an LPC-induced focal demyelination model [74]. These results render metformin a promising remyelinating agent that could treat neural deficits and impaired social behavior, a common symptom of white-matter-demyelinating diseases.

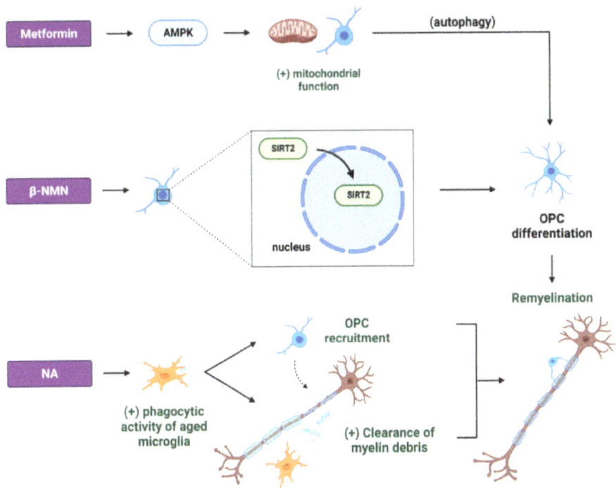

Figure 4. The effects of different CRMs on the aged central nervous system (CNS) after a demyelination insult. The administration of metformin improves the mitochondrial function of aged OPCs via the activation of AMPK, consequently facilitating the restoration of the CNS myelination, an effect that could be attributed to the induction of autophagy. Furthermore, β-NMN supplementation rescues SIRT2 nuclear localization in the OPCs of aged mice, thus enhancing remyelination by promoting the differentiation of aged OPCs. Finally, NA promotes remyelination by enhancing the phagocyting activity of middle-aged microglia. This process results in the removal of myelin debris from the lesion site and the recruitment and maturation of OPCs into myelinating OLs. β-NMN: β-nicotinamide mononucleotide; SIRT2: sirtuin 2; NA: nicotinic acid. Created with BioRender.com (accessed on 21 November 2023).

3. NAD+ Precursors

Nicotinic acid (NA), commonly referred to as niacin or vitamin B3, along with nicotinamide (NAM), its amide derivative, nicotinamide riboside (NR), and nicotinamide mononucleotide (NMN), serve as precursors for NAD+ (Figure 5). These compounds are available in various dietary products of both animal and plant origin, and they exhibit CRM-like properties [80,81]. NA is converted to NAD+ via the Preiss–Handler pathway, while NAM and NR enter the NAD+ salvage pathway, playing a pivotal role in the maintenance of cellular NAD+ levels [82]. NMN is synthesized from NAM by nicotinamide phosphoribosyltransferase (NAMPT), the rate-limiting NAD+ biosynthetic enzyme in mammals, as well as from NR by nicotinamide riboside kinases (NRKs), effectively bypassing the need for NAMPT (Figure 5) [83]. Accumulating evidence suggests that NAD+ intermediates not only prolong healthspan and/or lifespan [84–86], compensating for reduced NAD+ levels during aging, but also seem to be an effective intervention for various age-associated diseases, including cardiovascular diseases [87,88], cancer [89,90], and neurodegenerative disorders [91].

NAD+ plays a dual and pivotal role in cellular responses, serving as an essential coenzyme for enzymes facilitating oxidation–reduction reactions and as a co-substrate for NAD+-consuming enzymes. These enzymes compete for bioavailable NAD+ and belong into three classes: the cyclic ADP-ribose (cADPR) synthases, such as CD38; the poly (ADP-ribose) polymerase (PARP) protein family; and the sirtuin family of deacetylases (Figure 5) [92,93].

Specifically, CD38 plays important roles in many physiological processes, including glucose homeostasis, inflammation, and neuroprotection. Its deletion and the subsequent elevation in NAD+ levels protect against high-fat diet (HFD)-induced obesity [94], inflammatory reactions of microglia and astrocytes, and ROS, while it improves CPZ-induced demyelination and neurodegeneration [95,96]. PARP proteins mediate ADP-ribosylation and act as DNA-damage sensors [97]. It has been reported that the upregulation of PARP induces OL death, whereas its inhibition reduces CPZ-induced demyelination by suppressing p38 mitogen-activated protein kinases (p-38-MAPK) and JNK activation and increasing the activation of the PI3K/Akt pathway [98].

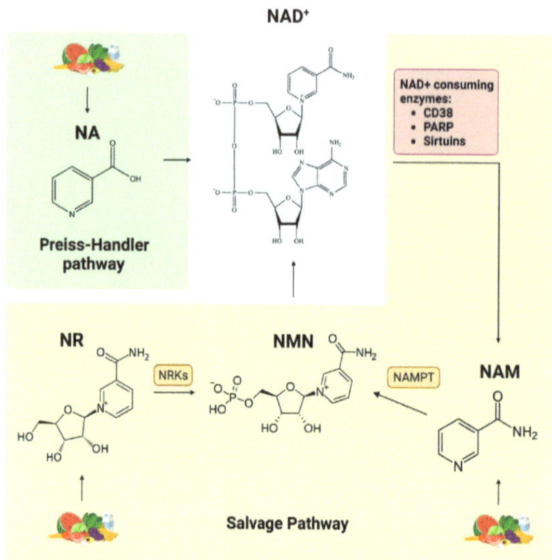

Figure 5. NAD+ biosynthetic pathways. NA is converted to NAD+ via the Preiss–Handler pathway, whereas NAM and NR enter the salvage pathway to produce NAD+. The NAD+ salvage pathway recycles NAM that is generated as a byproduct of the activity of NAD+-consuming enzymes: CD38, PARP, and sirtuins. NMN is synthesized from NAM by NAMPT as well as from NR by NRKs. PARP: poly (ADP-ribose) polymerase; NMN: nicotinamide mononucleotide; NAMPT: nicotinamide phosphoribosyltransferase; NRKs: nicotinamide riboside kinases. Created with BioRender.com (accessed on 21 November 2023).

Among the three classes of NAD+-consuming enzymes, sirtuins are the most well studied. Upon increased NAD+ levels, SIRT1 is activated, leading to the deacetylation of critical proteins of the autophagic pathway, including autophagy-related gene 5 (Atg5), Atg7, and microtubule-associated protein 1 light chain 3 (LC3), thus inducing autophagy, as well as to the deacetylation of transcription factors, like NF-κB, thus regulating inflammatory signaling [99,100]. Additionally, the administration of NA has been shown to inhibit vascular inflammation in vivo along with the suppression of the NOD-like receptor family pyrin domain-containing 3 (NLRP3) inflammasome in vascular endothelial cells in vitro via SIRT1 upregulation [101,102]. Apart from SIRT1, NAD+ supplementation has also been found to mediate the activation of sirtuin 2 (SIRT2). Specifically, NAD+ administration increased intracellular ATP levels via the activation of SIRT2, which regulates Akt phosphorylation in BV2 microglial cells [103], while NR treatment alleviated cisplatin-induced peripheral neuropathy in a SIRT2-dependent manner [104].

NAD+ supplementation was demonstrated to exert neuroprotective effects on various neurodegenerative diseases, including AD, PD, and HD. NR treatment reduced neuroinflammation in an APP/PS1 mouse model of AD, promoting the protective, phagocyting phenotype of microglia, while it also improved cognitive and synaptic functions [105]. A very recent study has highlighted NMN as a regulator of the gut microbiota, which exerted positive effects on AD [106]. Furthermore, NAM administration significantly protected against neuronal loss and attenuated motor dysfunction, oxidative stress, and neuroinflammation in a 1-methyl-4-phenyl-1,2,3,6-tetrahydropyridine (MPTP)-induced mouse model of PD [107], while it also provided neuroprotection in the 3-nitropropionic acid-induced animal model of HD [108].

Apart from these pre-clinical studies, multiple clinical trials are currently being conducted to evaluate the safety and the effects of NAD+ precursors on neurological disorders. In particular, NR has been demonstrated to be orally bio-available without serious adverse effects [109,110]. A recent randomized, placebo-controlled, crossover trial of oral NR supplementation has indicated increased levels of NAD+ in plasma extracellular vesicles enriched for neuronal origin (NEVs). Increased NAD+ levels were accompanied by decreased levels of Aβ42 and of the activated kinases pJNK and pERK1/2, which are implicated in AD [111]. Furthermore, in a randomized, placebo-controlled, phase I clinical trial, oral NR administration increased cerebral NAD levels in individuals with PD, an effect that was associated with the downregulation of inflammatory cytokines and general clinical improvement [112]. Regarding NAM, a new clinical trial (NCT03061474) is investigating whether NAM can reduce the phosphorylation of the tau protein found in cerebrospinal fluid (CSF) in people with mild cognitive impairment or mild AD [113].

In the same context of neurodegenerative conditions, NAD+ precursors have been shown to exert beneficial effects on demyelinating, neuroinflammatory diseases, like MS. NAD+ treatment was shown to alleviate demyelination and neuroinflammation in both the spinal cord [114] and the optic nerve [115] of a murine EAE model. Its administration exhibited a marked reduction in the activation of microglia and astrocytes, as well as in the expression of pro-inflammatory cytokines, while it facilitated the expression of anti-inflammatory cytokines, thereby fostering a less inflammatory milieu in vivo, which could support the remyelination process (Figures 1 and 2) [114,115]. Notably, successful remyelination hinges upon the activities of OPCs. In response to myelin damage, these cells proliferate and migrate to lesion sites, where they mature to myelin-forming cells [116]. Guo et al. demonstrated that NAD+ supplementation effectively mitigates apoptosis among OLs and concurrently facilitates the recruitment and proliferation of OPCs in the optic nerve of mice with EAE. These beneficial effects of NAD+ in optic neuritis were orchestrated through the activation of the SIRT1-signaling pathway (Figure 3) [115]. Additionally, Wang et al. attributed the beneficial outcomes of NAD+ administration to the induction of autophagy because its inhibition abolished the protective effects of NAD+ [114]. Given the established role of SIRT1 deacetylase as an autophagy inducer [100], both studies converge on the critical role of the autophagic pathway in ameliorating EAE symptoms after NAD+ treatment.

In addition to NAD+ supplementation, numerous pre-clinical investigations have explored NAD+ precursors as potential therapeutic strategies for alleviating symptoms associated with MS. A recent study from our laboratory has revealed that NAM treatment resulted in a substantial augmentation in myelin production at the lesion site in the cc of an LPC-induced focal demyelination mouse model, concurrently with a reduction in microgliosis and astrogliosis (Figures 1 and 2). Importantly, NAM treatment did not exert a direct influence on oligodendrocyte lineage cells, thereby suggesting that it accelerated the overall myelin production under demyelinating conditions by mitigating both microgliosis and astrogliosis [117]. Furthermore, the same study indicated that NAM directly affected microglial and astrocyte polarization toward their anti-inflammatory phenotypes, thus fostering a beneficial, less inflammatory microenvironment for remyelination. In addition to NAM, NR pre-treatment attenuated inflammatory responses, glial activation, and subsequent neurodegeneration in the brain of a lipopolysaccharide (LPS)-injected mouse model (Figures 1 and 2) [118]. Despite these promising findings, the precise molecular mechanisms underpinning the NAD+-mediated regulation of glial activity remain elusive. Kaplanis et al. suggested that the shift in astrocytes toward their anti-inflammatory phenotype arises, at least in part, from the induction of autophagy, as observed in primary astrocyte cultures following NAM treatment (Figure 1) [117]. Notably, a recent study has identified a correlation between the induction of autophagy and the suppression of the inflammatory phenotype in astrocytes [119]. Regarding microglia, it appears that NAD+-dependent deacetylase SIRT2 inhibits pro-inflammatory responses through the deacetylation of NF-κB [120], indicating the participation of different NAD+-dependent pathways in glial phenotype commitment.

Among all seven sirtuins, SIRT2 is the most abundantly expressed in the brain, primarily residing in the cytoplasm of mature OLs but also present in neurons, astrocytes, and microglia [121,122]. Ma et al. further demonstrated that SIRT2 is predominantly expressed in the nuclei of postnatal OPCs during myelin development and changes its expression pattern in mature OLs, where it is found in the cytoplasm. Following a demyelination injury induced by LPC, SIRT2 is re-expressed in the majority of OPCs, primarily localizing within the OPC nuclear compartment in young adult mice. However, this re-expression and nuclear localization of SIRT2 declines with aging. Interestingly, β-NMN supplementation rescues SIRT2 nuclear localization in aged mice and affects the myelin status. In particular, it delays myelin aging under normal aging conditions and influences myelin compaction and thickness after a focal demyelinating LPC-induced lesion, thus enhancing remyelination by promoting the differentiation of OPCs (Figure 4) [123].

Enhanced remyelination was also observed in middle-aged animals upon niacin (NA) treatment in an LPC-induced focal demyelination mouse model [124]. Notably, the aging process is associated with delayed microglial recruitment to the lesion site and deficient phagocytosis, contributing to the establishment of an inhibitory microenvironment [125,126]. Rawji et al. demonstrated that NA administration enhanced the phagocytic activity of microglia in middle-aged animals, thus promoting the clearance of myelin debris from the lesion site and the recruitment of OPCs in favor of the remyelination process (Figure 4) [124]. Finally, NAM treatment promoted the maturation of OPCs and enhanced remyelination after stroke. NAM-treated animals had increased motor, sensory, and cognitive functions, and this functional remyelination was mediated by the BDNF/tropomyosin receptor kinase B (TrkB) pathway (Figure 3) [127]. Because BDNF is reported to enhance myelination via a direct effect on OLs [128], it is plausible that BDNF mediates the maturation of OPCs during remyelination.

These investigations highlight the favorable impacts of NAD+ and its precursors in age-related diseases, particularly in neurodegenerative and demyelinating diseases, like MS, rendering them promising therapeutic agents. Nevertheless, it is evident that distinct NAD+ precursors manifest their beneficial effects by targeting diverse molecules/pathways in various cell types of the CNS and within different mouse models of MS. Hence, it becomes imperative to discern the optimal precursor based on the considerations of absorption, kinetics, and specific MS symptoms. Finally, given that the majority of research efforts have centered on SIRT1 activation upon NAD+ treatment, it is equally important to delve into the roles of the other two classes of NAD+-depleting enzymes under demyelinating conditions.

4. Resveratrol

Resveratrol (3,4′,5-trihydroxystilbene) is a natural polyphenol that acts as a phytoalexin and is found in a wide variety of foods, including blueberries and peanuts, as well as grapes and products derived from them, like red wine [129,130]. Ever since resveratrol's potent anticancer properties were highlighted by Jang in 1997 [131], both experimental and epidemiological studies have been conducted to elucidate its diverse bioactivities and, consequentially, its health advantages. Interestingly, resveratrol has a positive impact on a wide spectrum of diseases, including heart diseases [132], diabetes [133], cancer [134], obesity [135], and neurodegenerative diseases [136,137], while it also exerts beneficial effects on aging [138,139].

Mechanistically, resveratrol is mainly associated with the activation of the NAD+-dependent deacetylase SIRT1. Once activated, SIRT1 can deacetylate the core proteins of the autophagic pathway, like Atg5 and Atg7, leading to the induction of this pathway [100,140]. Furthermore, the induction of SIRT1 activation by resveratrol necessitates its phosphorylation by LKB1 in multiple cell lines, subsequently resulting in the deacetylation of the peroxisome proliferator-activated receptor-gamma coactivator-1-alpha (PGC-1a) transcriptional co-activator, which regulates mitochondrial biogenesis and respiration [141,142].

Beyond SIRT1, resveratrol also engages AMPK as a target [143]. Its activation upon resveratrol treatment was found to rescue Aβ-mediated neurotoxicity in human neural stem cells (hNSCs) [144] as well as oxygen and glucose deprivation in human SH-SY5Y neuroblastoma cells [145]. Because AMPK has been shown to activate SIRT1 through an indirect increase in cellular NAD+ levels [146], there is clearly a dynamic interaction between the two pathways. Finally, it is worth mentioning that resveratrol exhibits anti-inflammatory properties by suppressing the production of ROS and downregulating NF-κB [147].

Resveratrol has been documented for its neuroprotective potential in various CNS disorders, notably AD and PD. In particular, resveratrol treatment has been shown to mitigate neuroinflammation and reduce Aβ accumulation in the brains of 3×Tg-AD mice [148]. Furthermore, it inhibited tau aggregation and cytotoxicity in vitro, and it reduced the levels of phosphorylated tau, neuroinflammation, and synapse loss in the brain of a PS19 mouse model of AD, thus rescuing the cognitive deficits [149]. Resveratrol treatment was also able to ameliorate motor and cognitive impairments in an A53T α-synuclein mouse model of PD by diminishing the levels of α-synuclein aggregates and reducing microgliosis, astrocytosis, and oxidative-stress levels within the brain [150].

Meanwhile, the effects of resveratrol on neurological disorders are evaluated through clinical trials. One of the first studies evaluating the effects of resveratrol on individuals with mild to moderate AD was conducted by Turner et al. in 2015. This randomized, double-blinded, placebo-controlled phase II study indicated that resveratrol is safe and well tolerated by patients, while it could also penetrate the blood–brain barrier because it was detectable in the CSF. However, neuroprotective benefits could not be detected in this study, while the longer AD duration, measured in years from the diagnosis, in the placebo-treated group should be taken into consideration [151]. In the next step, the same research group analyzed samples of CSF and plasma from a subset of AD subjects with CSF Aβ 42 concentrations of <600 ng/mL. In this subset analysis, resveratrol decreased the levels of metalloproteinase (MMP) 9 in the CSF, suggesting increased maintenance of the blood–brain barrier and reduced infiltration of immune cells, while it also regulated neuroinflammation, induced adaptive immunity, and mitigated progressive cognitive decline [152].

The established capacity of resveratrol to mitigate inflammation and attenuate gliosis in the context of neurodegenerative pathologies endows it with substantial therapeutic potential for addressing demyelinating diseases, like MS. MS is predominantly characterized by pronounced inflammatory responses orchestrated by microglia, which can participate in mechanisms of tissue repair and injury depending on their activation state [14,153]. Traditionally, microglia have been categorized into pro-inflammatory (M1) and anti-inflammatory (M2) phenotypes; however, this categorization appears to be simplistic. The use of new technologies, including single-cell RNA sequencing, has led to the identification of intermediate subpopulations that display a combination of pro- and anti-inflammatory markers, suggesting that microglial activation is a dynamic process [154–156]. A crucial requirement for the achievement of successful remyelination in MS is a switch toward the M2 activation state [157].

Resveratrol was shown to not only suppress microglial polarization toward the M1 phenotype but also promote the M2 phenotype of LPS-stimulated BV2 microglial cells in vitro and of microglial cells in vivo, in a model of systemic LPS administration that leads to brain inflammation (Figure 1) [158]. The neuroprotective role of resveratrol in microglial polarization was mainly attributed to PGC-1a activation, which can not only halt M1 polarization by suppressing NF-κB phosphorylation and the expression of inflammatory cytokines, like tumor necrosis factor alpha (TNF-α), but also interact with transcription factor signal transducer and activator of transcription 3 (STAT3) and STAT6, promoting the expression of the anti-inflammatory M2 markers arginase 1 (Arg1) and IL-10 [158]. A recent study has also indicated that resveratrol can promote the M2 microglial phenotype and reduce the degree of neuroinflammation after cerebral ischemia by inhibiting miR-155, a molecule linked to inflammatory processes and to the promotion of M1 polarization [159].

Interestingly, resveratrol-loaded macrophage exosomes, which addressed the low solubility of resveratrol, alleviated inflammation and symptom severity in EAE mice by targeting microglia [160]. These results indicate that resveratrol promotes the M2 microglial phenotype by mitigating inflammation, which is the main impediment of the remyelination process.

Like microglia, astrocytes can exert both detrimental and beneficial effects on remyelination depending on their neurotoxic (A1) or their neuroprotective (A2) phenotype, respectively [161]. Resveratrol treatment inhibited the expression of LPS-induced pro-inflammatory cytokines in both primary murine microglia and astrocytes, while it also reduced the expression of iNOS and the production of nitric oxide (NO) in these glial cell types (Figures 1 and 2) [162]. It is well established that in response to CNS demyelination, astrocytes become activated, proliferate, and form the glial scar, which impedes the remyelination process and is STAT3 dependent [163]. Resveratrol was found to attenuate reactive astrocyte proliferation and activation by downregulating STAT3 signaling in primary rat astrocyte cultures (Figure 2) [164]. These in vitro results suggest that resveratrol could be a promising agent for facilitating remyelination in vivo by regulating the glial scar and establishing a less inflammatory microenvironment.

Reduced inflammation following the administration of resveratrol was further observed in a mouse model of CPZ-induced demyelination. In this context, resveratrol also reduced lipid peroxidation and countered the negative impact of CPZ on the mitochondrial respiratory chain, as assayed by increased cytochrome oxidase activity and ATP levels [165]. Recent studies have established a connection between oxidative stress and the compromised differentiation capacity of OLs, consequently contributing to the process of demyelination [166]. Thus, resveratrol's effect on the alleviation of oxidative stress could be correlated with the myelin status recovery. Indeed, Ghaiad et al. showed that resveratrol increased myelin basic protein (MBP) expression levels and the stain intensity of Luxol fast blue (LFB), while it also improved balance and motor coordination that were impaired in CPZ-intoxicated mice. These biochemical, histological, and behavioral results indicate that resveratrol reversed CPZ-induced demyelination and enhanced the remyelination process (Figure 3) [165].

Similar effects of resveratrol on balance and motor coordination as well as on enhanced myelin repair in CPZ-treated mice were reported by Samy et al. in 2023. However, the significant improvement in behavioral tests was incomplete compared to control animals, whereas despite the increased number of myelinated axons in the cc, not all the repaired myelin was compacted, and resveratrol failed to upregulate MBP expression levels. These conflicting effects of resveratrol were attributed to different disease-induction and treatment protocols [167]. Interestingly, Samy et al. correlated the positive effects of resveratrol with the induction of autophagy, which is the main result of CR and was interrupted at a late stage in CPZ-treated mice. The induction of the autophagic flux and the successful autophagic degradation upon resveratrol administration involved the activation of the SIRT1/forkhead box protein O1 (FOXO1) pathway [167]. However, the cell-autonomous effect of resveratrol regarding the induction of autophagy and its beneficial effects on remyelination are yet to be determined.

Previous studies have highlighted the advantageous impact of resveratrol on myelination within the PNS. Using an in vitro system comprising a dorsal root ganglion (DRG)/SC co-culture, researchers discerned that resveratrol enhanced myelination, an effect that was mediated, at least in part, by SIRT1 activation in SCs, which serve as the myelinating cells of the PNS [168]. Furthermore, resveratrol induced autophagy in SCs, leading to myelin sheath degeneration in the early stages of nerve injury and, thus, promoting recovery from sciatic nerve crush injury [169]. It is important to acknowledge that myelin clearance represents a critical phase in the regeneration process following peripheral nerve injury [170].

In the context of the CNS, resveratrol mediates protective effects on OLs by preventing LPS-mediated cytotoxicity and reducing the abundance of ROS [171], while it also promotes the survival, migration, proliferation, and differentiation of OPCs in a rat model of ischemic cerebral injury (Figure 3) [172]. Furthermore, resveratrol has demonstrated neuroprotective effects on a chronic EAE mouse model because its administration attenuated the neuronal loss of retinal ganglion cells (RGCs) [173]. Correspondingly, recent research has corroborated resveratrol's neuroprotective effects, which were attributed to its capacity to promote autophagic activity in a mouse spinal cord injury model [174]. Although the existing evidence pertaining to the roles of resveratrol in myelination and regeneration in the CNS is limited, it is plausible that these processes are regulated, similarly to PNS, by the induction of the autophagic pathway in OLs, which are the myelinating cells of the CNS.

Recent research has emphasized the significance of oligodendroglial autophagy in OL maturation and the maintenance of CNS myelin [21,22]. The activation of the autophagy inducer SIRT1 has been shown to mediate the proliferation and regeneration of OPCs in the white matter of neonatal mice under hypoxic conditions [175]. During adulthood, on the other hand, the genetic ablation of SIRT1 increased the pool of OPCs after focal demyelination, promoting the remyelination process and, thus, indicating the temporally restricted role of SIRT1 in glial regeneration following brain injury [176]. Furthermore, recent findings have suggested that SIRT1 is upregulated in OPCs in EAE and likely plays a role in remyelination [177]. Given that resveratrol is predominantly associated with SIRT1 activation, these pieces of evidence underscore the importance for investigating the cell-autonomous effects of resveratrol on OLs under demyelinating conditions and its potent role as a therapeutic agent for MS.

5. Conclusions

CRMs have gained significant attention within the scientific community, emerging as promising agents capable of emulating numerous effects that are typically induced by CR. Notably, many CRM candidates can induce autophagy, prolong lifespan and/or healthspan, and mitigate the symptoms of age-related diseases, all without the subjective discomfort associated with CR. In addition, CRMs have been shown to exert beneficial effects on demyelinating neuroinflammatory diseases, like MS, by modulating the profile of glial cells, ultimately facilitating the remyelination process. In particular, apart from targeting the migration, proliferation, and differentiation of OLs, CRMs affect microglia and astrocytes by promoting their protective phenotypes, thereby establishing a less inflammatory microenvironment that supports remyelination.

This translational research on CRMs has now progressed to the clinical phase because there is an unmet need to verify their favorable effects through clinical trials. Presently, there are ongoing clinical trials investigating the effects of metformin on endogenous neural progenitor cells in children or young adults with MS (NCT04121468) [178], as well as the safety of metformin for the treatment of progressive MS (NCT05349474) [179]. There is also a clinical trial (NCT05740722), currently recruiting patients, that aims to evaluate the safety and efficacy of NR in the treatment of patients with progressive MS [180]. Despite the large number of in vitro and in vivo studies using animal models of MS, clinical evidence for the protective role of polyphenols in MS patients is restricted, encompassing only a few compounds, like curcumin [181]. However, taking into consideration the beneficial effects of resveratrol on mouse models of MS, as well as its established safety and its ability to modulate neuroinflammation in patients with AD, clinical trials need to be conducted to evaluate the potential of resveratrol to mitigate the symptoms of patients with MS. It is important, though, that aspects such as bioavailability, cellular uptake, systemic distribution, and organ-specific effects are settled. A recent study has used resveratrol nanoparticles to address the poor water solubility and bioavailability of resveratrol in an EAE mouse model. The results have suggested that the nanoparticles increased the bioavailability of the resveratrol and exerted neuroprotective effects by reducing the loss of retinal ganglion cells [182]. Moreover, it is possible that the combination of mechanistically different CRMs will have synergistic effects, thereby maximizing their positive impact.

Additional research also needs to be undertaken to elucidate the influences of distinct CRMs on the myelin sheaths of the elderly. As the human brain ages, the capacity of OPCs to differentiate in mature myelinating OLs significantly declines [183,184]. Notably, the transition from relapsing–remitting to progressive MS takes place at around the same age in MS patients, indicating that it is mostly age rather that disease-duration dependent [185]. Apart from aging, both the disease duration and anatomic sites of lesions affect the remyelination potential of MS patients. It is suggested that remyelination is a more frequent event at the beginning of the disease than in the chronic phase, when remyelination is scarce and predominantly confined to the peripheries of lesions [186]. Regarding the location, cortical lesions are more extensively remyelinated than white-matter ones [187]. Thus, it becomes evident that even though remyelination is highly efficient in animal models and is commonly observed in MS patients, it varies considerably between lesions and between individuals, and these facts should be taken into account during the design of clinical trials. Finally, neuropathological studies reveal that some lesions of MS patients lack OPCs [188], whereas other lesions are characterized by a great number of OPCs with an impaired differentiation capacity [189], indicating that proliferating or differentiating agents should be used according to the lesion status. Consequently, even though spontaneous remyelination exists in humans following a demyelination insult, many obstacles need to be overcome not only for the development of efficient MS treatments based on CRMs but also for the proper evaluation of remyelination. However, despite the imperative for validating CRMs as therapeutic approaches, the existing body of evidence corroborates the considerable potential of these autophagy inducers against MS and multiple age-related diseases.

Author Contributions: D.K. (Despoina Kaffe), writing—original draft preparation and visualization; S.I.K., writing—review and editing; D.K. (Domna Karagogeos), conceptualization, supervision and editing; D.K. (Despoina Kaffe), S.I.K. and D.K. (Domna Karagogeos), funding acquisition. All authors have read and agreed to the published version of the manuscript.

Funding: This research was funded by the Hellenic Foundation for Research and Innovation (HFRI) under grant agreement No. 1676, the Hellenic Academy of Neuroimmunology (HELANI), and the Fondation Sante (The Sidney Altman Scholarship Program). De.K was supported by an Onassis Foundation Scholarship (G ZS 004-1/2022-2023).

Institutional Review Board Statement: Not applicable.

Informed Consent Statement: Not applicable.

Data Availability Statement: Not applicable.

Acknowledgments: The authors would like to thank all the members of the Karagogeos laboratory for helpful and thought-provoking conversations.

Conflicts of Interest: The authors declare no conflict of interest.

References

1. Williams, K.A.; Deber, C.M. The structure and function of central nervous system myelin. *Crit. Rev. Clin. Lab. Sci.* **1993**, *30*, 29–64. [CrossRef] [PubMed]
2. Stadelmann, C.; Timmler, S.; Barrantes-Freer, A.; Simons, M. Myelin in the Central Nervous System: Structure, Function, and Pathology. *Physiol. Rev.* **2019**, *99*, 1381–1431. [CrossRef] [PubMed]
3. Poliak, S.; Peles, E. The local differentiation of myelinated axons at nodes of Ranvier. *Nat. Rev. Neurosci.* **2003**, *4*, 968–980. [CrossRef] [PubMed]
4. Chen, J.F.; Wang, F.; Huang, N.X.; Xiao, L.; Mei, F. Oligodendrocytes and myelin: Active players in neurodegenerative brains? *Dev. Neurobiol.* **2022**, *82*, 160–174. [CrossRef] [PubMed]
5. Neely, S.A.; Williamson, J.M.; Klingseisen, A.; Zoupi, L.; Early, J.J.; Williams, A.; Lyons, D.A. New oligodendrocytes exhibit more abundant and accurate myelin regeneration than those that survive demyelination. *Nat. Neurosci.* **2022**, *25*, 415–420. [CrossRef] [PubMed]
6. Baaklini, C.S.; Rawji, K.S.; Duncan, G.J.; Ho, M.F.S.; Plemel, J.R. Central Nervous System Remyelination: Roles of Glia and Innate Immune Cells. *Front. Mol. Neurosci.* **2019**, *12*, 225. [CrossRef]
7. Djannatian, M.; Radha, S.; Weikert, U.; Safaiyan, S.; Wrede, C.; Deichsel, C.; Kislinger, G.; Rhomberg, A.; Ruhwedel, T.; Campbell, D.S.; et al. Myelination generates aberrant ultrastructure that is resolved by microglia. *J. Cell Biol.* **2023**, *222*, e202204010. [CrossRef]

8. Nave, K.A.; Werner, H.B. Myelination of the nervous system: Mechanisms and functions. *Annu. Rev. Cell Dev. Biol.* **2014**, *30*, 503–533. [CrossRef]
9. Yamasaki, R.; Lu, H.; Butovsky, O.; Ohno, N.; Rietsch, A.M.; Cialic, R.; Wu, P.M.; Doykan, C.E.; Lin, J.; Cotleur, A.C.; et al. Differential roles of microglia and monocytes in the inflamed central nervous system. *J. Exp. Med.* **2014**, *211*, 1533–1549. [CrossRef]
10. Lloyd, A.F.; Miron, V.E. The pro-remyelination properties of microglia in the central nervous system. *Nat. Rev. Neurol.* **2019**, *15*, 447–458. [CrossRef]
11. Miron, V.E. Microglia-driven regulation of oligodendrocyte lineage cells, myelination, and remyelination. *J. Leukoc. Biol.* **2017**, *101*, 1103–1108. [CrossRef] [PubMed]
12. Lampron, A.; Larochelle, A.; Laflamme, N.; Préfontaine, P.; Plante, M.M.; Sánchez, M.G.; Yong, V.W.; Stys, P.K.; Tremblay, M.; Rivest, S. Inefficient clearance of myelin debris by microglia impairs remyelinating processes. *J. Exp. Med.* **2015**, *212*, 481–495. [CrossRef] [PubMed]
13. Ghorbani, S.; Yong, V.W. The extracellular matrix as modifier of neuroinflammation and remyelination in multiple sclerosis. *Brain A J. Neurol.* **2021**, *144*, 1958–1973. [CrossRef] [PubMed]
14. Kalafatakis, I.; Karagogeos, D. Oligodendrocytes and Microglia: Key Players in Myelin Development, Damage and Repair. *Biomolecules* **2021**, *11*, 1058. [CrossRef]
15. Zamanian, J.L.; Xu, L.; Foo, L.C.; Nouri, N.; Zhou, L.; Giffard, R.G.; Barres, B.A. Genomic analysis of reactive astrogliosis. *J. Neurosci. Off. J. Soc. Neurosci.* **2012**, *32*, 6391–6410. [CrossRef]
16. Liddelow, S.A.; Guttenplan, K.A.; Clarke, L.E.; Bennett, F.C.; Bohlen, C.J.; Schirmer, L.; Bennett, M.L.; Münch, A.E.; Chung, W.S.; Peterson, T.C.; et al. Neurotoxic reactive astrocytes are induced by activated microglia. *Nature* **2017**, *541*, 481–487. [CrossRef]
17. Liddelow, S.A.; Barres, B.A. Reactive Astrocytes: Production, Function, and Therapeutic Potential. *Immunity* **2017**, *46*, 957–967. [CrossRef]
18. Skripuletz, T.; Hackstette, D.; Bauer, K.; Gudi, V.; Pul, R.; Voss, E.; Berger, K.; Kipp, M.; Baumgärtner, W.; Stangel, M. Astrocytes regulate myelin clearance through recruitment of microglia during cuprizone-induced demyelination. *Brain A J. Neurol.* **2013**, *136*, 147–167. [CrossRef]
19. Pu, A.; Stephenson, E.L.; Yong, V.W. The extracellular matrix: Focus on oligodendrocyte biology and targeting CSPGs for remyelination therapies. *Glia* **2018**, *66*, 1809–1825. [CrossRef]
20. Bankston, A.N.; Forston, M.D.; Howard, R.M.; Andres, K.R.; Smith, A.E.; Ohri, S.S.; Bates, M.L.; Bunge, M.B.; Whittemore, S.R. Autophagy is essential for oligodendrocyte differentiation, survival, and proper myelination. *Glia* **2019**, *67*, 1745–1759. [CrossRef]
21. Aber, E.R.; Griffey, C.J.; Davies, T.; Li, A.M.; Yang, Y.J.; Croce, K.R.; Goldman, J.E.; Grutzendler, J.; Canman, J.C.; Yamamoto, A. Oligodendroglial macroautophagy is essential for myelin sheath turnover to prevent neurodegeneration and death. *Cell Rep.* **2022**, *41*, 111480. [CrossRef]
22. Ktena, N.; Kaplanis, S.I.; Kolotuev, I.; Georgilis, A.; Kallergi, E.; Stavroulaki, V.; Nikoletopoulou, V.; Savvaki, M.; Karagogeos, D. Autophagic degradation of CNS myelin maintains axon integrity. *Cell Stress* **2022**, *6*, 93–107. [CrossRef]
23. Piccio, L.; Stark, J.L.; Cross, A.H. Chronic calorie restriction attenuates experimental autoimmune encephalomyelitis. *J. Leukoc. Biol.* **2008**, *84*, 940–948. [CrossRef]
24. Mojaverrostami, S.; Pasbakhsh, P.; Madadi, S.; Nekoonam, S.; Zarini, D.; Noori, L.; Shiri, E.; Salama, M.; Zibara, K.; Kashani, I.R. Calorie restriction promotes remyelination in a Cuprizone-Induced demyelination mouse model of multiple sclerosis. *Metab. Brain Dis.* **2020**, *35*, 1211–1224. [CrossRef]
25. Masoro, E.J. Overview of caloric restriction and ageing. *Mech. Ageing Dev.* **2005**, *126*, 913–922. [CrossRef]
26. Fontana, L.; Partridge, L.; Longo, V.D. Extending healthy life span—From yeast to humans. *Science* **2010**, *328*, 321–326. [CrossRef]
27. Mariño, G.; Pietrocola, F.; Eisenberg, T.; Kong, Y.; Malik, S.A.; Andryushkova, A.; Schroeder, S.; Pendl, T.; Harger, A.; Niso-Santano, M.; et al. Regulation of autophagy by cytosolic acetyl-coenzyme A. *Mol. Cell* **2014**, *53*, 710–725. [CrossRef]
28. Menzies, F.M.; Fleming, A.; Caricasole, A.; Bento, C.F.; Andrews, S.P.; Ashkenazi, A.; Füllgrabe, J.; Jackson, A.; Jimenez Sanchez, M.; Karabiyik, C.; et al. Autophagy and Neurodegeneration: Pathogenic Mechanisms and Therapeutic Opportunities. *Neuron* **2017**, *93*, 1015–1034. [CrossRef] [PubMed]
29. Yang, S.; Moon, S.; Hur, S.C.; Jeong, S.M. Fatty acid oxidation regulates cellular senescence by modulating the autophagy-SIRT1 axis. *BMB Rep.* **2023**, 5938. [CrossRef]
30. Lv, S.; Zhang, Y.; Lin, Y.; Fang, W.; Wang, Y.; Li, Z.; Lin, A.; Dai, X.; Ye, Q.; Zhang, J.; et al. ApoE4 exacerbates the senescence of hippocampal neurons and spatial cognitive impairment by downregulating acetyl-CoA level. *Aging Cell* **2023**, *22*, e13932. [CrossRef] [PubMed]
31. Ren, J.; Zhang, Y. Targeting Autophagy in Aging and Aging-Related Cardiovascular Diseases. *Trends Pharmacol. Sci.* **2018**, *39*, 1064–1076. [CrossRef]
32. Bosi, E. Metformin--the gold standard in type 2 diabetes: What does the evidence tell us? *Diabetes Obes. Metab.* **2009**, *11* (Suppl. S2), 3–8. [CrossRef]
33. Madeo, F.; Carmona-Gutierrez, D.; Hofer, S.J.; Kroemer, G. Caloric Restriction Mimetics against Age-Associated Disease: Targets, Mechanisms, and Therapeutic Potential. *Cell Metab.* **2019**, *29*, 592–610. [CrossRef]
34. LaMoia, T.E.; Shulman, G.I. Cellular and Molecular Mechanisms of Metformin Action. *Endocr. Rev.* **2021**, *42*, 77–96. [CrossRef]

35. Wang, J.C.; Li, G.Y.; Wang, B.; Han, S.X.; Sun, X.; Jiang, Y.N.; Shen, Y.W.; Zhou, C.; Feng, J.; Lu, S.Y.; et al. Metformin inhibits metastatic breast cancer progression and improves chemosensitivity by inducing vessel normalization via PDGF-B downregulation. *J. Exp. Clin. Cancer Res.* **2019**, *38*, 235. [CrossRef]
36. Sugiura, K.; Okabayashi, K.; Seishima, R.; Ishida, T.; Shigeta, K.; Tsuruta, M.; Hasegawa, H.; Kitagawa, Y. Metformin inhibits the development and metastasis of colorectal cancer. *Med. Oncol.* **2022**, *39*, 136. [CrossRef]
37. Zhang, J.; Huang, L.; Shi, X.; Yang, L.; Hua, F.; Ma, J.; Zhu, W.; Liu, X.; Xuan, R.; Shen, Y.; et al. Metformin protects against myocardial ischemia-reperfusion injury and cell pyroptosis via AMPK/NLRP3 inflammasome pathway. *Aging* **2020**, *12*, 24270–24287. [CrossRef]
38. Yerevanian, A.; Soukas, A.A. Metformin: Mechanisms in Human Obesity and Weight Loss. *Curr. Obes. Rep.* **2019**, *8*, 156–164. [CrossRef] [PubMed]
39. Du, M.R.; Gao, Q.Y.; Liu, C.L.; Bai, L.Y.; Li, T.; Wei, F.L. Exploring the Pharmacological Potential of Metformin for Neurodegenerative Diseases. *Front. Aging Neurosci.* **2022**, *14*, 838173. [CrossRef] [PubMed]
40. Chen, S.; Gan, D.; Lin, S.; Zhong, Y.; Chen, M.; Zou, X.; Shao, Z.; Xiao, G. Metformin in aging and aging-related diseases: Clinical applications and relevant mechanisms. *Theranostics* **2022**, *12*, 2722–2740. [CrossRef] [PubMed]
41. Lv, Z.; Guo, Y. Metformin and Its Benefits for Various Diseases. *Front. Endocrinol.* **2020**, *11*, 191. [CrossRef] [PubMed]
42. Owen, M.R.; Doran, E.; Halestrap, A.P. Evidence that metformin exerts its anti-diabetic effects through inhibition of complex 1 of the mitochondrial respiratory chain. *Biochem. J.* **2000**, *348 Pt 3*, 607–614. [CrossRef] [PubMed]
43. Zhou, G.; Myers, R.; Li, Y.; Chen, Y.; Shen, X.; Fenyk-Melody, J.; Wu, M.; Ventre, J.; Doebber, T.; Fujii, N.; et al. Role of AMP-activated protein kinase in mechanism of metformin action. *J. Clin. Investig.* **2001**, *108*, 1167–1174. [CrossRef]
44. Duca, F.A.; Côté, C.D.; Rasmussen, B.A.; Zadeh-Tahmasebi, M.; Rutter, G.A.; Filippi, B.M.; Lam, T.K. Metformin activates a duodenal Ampk-dependent pathway to lower hepatic glucose production in rats. *Nat. Med.* **2015**, *21*, 506–511. [CrossRef] [PubMed]
45. Lim, J.Y.; Oh, M.A.; Kim, W.H.; Sohn, H.Y.; Park, S.I. AMP-activated protein kinase inhibits TGF-β-induced fibrogenic responses of hepatic stellate cells by targeting transcriptional coactivator p300. *J. Cell. Physiol.* **2012**, *227*, 1081–1089. [CrossRef] [PubMed]
46. Caton, P.W.; Nayuni, N.K.; Kieswich, J.; Khan, N.Q.; Yaqoob, M.M.; Corder, R. Metformin suppresses hepatic gluconeogenesis through induction of SIRT1 and GCN5. *J. Endocrinol.* **2010**, *205*, 97–106. [CrossRef]
47. Zhang, C.S.; Li, M.; Ma, T.; Zong, Y.; Cui, J.; Feng, J.W.; Wu, Y.Q.; Lin, S.Y.; Lin, S.C. Metformin Activates AMPK through the Lysosomal Pathway. *Cell Metab.* **2016**, *24*, 521–522. [CrossRef]
48. Li, Y.; Chen, Y. AMPK and Autophagy. *Adv. Exp. Med. Biol.* **2019**, *1206*, 85–108. [CrossRef]
49. Wang, Y.; Zhao, J.; Guo, F.L.; Gao, X.; Xie, X.; Liu, S.; Yang, X.; Yang, X.; Zhang, L.; Ye, Y.; et al. Metformin Ameliorates Synaptic Defects in a Mouse Model of AD by Inhibiting Cdk5 Activity. *Front. Cell. Neurosci.* **2020**, *14*, 170. [CrossRef]
50. Chen, Y.; Zhao, S.; Fan, Z.; Li, Z.; Zhu, Y.; Shen, T.; Li, K.; Yan, Y.; Tian, J.; Liu, Z.; et al. Metformin attenuates plaque-associated tau pathology and reduces amyloid-β burden in APP/PS1 mice. *Alzheimers Res. Ther.* **2021**, *13*, 40. [CrossRef]
51. Saewanee, N.; Praputpittaya, T.; Malaiwong, N.; Chalorak, P.; Meemon, K. Neuroprotective effect of metformin on dopaminergic neurodegeneration and α-synuclein aggregation in *C. elegans* model of Parkinson's disease. *Neurosci. Res.* **2019**, *162*, 13–21. [CrossRef]
52. Sanchis, A.; García-Gimeno, M.A.; Cañada-Martínez, A.J.; Sequedo, M.D.; Millán, J.M.; Sanz, P.; Vázquez-Manrique, R.P. Metformin treatment reduces motor and neuropsychiatric phenotypes in the zQ175 mouse model of Huntington disease. *Exp. Mol. Med.* **2019**, *51*, 1–16. [CrossRef]
53. Samaras, K.; Makkar, S.; Crawford, J.D.; Kochan, N.A.; Wen, W.; Draper, B.; Trollor, J.N.; Brodaty, H.; Sachdev, P.S. Metformin Use Is Associated With Slowed Cognitive Decline and Reduced Incident Dementia in Older Adults With Type 2 Diabetes: The Sydney Memory and Ageing Study. *Diabetes Care* **2020**, *43*, 2691–2701. [CrossRef] [PubMed]
54. Koenig, A.M.; Mechanic-Hamilton, D.; Xie, S.X.; Combs, M.F.; Cappola, A.R.; Xie, L.; Detre, J.A.; Wolk, D.A.; Arnold, S.E. Effects of the Insulin Sensitizer Metformin in Alzheimer Disease: Pilot Data From a Randomized Placebo-controlled Crossover Study. *Alzheimer Dis. Assoc. Disord.* **2017**, *31*, 107–113. [CrossRef]
55. Moore, E.M.; Mander, A.G.; Ames, D.; Kotowicz, M.A.; Carne, R.P.; Brodaty, H.; Woodward, M.; Boundy, K.; Ellis, K.A.; Bush, A.I.; et al. Increased risk of cognitive impairment in patients with diabetes is associated with metformin. *Diabetes Care* **2013**, *36*, 2981–2987. [CrossRef]
56. Dziedzic, A.; Saluk-Bijak, J.; Miller, E.; Bijak, M. Metformin as a Potential Agent in the Treatment of Multiple Sclerosis. *Int. J. Mol. Sci.* **2020**, *21*, 5957. [CrossRef]
57. Thompson, A.J.; Baranzini, S.E.; Geurts, J.; Hemmer, B.; Ciccarelli, O. Multiple sclerosis. *Lancet* **2018**, *391*, 1622–1636. [CrossRef]
58. Largani, S.H.H.; Borhani-Haghighi, M.; Pasbakhsh, P.; Mahabadi, V.P.; Nekoonam, S.; Shiri, E.; Kashani, I.R.; Zendehdel, A. Oligoprotective effect of metformin through the AMPK-dependent on restoration of mitochondrial hemostasis in the cuprizone-induced multiple sclerosis model. *J. Mol. Histol.* **2019**, *50*, 263–271. [CrossRef]
59. Abdi, M.; Pasbakhsh, P.; Shabani, M.; Nekoonam, S.; Sadeghi, A.; Fathi, F.; Abouzaripour, M.; Mohamed, W.; Zibara, K.; Kashani, I.R.; et al. Metformin Therapy Attenuates Pro-inflammatory Microglia by Inhibiting NF-κB in Cuprizone Demyelinating Mouse Model of Multiple Sclerosis. *Neurotox. Res.* **2021**, *39*, 1732–1746. [CrossRef] [PubMed]
60. Ishihara, Y.; Itoh, K. Microglial inflammatory reactions regulated by oxidative stress. *J. Clin. Biochem. Nutr.* **2023**, *72*, 23–27. [CrossRef] [PubMed]

61. Nahirnyj, A.; Livne-Bar, I.; Guo, X.; Sivak, J.M. ROS detoxification and proinflammatory cytokines are linked by p38 MAPK signaling in a model of mature astrocyte activation. *PLoS ONE* **2013**, *8*, e83049. [CrossRef] [PubMed]
62. Nath, N.; Khan, M.; Paintlia, M.K.; Singh, I.; Hoda, M.N.; Giri, S. Metformin attenuated the autoimmune disease of the central nervous system in animal models of multiple sclerosis. *J. Immunol.* **2009**, *182*, 8005–8014. [CrossRef] [PubMed]
63. Wu, Y.Q.; Xiong, J.; He, Z.L.; Yuan, Y.; Wang, B.N.; Xu, J.Y.; Wu, M.; Zhang, S.S.; Cai, S.F.; Zhao, J.X.; et al. Metformin promotes microglial cells to facilitate myelin debris clearance and accelerate nerve repairment after spinal cord injury. *Acta Pharmacol. Sin.* **2022**, *43*, 1360–1371. [CrossRef] [PubMed]
64. Sanadgol, N.; Barati, M.; Houshmand, F.; Hassani, S.; Clarner, T.; Shahlaei, M.; Golab, F. Metformin accelerates myelin recovery and ameliorates behavioral deficits in the animal model of multiple sclerosis via adjustment of AMPK/Nrf2/mTOR signaling and maintenance of endogenous oligodendrogenesis during brain self-repairing period. *Pharmacol. Rep.* **2020**, *72*, 641–658. [CrossRef] [PubMed]
65. Bercury, K.K.; Dai, J.; Sachs, H.H.; Ahrendsen, J.T.; Wood, T.L.; Macklin, W.B. Conditional ablation of raptor or rictor has differential impact on oligodendrocyte differentiation and CNS myelination. *J. Neurosci.* **2014**, *34*, 4466–4480. [CrossRef] [PubMed]
66. Ishii, A.; Furusho, M.; Macklin, W.; Bansal, R. Independent and cooperative roles of the Mek/ERK1/2-MAPK and PI3K/Akt/mTOR pathways during developmental myelination and in adulthood. *Glia* **2019**, *67*, 1277–1295. [CrossRef]
67. Carson, R.P.; Van Nielen, D.L.; Winzenburger, P.A.; Ess, K.C. Neuronal and glia abnormalities in Tsc1-deficient forebrain and partial rescue by rapamycin. *Neurobiol. Dis.* **2012**, *45*, 369–380. [CrossRef] [PubMed]
68. McLane, L.E.; Bourne, J.N.; Evangelou, A.V.; Khandker, L.; Macklin, W.B.; Wood, T.L. Loss of Tuberous Sclerosis Complex1 in Adult Oligodendrocyte Progenitor Cells Enhances Axon Remyelination and Increases Myelin Thickness after a Focal Demyelination. *J. Neurosci.* **2017**, *37*, 7534–7546. [CrossRef]
69. Manwani, B.; McCullough, L.D. Function of the master energy regulator adenosine monophosphate-activated protein kinase in stroke. *J. Neurosci. Res.* **2013**, *91*, 1018–1029. [CrossRef]
70. Narine, M.; Azmi, M.A.; Umali, M.; Volz, A.; Colognato, H. The AMPK activator metformin improves recovery from demyelination by shifting oligodendrocyte bioenergetics and accelerating OPC differentiation. *Front. Cell. Neurosci.* **2023**, *17*, 1254303. [CrossRef]
71. Paintlia, A.S.; Paintlia, M.K.; Mohan, S.; Singh, A.K.; Singh, I. AMP-activated protein kinase signaling protects oligodendrocytes that restore central nervous system functions in an experimental autoimmune encephalomyelitis model. *Am. J. Pathol.* **2013**, *183*, 526–541. [CrossRef]
72. Houshmand, F.; Barati, M.; Golab, F.; Ramezani-Sefidar, S.; Tanbakooie, S.; Tabatabaei, M.; Amiri, M.; Sanadgol, N. Metformin-induced AMPK activation stimulates remyelination through induction of neurotrophic factors, downregulation of NogoA and recruitment of $Olig^{2+}$ precursor cells in the cuprizone murine model of multiple sclerosis. *Daru* **2019**, *27*, 583–592. [CrossRef]
73. Pöyhönen, S.; Er, S.; Domanskyi, A.; Airavaara, M. Effects of Neurotrophic Factors in Glial Cells in the Central Nervous System: Expression and Properties in Neurodegeneration and Injury. *Front. Physiol.* **2019**, *10*, 486. [CrossRef]
74. Kosaraju, J.; Seegobin, M.; Gouveia, A.; Syal, C.; Sarma, S.N.; Lu, K.J.; Ilin, J.; He, L.; Wondisford, F.E.; Lagace, D.; et al. Metformin promotes CNS remyelination and improves social interaction following focal demyelination through CBP Ser436 phosphorylation. *Exp. Neurol.* **2020**, *334*, 113454. [CrossRef]
75. Franklin, R.J.; Ffrench-Constant, C.; Edgar, J.M.; Smith, K.J. Neuroprotection and repair in multiple sclerosis. *Nat. Rev. Neurol.* **2012**, *8*, 624–634. [CrossRef]
76. Sim, F.J.; Zhao, C.; Penderis, J.; Franklin, R.J. The age-related decrease in CNS remyelination efficiency is attributable to an impairment of both oligodendrocyte progenitor recruitment and differentiation. *J. Neurosci.* **2002**, *22*, 2451–2459. [CrossRef]
77. Neumann, B.; Baror, R.; Zhao, C.; Segel, M.; Dietmann, S.; Rawji, K.S.; Foerster, S.; McClain, C.R.; Chalut, K.; van Wijngaarden, P.; et al. Metformin Restores CNS Remyelination Capacity by Rejuvenating Aged Stem Cells. *Cell Stem Cell* **2019**, *25*, 473–485.e8. [CrossRef]
78. Najafi, M.; Cheki, M.; Rezapoor, S.; Geraily, G.; Motevaseli, E.; Carnovale, C.; Clementi, E.; Shirazi, A. Metformin: Prevention of genomic instability and cancer: A review. *Mutat. Res. Genet. Toxicol. Environ. Mutagen.* **2018**, *827*, 1–8. [CrossRef]
79. Bharath, L.P.; Agrawal, M.; McCambridge, G.; Nicholas, D.A.; Hasturk, H.; Liu, J.; Jiang, K.; Liu, R.; Guo, Z.; Deeney, J.; et al. Metformin Enhances Autophagy and Normalizes Mitochondrial Function to Alleviate Aging-Associated Inflammation. *Cell Metab.* **2020**, *32*, 44–55.e6. [CrossRef]
80. Bogan, K.L.; Brenner, C. Nicotinic acid, nicotinamide, and nicotinamide riboside: A molecular evaluation of NAD^+ precursor vitamins in human nutrition. *Annu. Rev. Nutr.* **2008**, *28*, 115–130. [CrossRef]
81. Hofer, S.J.; Davinelli, S.; Bergmann, M.; Scapagnini, G.; Madeo, F. Caloric Restriction Mimetics in Nutrition and Clinical Trials. *Front. Nutr.* **2021**, *8*, 717343. [CrossRef]
82. Verdin, E. NAD^+ in aging, metabolism, and neurodegeneration. *Science* **2015**, *350*, 1208–1213. [CrossRef]
83. Yoshino, J.; Baur, J.A.; Imai, S.I. NAD^+ Intermediates: The Biology and Therapeutic Potential of NMN and NR. *Cell Metab.* **2018**, *27*, 513–528. [CrossRef]
84. Fang, E.F.; Kassahun, H.; Croteau, D.L.; Scheibye-Knudsen, M.; Marosi, K.; Lu, H.; Shamanna, R.A.; Kalyanasundaram, S.; Bollineni, R.C.; Wilson, M.A.; et al. NAD^+ Replenishment Improves Lifespan and Healthspan in Ataxia Telangiectasia Models via Mitophagy and DNA Repair. *Cell Metab.* **2016**, *24*, 566–581. [CrossRef]

85. Zhang, H.; Ryu, D.; Wu, Y.; Gariani, K.; Wang, X.; Luan, P.; D'Amico, D.; Ropelle, E.R.; Lutolf, M.P.; Aebersold, R.; et al. NAD$^+$ repletion improves mitochondrial and stem cell function and enhances life span in mice. *Science* **2016**, *352*, 1436–1443. [CrossRef]
86. Mitchell, S.J.; Bernier, M.; Aon, M.A.; Cortassa, S.; Kim, E.Y.; Fang, E.F.; Palacios, H.H.; Ali, A.; Navas-Enamorado, I.; Di Francesco, A.; et al. Nicotinamide Improves Aspects of Healthspan, but Not Lifespan, in Mice. *Cell Metab.* **2018**, *27*, 667–676.e4. [CrossRef]
87. Abdellatif, M.; Trummer-Herbst, V.; Koser, F.; Durand, S.; Adão, R.; Vasques-Nóvoa, F.; Freundt, J.K.; Voglhuber, J.; Pricolo, M.R.; Kasa, M.; et al. Nicotinamide for the treatment of heart failure with preserved ejection fraction. *Sci. Transl. Med.* **2021**, *13*, eabd7064. [CrossRef]
88. Wu, K.; Li, B.; Lin, Q.; Xu, W.; Zuo, W.; Li, J.; Liu, N.; Tu, T.; Zhang, B.; Xiao, Y.; et al. Nicotinamide mononucleotide attenuates isoproterenol-induced cardiac fibrosis by regulating oxidative stress and Smad3 acetylation. *Life Sci.* **2021**, *274*, 119299. [CrossRef]
89. Scatozza, F.; Moschella, F.; D'Arcangelo, D.; Rossi, S.; Tabolacci, C.; Giampietri, C.; Proietti, E.; Facchiano, F.; Facchiano, A. Nicotinamide inhibits melanoma in vitro and in vivo. *J. Exp. Clin. Cancer Res.* **2020**, *39*, 211. [CrossRef]
90. Jung, M.; Lee, K.M.; Im, Y.; Seok, S.H.; Chung, H.; Kim, D.Y.; Han, D.; Lee, C.H.; Hwang, E.H.; Park, S.Y.; et al. Nicotinamide (niacin) supplement increases lipid metabolism and ROS-induced energy disruption in triple-negative breast cancer: Potential for drug repositioning as an anti-tumor agent. *Mol. Oncol.* **2022**, *16*, 1795–1815. [CrossRef]
91. Lautrup, S.; Sinclair, D.A.; Mattson, M.P.; Fang, E.F. NAD$^+$ in Brain Aging and Neurodegenerative Disorders. *Cell Metab.* **2019**, *30*, 630–655. [CrossRef]
92. Fang, E.F.; Lautrup, S.; Hou, Y.; Demarest, T.G.; Croteau, D.L.; Mattson, M.P.; Bohr, V.A. NAD$^+$ in Aging: Molecular Mechanisms and Translational Implications. *Trends Mol. Med.* **2017**, *23*, 899–916. [CrossRef] [PubMed]
93. Katsyuba, E.; Romani, M.; Hofer, D.; Auwerx, J. NAD$^+$ homeostasis in health and disease. *Nat. Metab.* **2020**, *2*, 9–31. [CrossRef] [PubMed]
94. Barbosa, M.T.; Soares, S.M.; Novak, C.M.; Sinclair, D.; Levine, J.A.; Aksoy, P.; Chini, E.N. The enzyme CD38 (a NAD glycohydrolase, EC 3.2.2.5) is necessary for the development of diet-induced obesity. *FASEB J.* **2007**, *21*, 3629–3639. [CrossRef] [PubMed]
95. Langley, M.R.; Choi, C.I.; Peclat, T.R.; Guo, Y.; Simon, W.L.; Yoon, H.; Kleppe, L.; Lucchinetti, C.F.; Chini, C.C.S.; Chini, E.N.; et al. Critical Role of Astrocyte NAD$^+$ Glycohydrolase in Myelin Injury and Regeneration. *J. Neurosci.* **2021**, *41*, 8644–8667. [CrossRef] [PubMed]
96. Roboon, J.; Hattori, T.; Ishii, H.; Takarada-Iemata, M.; Le, T.M.; Shiraishi, Y.; Ozaki, N.; Yamamoto, Y.; Sugawara, A.; Okamoto, H.; et al. Deletion of CD38 Suppresses Glial Activation and Neuroinflammation in a Mouse Model of Demyelination. *Front. Cell. Neurosci.* **2019**, *13*, 258. [CrossRef] [PubMed]
97. Rouleau, M.; Patel, A.; Hendzel, M.J.; Kaufmann, S.H.; Poirier, G.G. PARP inhibition: PARP1 and beyond. *Nat. Rev. Cancer* **2010**, *10*, 293–301. [CrossRef]
98. Veto, S.; Acs, P.; Bauer, J.; Lassmann, H.; Berente, Z.; Setalo, G., Jr.; Borgulya, G.; Sumegi, B.; Komoly, S.; Gallyas, F., Jr.; et al. Inhibiting poly(ADP-ribose) polymerase: A potential therapy against oligodendrocyte death. *Brain A J. Neurol.* **2010**, *133*, 822–834. [CrossRef]
99. Lee, I.H.; Cao, L.; Mostoslavsky, R.; Lombard, D.B.; Liu, J.; Bruns, N.E.; Tsokos, M.; Alt, F.W.; Finkel, T. A role for the NAD-dependent deacetylase Sirt1 in the regulation of autophagy. *Proc. Natl. Acad. Sci. USA* **2008**, *105*, 3374–3379. [CrossRef]
100. Kitada, M.; Ogura, Y.; Koya, D. Chapter 3—Role of Sirt1 as a Regulator of Autophagy. In *Autophagy: Cancer, Other Pathologies, Inflammation, Immunity, Infection, and Aging*; Hayat, M.A., Ed.; Academic Press: San Diego, CA, USA, 2016; pp. 89–100. [CrossRef]
101. Li, Y.; Yang, G.; Yang, X.; He, Y.; Wang, W.; Zhang, J.; Li, T.; Zhang, W.; Lin, R. Nicotinic acid inhibits vascular inflammation via the SIRT1-dependent signaling pathway. *J. Nutr. Biochem.* **2015**, *26*, 1338–1347. [CrossRef]
102. Li, Y.; Yang, G.; Yang, X.; Wang, W.; Zhang, J.; He, Y.; Zhang, W.; Jing, T.; Lin, R. Nicotinic acid inhibits NLRP3 inflammasome activation via SIRT1 in vascular endothelial cells. *Int. Immunopharmacol.* **2016**, *40*, 211–218. [CrossRef] [PubMed]
103. Zhang, J.; Wang, C.; Ying, W. SIRT2 and Akt mediate NAD$^+$-induced and NADH-induced increases in the intracellular ATP levels of BV2 microglia under basal conditions. *Neuroreport* **2018**, *29*, 65–70. [CrossRef] [PubMed]
104. Acklin, S.; Sadhukhan, R.; Du, W.; Patra, M.; Cholia, R.; Xia, F. Nicotinamide riboside alleviates cisplatin-induced peripheral neuropathy via SIRT2 activation. *Neurooncol. Adv.* **2022**, *4*, vdac101. [CrossRef] [PubMed]
105. Hou, Y.; Wei, Y.; Lautrup, S.; Yang, B.; Wang, Y.; Cordonnier, S.; Mattson, M.P.; Croteau, D.L.; Bohr, V.A. NAD(+) supplementation reduces neuroinflammation and cell senescence in a transgenic mouse model of Alzheimer's disease via cGAS-STING. *Proc. Natl. Acad. Sci. USA* **2021**, *118*, e2011226118. [CrossRef] [PubMed]
106. Zhao, X.; Kong, M.; Wang, Y.; Mao, Y.; Xu, H.; He, W.; He, Y.; Gu, J. Nicotinamide mononucleotide improves the Alzheimer's disease by regulating intestinal microbiota. *Biochem. Biophys. Res. Commun.* **2023**, *670*, 27–35. [CrossRef] [PubMed]
107. Rehman, I.U.; Khan, A.; Ahmad, R.; Choe, K.; Park, H.Y.; Lee, H.J.; Atiq, A.; Park, J.; Hahm, J.R.; Kim, M.O. Neuroprotective Effects of Nicotinamide against MPTP-Induced Parkinson's Disease in Mice: Impact on Oxidative Stress, Neuroinflammation, Nrf2/HO-1 and TLR4 Signaling Pathways. *Biomedicines* **2022**, *10*, 2929. [CrossRef] [PubMed]
108. Sidhu, A.; Diwan, V.; Kaur, H.; Bhateja, D.; Singh, C.K.; Sharma, S.; Padi, S.S.V. Nicotinamide reverses behavioral impairments and provides neuroprotection in 3-nitropropionic acid induced animal model ofHuntington's disease: Implication of oxidative stress- poly(ADP- ribose) polymerase pathway. *Metab. Brain Dis.* **2018**, *33*, 1911–1921. [CrossRef]
109. Trammell, S.A.; Schmidt, M.S.; Weidemann, B.J.; Redpath, P.; Jaksch, F.; Dellinger, R.W.; Li, Z.; Abel, E.D.; Migaud, M.E.; Brenner, C. Nicotinamide riboside is uniquely and orally bioavailable in mice and humans. *Nat. Commun.* **2016**, *7*, 12948. [CrossRef]

110. Martens, C.R.; Denman, B.A.; Mazzo, M.R.; Armstrong, M.L.; Reisdorph, N.; McQueen, M.B.; Chonchol, M.; Seals, D.R. Chronic nicotinamide riboside supplementation is well-tolerated and elevates NAD$^+$ in healthy middle-aged and older adults. *Nat. Commun.* **2018**, *9*, 1286. [CrossRef]
111. Vreones, M.; Mustapic, M.; Moaddel, R.; Pucha, K.A.; Lovett, J.; Seals, D.R.; Kapogiannis, D.; Martens, C.R. Oral nicotinamide riboside raises NAD$^+$ and lowers biomarkers of neurodegenerative pathology in plasma extracellular vesicles enriched for neuronal origin. *Aging Cell* **2023**, *22*, e13754. [CrossRef]
112. Brakedal, B.; Dölle, C.; Riemer, F.; Ma, Y.; Nido, G.S.; Skeie, G.O.; Craven, A.R.; Schwarzlmüller, T.; Brekke, N.; Diab, J.; et al. The NADPARK study: A randomized phase I trial of nicotinamide riboside supplementation in Parkinson's disease. *Cell Metab.* **2022**, *34*, 396–407.e6. [CrossRef] [PubMed]
113. Nicotinamide as an Early Alzheimer's Disease Treatment. Available online: https://clinicaltrials.gov/study/NCT03061474 (accessed on 8 November 2023).
114. Wang, X.; Li, B.; Liu, L.; Zhang, L.; Ma, T.; Guo, L. Nicotinamide adenine dinucleotide treatment alleviates the symptoms of experimental autoimmune encephalomyelitis by activating autophagy and inhibiting the NLRP3 inflammasome. *Int. Immunopharmacol.* **2021**, *90*, 107092. [CrossRef] [PubMed]
115. Guo, J.; Li, B.; Wang, J.; Guo, R.; Tian, Y.; Song, S.; Guo, L. Protective effect and mechanism of nicotinamide adenine dinucleotide against optic neuritis in mice with experimental autoimmune encephalomyelitis. *Int. Immunopharmacol.* **2021**, *98*, 107846. [CrossRef] [PubMed]
116. Franklin, R.J.; Ffrench-Constant, C. Remyelination in the CNS: From biology to therapy. *Nat. Rev. Neurosci.* **2008**, *9*, 839–855. [CrossRef] [PubMed]
117. Kaplanis, S.I.; Kaffe, D.; Ktena, N.; Lygeraki, A.; Kolliniati, O.; Savvaki, M.; Karagogeos, D. Nicotinamide enhances myelin production after demyelination through reduction of astrogliosis and microgliosis. *Front. Cell. Neurosci.* **2023**, *17*, 1201317. [CrossRef] [PubMed]
118. Roboon, J.; Hattori, T.; Ishii, H.; Takarada-Iemata, M.; Nguyen, D.T.; Heer, C.D.; O'Meally, D.; Brenner, C.; Yamamoto, Y.; Okamoto, H.; et al. Inhibition of CD38 and supplementation of nicotinamide riboside ameliorate lipopolysaccharide-induced microglial and astrocytic neuroinflammation by increasing NAD$^+$. *J. Neurochem.* **2021**, *158*, 311–327. [CrossRef] [PubMed]
119. Hong, Y.; Liu, Y.; Zhang, G.; Wu, H.; Hou, Y. Progesterone suppresses Aβ(42)-induced neuroinflammation by enhancing autophagy in astrocytes. *Int. Immunopharmacol.* **2018**, *54*, 336–343. [CrossRef]
120. Pais, T.F.; Szegő, É.M.; Marques, O.; Miller-Fleming, L.; Antas, P.; Guerreiro, P.; de Oliveira, R.M.; Kasapoglu, B.; Outeiro, T.F. The NAD-dependent deacetylase sirtuin 2 is a suppressor of microglial activation and brain inflammation. *EMBO J.* **2013**, *32*, 2603–2616. [CrossRef]
121. Li, W.; Zhang, B.; Tang, J.; Cao, Q.; Wu, Y.; Wu, C.; Guo, J.; Ling, E.A.; Liang, F. Sirtuin 2, a mammalian homolog of yeast silent information regulator-2 longevity regulator, is an oligodendroglial protein that decelerates cell differentiation through deacetylating alpha-tubulin. *J. Neurosci.* **2007**, *27*, 2606–2616. [CrossRef]
122. Jayasena, T.; Poljak, A.; Braidy, N.; Zhong, L.; Rowlands, B.; Muenchhoff, J.; Grant, R.; Smythe, G.; Teo, C.; Raftery, M.; et al. Application of Targeted Mass Spectrometry for the Quantification of Sirtuins in the Central Nervous System. *Sci. Rep.* **2016**, *6*, 35391. [CrossRef]
123. Ma, X.R.; Zhu, X.; Xiao, Y.; Gu, H.M.; Zheng, S.S.; Li, L.; Wang, F.; Dong, Z.J.; Wang, D.X.; Wu, Y.; et al. Restoring nuclear entry of Sirtuin 2 in oligodendrocyte progenitor cells promotes remyelination during ageing. *Nat. Commun.* **2022**, *13*, 1225. [CrossRef] [PubMed]
124. Rawji, K.S.; Young, A.M.H.; Ghosh, T.; Michaels, N.J.; Mirzaei, R.; Kappen, J.; Kolehmainen, K.L.; Alaeiilkhchi, N.; Lozinski, B.; Mishra, M.K.; et al. Niacin-mediated rejuvenation of macrophage/microglia enhances remyelination of the aging central nervous system. *Acta Neuropathol.* **2020**, *139*, 893–909. [CrossRef] [PubMed]
125. Zhao, C.; Li, W.W.; Franklin, R.J. Differences in the early inflammatory responses to toxin-induced demyelination are associated with the age-related decline in CNS remyelination. *Neurobiol. Aging* **2006**, *27*, 1298–1307. [CrossRef] [PubMed]
126. Natrajan, M.S.; de la Fuente, A.G.; Crawford, A.H.; Linehan, E.; Nuñez, V.; Johnson, K.R.; Wu, T.; Fitzgerald, D.C.; Ricote, M.; Bielekova, B.; et al. Retinoid X receptor activation reverses age-related deficiencies in myelin debris phagocytosis and remyelination. *Brain A J. Neurol.* **2015**, *138*, 3581–3597. [CrossRef] [PubMed]
127. Wang, C.; Zhang, Y.; Ding, J.; Zhao, Z.; Qian, C.; Luan, Y.; Teng, G.J. Nicotinamide Administration Improves Remyelination after Stroke. *Neural Plast.* **2017**, *2017*, 7019803. [CrossRef] [PubMed]
128. Xiao, J.; Wong, A.W.; Willingham, M.M.; van den Buuse, M.; Kilpatrick, T.J.; Murray, S.S. Brain-derived neurotrophic factor promotes central nervous system myelination via a direct effect upon oligodendrocytes. *Neurosignals* **2010**, *18*, 186–202. [CrossRef]
129. Pirola, L.; Fröjdö, S. Resveratrol: One molecule, many targets. *IUBMB Life* **2008**, *60*, 323–332. [CrossRef]
130. Meng, X.; Zhou, J.; Zhao, C.N.; Gan, R.Y.; Li, H.B. Health Benefits and Molecular Mechanisms of Resveratrol: A Narrative Review. *Foods* **2020**, *9*, 340. [CrossRef]
131. Jang, M.; Cai, L.; Udeani, G.O.; Slowing, K.V.; Thomas, C.F.; Beecher, C.W.; Fong, H.H.; Farnsworth, N.R.; Kinghorn, A.D.; Mehta, R.G.; et al. Cancer chemopreventive activity of resveratrol, a natural product derived from grapes. *Science* **1997**, *275*, 218–220. [CrossRef]
132. Li, T.; Tan, Y.; Ouyang, S.; He, J.; Liu, L. Resveratrol protects against myocardial ischemia-reperfusion injury via attenuating ferroptosis. *Gene* **2022**, *808*, 145968. [CrossRef]

133. Mahjabeen, W.; Khan, D.A.; Mirza, S.A. Role of resveratrol supplementation in regulation of glucose hemostasis, inflammation and oxidative stress in patients with diabetes mellitus type 2: A randomized, placebo-controlled trial. *Complement. Ther. Med.* **2022**, *66*, 102819. [CrossRef] [PubMed]
134. Sun, Y.; Zhou, Q.M.; Lu, Y.Y.; Zhang, H.; Chen, Q.L.; Zhao, M.; Su, S.B. Resveratrol Inhibits the Migration and Metastasis of MDA-MB-231 Human Breast Cancer by Reversing TGF-β1-Induced Epithelial-Mesenchymal Transition. *Molecules* **2019**, *24*, 1131. [CrossRef] [PubMed]
135. Wang, P.; Gao, J.; Ke, W.; Wang, J.; Li, D.; Liu, R.; Jia, Y.; Wang, X.; Chen, X.; Chen, F.; et al. Resveratrol reduces obesity in high-fat diet-fed mice via modulating the composition and metabolic function of the gut microbiota. *Free Radic. Biol. Med.* **2020**, *156*, 83–98. [CrossRef] [PubMed]
136. Yan, Y.; Yang, H.; Xie, Y.; Ding, Y.; Kong, D.; Yu, H. Research Progress on Alzheimer's Disease and Resveratrol. *Neurochem. Res.* **2020**, *45*, 989–1006. [CrossRef] [PubMed]
137. Dos Santos, M.G.; Schimith, L.E.; André-Miral, C.; Muccillo-Baisch, A.L.; Arbo, B.D.; Hort, M.A. Neuroprotective Effects of Resveratrol in In vivo and In vitro Experimental Models of Parkinson's Disease: A Systematic Review. *Neurotox. Res.* **2022**, *40*, 319–345. [CrossRef] [PubMed]
138. Ginés, C.; Cuesta, S.; Kireev, R.; García, C.; Rancan, L.; Paredes, S.D.; Vara, E.; Tresguerres, J.A.F. Protective effect of resveratrol against inflammation, oxidative stress and apoptosis in pancreas of aged SAMP8 mice. *Exp. Gerontol.* **2017**, *90*, 61–70. [CrossRef] [PubMed]
139. Wang, N.; Luo, Z.; Jin, M.; Sheng, W.; Wang, H.T.; Long, X.; Wu, Y.; Hu, P.; Xu, H.; Zhang, X. Exploration of age-related mitochondrial dysfunction and the anti-aging effects of resveratrol in zebrafish retina. *Aging* **2019**, *11*, 3117–3137. [CrossRef]
140. Morselli, E.; Maiuri, M.C.; Markaki, M.; Megalou, E.; Pasparaki, A.; Palikaras, K.; Criollo, A.; Galluzzi, L.; Malik, S.A.; Vitale, I.; et al. Caloric restriction and resveratrol promote longevity through the Sirtuin-1-dependent induction of autophagy. *Cell Death Dis.* **2010**, *1*, e10. [CrossRef]
141. Price, N.L.; Gomes, A.P.; Ling, A.J.; Duarte, F.V.; Martin-Montalvo, A.; North, B.J.; Agarwal, B.; Ye, L.; Ramadori, G.; Teodoro, J.S.; et al. SIRT1 is required for AMPK activation and the beneficial effects of resveratrol on mitochondrial function. *Cell Metab.* **2012**, *15*, 675–690. [CrossRef]
142. Huang, Y.; Lu, J.; Zhan, L.; Wang, M.; Shi, R.; Yuan, X.; Gao, X.; Liu, X.; Zang, J.; Liu, W.; et al. Resveratrol-induced Sirt1 phosphorylation by LKB1 mediates mitochondrial metabolism. *J. Biol. Chem.* **2021**, *297*, 100929. [CrossRef]
143. Um, J.H.; Park, S.J.; Kang, H.; Yang, S.; Foretz, M.; McBurney, M.W.; Kim, M.K.; Viollet, B.; Chung, J.H. AMP-activated protein kinase-deficient mice are resistant to the metabolic effects of resveratrol. *Diabetes* **2010**, *59*, 554–563. [CrossRef] [PubMed]
144. Chiang, M.C.; Nicol, C.J.; Cheng, Y.C. Resveratrol activation of AMPK-dependent pathways is neuroprotective in human neural stem cells against amyloid-beta-induced inflammation and oxidative stress. *Neurochem. Int.* **2018**, *115*, 1–10. [CrossRef] [PubMed]
145. Lin, C.H.; Nicol, C.J.B.; Cheng, Y.C.; Yen, C.; Wang, Y.S.; Chiang, M.C. Neuroprotective effects of resveratrol against oxygen glucose deprivation induced mitochondrial dysfunction by activation of AMPK in SH-SY5Y cells with 3D gelatin scaffold. *Brain Res.* **2020**, *1726*, 146492. [CrossRef] [PubMed]
146. Cantó, C.; Gerhart-Hines, Z.; Feige, J.N.; Lagouge, M.; Noriega, L.; Milne, J.C.; Elliott, P.J.; Puigserver, P.; Auwerx, J. AMPK regulates energy expenditure by modulating NAD^+ metabolism and SIRT1 activity. *Nature* **2009**, *458*, 1056–1060. [CrossRef] [PubMed]
147. Meng, T.; Xiao, D.; Muhammed, A.; Deng, J.; Chen, L.; He, J. Anti-Inflammatory Action and Mechanisms of Resveratrol. *Molecules* **2021**, *26*, 229. [CrossRef]
148. Broderick, T.L.; Rasool, S.; Li, R.; Zhang, Y.; Anderson, M.; Al-Nakkash, L.; Plochocki, J.H.; Geetha, T.; Babu, J.R. Neuroprotective Effects of Chronic Resveratrol Treatment and Exercise Training in the 3xTg-AD Mouse Model of Alzheimer's Disease. *Int. J. Mol. Sci.* **2020**, *21*, 7337. [CrossRef] [PubMed]
149. Sun, X.Y.; Dong, Q.X.; Zhu, J.; Sun, X.; Zhang, L.F.; Qiu, M.; Yu, X.L.; Liu, R.T. Resveratrol Rescues Tau-Induced Cognitive Deficits and Neuropathology in a Mouse Model of Tauopathy. *Curr. Alzheimer Res.* **2019**, *16*, 710–722. [CrossRef] [PubMed]
150. Zhang, L.F.; Yu, X.L.; Ji, M.; Liu, S.Y.; Wu, X.L.; Wang, Y.J.; Liu, R.T. Resveratrol alleviates motor and cognitive deficits and neuropathology in the A53T α-synuclein mouse model of Parkinson's disease. *Food Funct.* **2018**, *9*, 6414–6426. [CrossRef]
151. Turner, R.S.; Thomas, R.G.; Craft, S.; van Dyck, C.H.; Mintzer, J.; Reynolds, B.A.; Brewer, J.B.; Rissman, R.A.; Raman, R.; Aisen, P.S. A randomized, double-blind, placebo-controlled trial of resveratrol for Alzheimer disease. *Neurology* **2015**, *85*, 1383–1391. [CrossRef]
152. Moussa, C.; Hebron, M.; Huang, X.; Ahn, J.; Rissman, R.A.; Aisen, P.S.; Turner, R.S. Resveratrol regulates neuro-inflammation and induces adaptive immunity in Alzheimer's disease. *J. Neuroinflamm.* **2017**, *14*, 1. [CrossRef]
153. Wang, J.; Wang, J.; Wang, J.; Yang, B.; Weng, Q.; He, Q. Targeting Microglia and Macrophages: A Potential Treatment Strategy for Multiple Sclerosis. *Front. Pharmacol.* **2019**, *10*, 286. [CrossRef] [PubMed]
154. Jha, M.K.; Lee, W.H.; Suk, K. Functional polarization of neuroglia: Implications in neuroinflammation and neurological disorders. *Biochem. Pharmacol.* **2016**, *103*, 1–16. [CrossRef] [PubMed]
155. Hammond, T.R.; Dufort, C.; Dissing-Olesen, L.; Giera, S.; Young, A.; Wysoker, A.; Walker, A.J.; Gergits, F.; Segel, M.; Nemesh, J.; et al. Single-Cell RNA Sequencing of Microglia throughout the Mouse Lifespan and in the Injured Brain Reveals Complex Cell-State Changes. *Immunity* **2019**, *50*, 253–271.e6. [CrossRef] [PubMed]

156. Plemel, J.R.; Stratton, J.A.; Michaels, N.J.; Rawji, K.S.; Zhang, E.; Sinha, S.; Baaklini, C.S.; Dong, Y.; Ho, M.; Thorburn, K.; et al. Microglia response following acute demyelination is heterogeneous and limits infiltrating macrophage dispersion. *Sci. Adv.* **2020**, *6*, eaay6324. [CrossRef]
157. Lombardi, M.; Parolisi, R.; Scaroni, F.; Bonfanti, E.; Gualerzi, A.; Gabrielli, M.; Kerlero de Rosbo, N.; Uccelli, A.; Giussani, P.; Viani, P.; et al. Detrimental and protective action of microglial extracellular vesicles on myelin lesions: Astrocyte involvement in remyelination failure. *Acta Neuropathol.* **2019**, *138*, 987–1012. [CrossRef] [PubMed]
158. Yang, X.; Xu, S.; Qian, Y.; Xiao, Q. Resveratrol regulates microglia M1/M2 polarization via PGC-1α in conditions of neuroinflammatory injury. *Brain Behav. Immun.* **2017**, *64*, 162–172. [CrossRef]
159. Ma, S.; Fan, L.; Li, J.; Zhang, B.; Yan, Z. Resveratrol promoted the M2 polarization of microglia and reduced neuroinflammation after cerebral ischemia by inhibiting miR-155. *Int. J. Neurosci.* **2020**, *130*, 817–825. [CrossRef]
160. Zheng, X.; Sun, K.; Liu, Y.; Yin, X.; Zhu, H.; Yu, F.; Zhao, W. Resveratrol-loaded macrophage exosomes alleviate multiple sclerosis through targeting microglia. *J. Control. Release* **2023**, *353*, 675–684. [CrossRef]
161. Quan, L.; Uyeda, A.; Muramatsu, R. Central nervous system regeneration: The roles of glial cells in the potential molecular mechanism underlying remyelination. *Inflamm. Regen.* **2022**, *42*, 7. [CrossRef]
162. Lu, X.; Ma, L.; Ruan, L.; Kong, Y.; Mou, H.; Zhang, Z.; Wang, Z.; Wang, J.M.; Le, Y. Resveratrol differentially modulates inflammatory responses of microglia and astrocytes. *J. Neuroinflamm.* **2010**, *7*, 46. [CrossRef]
163. Fan, Y.Y.; Huo, J. A1/A2 astrocytes in central nervous system injuries and diseases: Angels or devils? *Neurochem. Int.* **2021**, *148*, 105080. [CrossRef] [PubMed]
164. Wu, M.; Wang, L.; Li, F.; Hu, R.; Ma, J.; Zhang, K.; Cheng, X. Resveratrol Downregulates STAT3 Expression and Astrocyte Activation in Primary Astrocyte Cultures of Rat. *Neurochem. Res.* **2020**, *45*, 455–464. [CrossRef] [PubMed]
165. Ghaiad, H.R.; Nooh, M.M.; El-Sawalhi, M.M.; Shaheen, A.A. Resveratrol Promotes Remyelination in Cuprizone Model of Multiple Sclerosis: Biochemical and Histological Study. *Mol. Neurobiol.* **2017**, *54*, 3219–3229. [CrossRef] [PubMed]
166. Spaas, J.; van Veggel, L.; Schepers, M.; Tiane, A.; van Horssen, J.; Wilson, D.M., 3rd; Moya, P.R.; Piccart, E.; Hellings, N.; Eijnde, B.O.; et al. Oxidative stress and impaired oligodendrocyte precursor cell differentiation in neurological disorders. *Cell. Mol. Life Sci.* **2021**, *78*, 4615–4637. [CrossRef] [PubMed]
167. Samy, D.M.; Zaki, E.I.; Hassaan, P.S.; Abdelmonsif, D.A.; Mohamed, D.Y.; Saleh, S.R. Neurobehavioral, biochemical and histological assessment of the effects of resveratrol on cuprizone-induced demyelination in mice: Role of autophagy modulation. *J. Physiol. Biochem.* **2023**, *79*, 583–596. [CrossRef] [PubMed]
168. Stettner, M.; Wolffram, K.; Mausberg, A.K.; Albrecht, P.; Derksen, A.; Methner, A.; Dehmel, T.; Hartung, H.P.; Dietrich, H.; Kieseier, B.C. Promoting myelination in an in vitro mouse model of the peripheral nervous system: The effect of wine ingredients. *PLoS ONE* **2013**, *8*, e66079. [CrossRef]
169. Zhang, J.; Ren, J.; Liu, Y.; Huang, D.; Lu, L. Resveratrol regulates the recovery of rat sciatic nerve crush injury by promoting the autophagy of Schwann cells. *Life Sci.* **2020**, *256*, 117959. [CrossRef]
170. Yuan, Y.; Wang, Y.; Wu, S.; Zhao, M.Y. Review: Myelin clearance is critical for regeneration after peripheral nerve injury. *Front. Neurol.* **2022**, *13*, 908148. [CrossRef]
171. Rosa, P.M.; Martins, L.A.M.; Souza, D.O.; Quincozes-Santos, A. Glioprotective Effect of Resveratrol: An Emerging Therapeutic Role for Oligodendroglial Cells. *Mol. Neurobiol.* **2018**, *55*, 2967–2978. [CrossRef]
172. Yu, P.; Wang, L.; Tang, F.; Guo, S.; Liao, H.; Fan, C.; Yang, Q. Resveratrol-mediated neurorestoration after cerebral ischemic injury—Sonic Hedgehog signaling pathway. *Life Sci.* **2021**, *280*, 119715. [CrossRef]
173. Fonseca-Kelly, Z.; Nassrallah, M.; Uribe, J.; Khan, R.S.; Dine, K.; Dutt, M.; Shindler, K.S. Resveratrol neuroprotection in a chronic mouse model of multiple sclerosis. *Front. Neurol.* **2012**, *3*, 84. [CrossRef] [PubMed]
174. Hu, J.; Han, H.; Cao, P.; Yu, W.; Yang, C.; Gao, Y.; Yuan, W. Resveratrol improves neuron protection and functional recovery through enhancement of autophagy after spinal cord injury in mice. *Am. J. Transl. Res.* **2017**, *9*, 4607–4616. [PubMed]
175. Jablonska, B.; Gierdalski, M.; Chew, L.J.; Hawley, T.; Catron, M.; Lichauco, A.; Cabrera-Luque, J.; Yuen, T.; Rowitch, D.; Gallo, V. Sirt1 regulates glial progenitor proliferation and regeneration in white matter after neonatal brain injury. *Nat. Commun.* **2016**, *7*, 13866. [CrossRef] [PubMed]
176. Rafalski, V.A.; Ho, P.P.; Brett, J.O.; Ucar, D.; Dugas, J.C.; Pollina, E.A.; Chow, L.M.; Ibrahim, A.; Baker, S.J.; Barres, B.A.; et al. Expansion of oligodendrocyte progenitor cells following SIRT1 inactivation in the adult brain. *Nat. Cell Biol.* **2013**, *15*, 614–624. [CrossRef] [PubMed]
177. Prozorovski, T.; Ingwersen, J.; Lukas, D.; Göttle, P.; Koop, B.; Graf, J.; Schneider, R.; Franke, K.; Schumacher, S.; Britsch, S.; et al. Regulation of sirtuin expression in autoimmune neuroinflammation: Induction of SIRT1 in oligodendrocyte progenitor cells. *Neurosci. Lett.* **2019**, *704*, 116–125. [CrossRef] [PubMed]
178. A Phase I Double Blind Study of Metformin Acting on Endogenous Neural Progenitor Cells in Children with Multiple Sclerosis. Available online: https://clinicaltrials.gov/study/NCT04121468 (accessed on 8 November 2023).
179. Metformin Treatment in Progressive Multiple Sclerosis. Available online: https://www.clinicaltrials.gov/study/NCT05349474 (accessed on 8 November 2023).
180. Nicotinamide Riboside Supplementation in Progressive Multiple Sclerosis. Available online: https://clinicaltrials.gov/study/NCT05740722 (accessed on 8 November 2023).

181. La Rosa, G.; Lonardo, M.S.; Cacciapuoti, N.; Muscariello, E.; Guida, B.; Faraonio, R.; Santillo, M.; Damiano, S. Dietary Polyphenols, Microbiome, and Multiple Sclerosis: From Molecular Anti-Inflammatory and Neuroprotective Mechanisms to Clinical Evidence. *Int. J. Mol. Sci.* **2023**, *24*, 7247. [CrossRef]
182. Shamsher, E.; Khan, R.S.; Davis, B.M.; Dine, K.; Luong, V.; Somavarapu, S.; Cordeiro, M.F.; Shindler, K.S. Nanoparticles Enhance Solubility and Neuroprotective Effects of Resveratrol in Demyelinating Disease. *Neurotherapeutics* **2023**, *20*, 1138–1153. [CrossRef]
183. Ruckh, J.M.; Zhao, J.W.; Shadrach, J.L.; van Wijngaarden, P.; Rao, T.N.; Wagers, A.J.; Franklin, R.J. Rejuvenation of regeneration in the aging central nervous system. *Cell Stem Cell* **2012**, *10*, 96–103. [CrossRef]
184. Shen, S.; Sandoval, J.; Swiss, V.A.; Li, J.; Dupree, J.; Franklin, R.J.; Casaccia-Bonnefil, P. Age-dependent epigenetic control of differentiation inhibitors is critical for remyelination efficiency. *Nat. Neurosci.* **2008**, *11*, 1024–1034. [CrossRef]
185. Tutuncu, M.; Tang, J.; Zeid, N.A.; Kale, N.; Crusan, D.J.; Atkinson, E.J.; Siva, A.; Pittock, S.J.; Pirko, I.; Keegan, B.M.; et al. Onset of progressive phase is an age-dependent clinical milestone in multiple sclerosis. *Mult. Scler.* **2013**, *19*, 188–198. [CrossRef]
186. Goldschmidt, T.; Antel, J.; König, F.B.; Brück, W.; Kuhlmann, T. Remyelination capacity of the MS brain decreases with disease chronicity. *Neurology* **2009**, *72*, 1914–1921. [CrossRef] [PubMed]
187. Strijbis, E.M.M.; Kooi, E.J.; van der Valk, P.; Geurts, J.J.G. Cortical Remyelination Is Heterogeneous in Multiple Sclerosis. *J. Neuropathol. Exp. Neurol.* **2017**, *76*, 390–401. [CrossRef] [PubMed]
188. Boyd, A.; Zhang, H.; Williams, A. Insufficient OPC migration into demyelinated lesions is a cause of poor remyelination in MS and mouse models. *Acta Neuropathol.* **2013**, *125*, 841–859. [CrossRef] [PubMed]
189. Kuhlmann, T.; Miron, V.; Cui, Q.; Wegner, C.; Antel, J.; Brück, W. Differentiation block of oligodendroglial progenitor cells as a cause for remyelination failure in chronic multiple sclerosis. *Brain A J. Neurol.* **2008**, *131*, 1749–1758. [CrossRef]

current issues in molecular biology

MDPI

Article

Testosterone Inhibits Secretion of the Pro-Inflammatory Chemokine CXCL1 from Astrocytes

Malgorzata Turniak-Kusy [1], Maciej Studzian [2,3], Piotr Szpakowski [1], Piotr Kuchta [4], Kaja Smietanka [1], Claudia Mattern [5,6], Lukasz Pulaski [2,3] and Bartosz Bielecki [7,*]

1 Department of Neurology and Stroke, Medical University of Lodz, 90-549 Lodz, Poland
2 Department of Oncobiology and Epigenetics, Faculty of Biology and Environmental Protection, University of Lodz, 90-237 Lodz, Poland
3 Laboratory of Transcriptional Regulation, Institute of Medical Biology, Polish Academy of Sciences, 90-364 Lodz, Poland
4 Faculty of Medicine, Medical University of Lodz, 90-419 Lodz, Poland
5 Oceanographic Center, Nova Southeastern University, Fort Lauderdale, FL 33314, USA
6 M&P Pharma AG, 6376 Emmetten, Switzerland
7 Department of Neurology, Laboratory of Neuroimmunology, Medical University of Lodz, 90-153 Lodz, Poland
* Correspondence: bartosz.bielecki@umed.lodz.pl

Abstract: Astrocytes play an important role in the regulation of the inflammatory response in the CNS, e.g., in demyelinating diseases. Since the chemokine CXCL1 is known to be secreted by astrocytes and to have a pro-inflammatory effect on immune cells in the CNS, we verified the effect of testosterone on its secretion in vitro (in the astrocytic cell line DI TNC1). Testosterone reduced the increase in CXCL1 production caused by the pro-inflammatory agent lysophosphatidylcholine and restored the basal production level of CXCL1. The androgen receptor (present and functional in the studied cell line) was strongly suggested to mediate this effect—its non-steroid ligand flutamide exerted an agonist-like effect, mimicking the activity of testosterone itself on CXCL1 secretion. This novel mechanism has important implications for the known immunomodulatory effect of testosterone and potentially other androgenic hormones. It provides a potential explanation on the molecular level and shows that astrocytes are important players in inflammatory homeostasis in the CNS and its hormonal regulation. Therefore, it suggests new directions for the development of the therapeutic intervention.

Keywords: astrocyte; inflammation; chemokine; CXCL1; testosterone; androgen; demyelination; LPC; neuroprotection; remyelination

1. Introduction

The inflammatory response in the central nervous system (CNS) is also known as neuroinflammation. This complex process is mediated by various cytokines and chemokines acting through specific receptors. Among the CNS resident cells, microglia and astrocytes are the most important sources of cytokines and chemokines. Astrocytes are considered a key element of neuroinflammation control by outside factors, including endocrine hormones. Following activation, astrocytes can become a potent source of proinflammatory cytokines such as TNFα, IL-12, IL-6, and IL-27, which are characteristic of the Th1 response. Upon a change of inflammatory milieu, astrocytes can also secrete the immunomodulatory cytokines IL-10 and IL-19, which are associated with the Th2 response [1–6]. Moreover, astrocytes secrete a repertoire of chemokines with different properties. Among them, CXCL1 is the most salient one, but others like CCL2, CCL3, and CXCL10 can also attract hematogenous cells such as T cells and macrophages, which may further enhance neuroinflammation. On the other hand, CXCL1, as well as CXCL2 and CXCL12, can promote repair by recruiting CNS resident cells such as oligodendrocyte progenitor cells (OPCs) [1,7–9].

We still do not understand well enough the mechanisms responsible for switching astrocyte function so that it promotes either damage to the CNS from excessive inflammation or its protection by anti-inflammatory mediator secretion. Deregulation of this response is strongly linked with the etiology of some demyelinating diseases of the CNS, including multiple sclerosis (MS) [1,10–12].

The chemokine (C-X-C motif) ligand 1 (CXCL1) is a small cytokine from the CXC chemokine family. CXCL1 is also known as melanoma growth-stimulating activity alpha (MGSA-α) and GRO-α in humans and as KC in mice [13]. Expression of CXCL1 has been observed in macrophages, neutrophils, epithelial cells, and glial cells [14–16]. Its effects are mediated through the chemokine receptor CXCR2 [16,17] and require binding to glycosaminoglycans (GAG) on endothelial and epithelial cells and the extracellular matrix [18]. High levels of CXCL1 are also able to stimulate the receptor CXCR1 [17].

When signaling through CXCR2, it bolsters the recruitment of neutrophils to the CNS. In other tissues, it is often a physiological response to microbial infection or tissue injury, but in the CNS, it is often pathological, e.g., in demyelinating diseases [19]. A recent report suggests that CXCL1 signaling is involved in microglia activation following brain injury [20]. While the role CXCL1 plays in OPC proliferation, migration, and differentiation into myelinating oligodendrocytes is multi-faceted [21–24], recent studies have identified mostly its negative effects, e.g., inhibition of the CXCL1/CXCR2 pathway, which promotes the differentiation of OPCs and consequently promotes myelin repair [25]. Astrocytes have also been reported to express CXCR2 receptors [26]. Since they are also a source of their ligand CXCL1, it suggests the possibility of an autocrine feedback loop regulating inflammation and remyelination.

Sex steroids influence not only the development and maintenance of reproductive systems but also several other organ systems, including the central nervous system (CNS) [27–29]. Among many functions, similarly to other steroid hormones, sex steroids (androgens, estrogens, and progestagens) exert several neuroprotective effects [30–32]. Within the context of immune response, particularly androgens and estrogens show effects on inflammatory cells and are potent modulators of immune responses within the CNS. It has become evident over last few decades that both the prevalence and severity of neuroinflammatory diseases of the brain and spinal cord are linked to sex hormones [33–36]. Epidemiological data from many studies show the higher prevalence of particularly demyelinating diseases of the CNS with neuroinflammation, such as MS, in women [37–39]. However, men with MS accumulate symptoms leading to a permanent neurological disability faster than female patients [40]. Moreover, men with testicular hypofunction are more likely to develop MS [41]. Testosterone is the major androgen with an important role in the physiology of both sexes. Testicles are the main source of testosterone in males; ovaries, adrenal glands, and adipocytes are the main source of this hormone in women. Testosterone and its metabolite dihydrotestosterone (DHT or 5αDHT) exert their principal function through a specific nuclear receptors—the androgen receptor (AR). Experimental data from animal models of MS further support androgens, particularly testosterone, as key players in alleviating inflammation-related pathological states in the CNS [42]. Experimental autoimmune encephalomyelitis (EAE) induced by the transfer of T cells shows a milder course when they are pre-treated with testosterone [43]. At the same time, testosterone has been shown to induce the production of anti-inflammatory IL-10 by T cells [44]. There is a large body of evidence pointing to resident and infiltrating immune cells as direct targets of androgen action in the CNS. However, despite the still-insufficient number of studies, the overall picture inexorably expands to include testosterone acting directly on astrocytes as well [45–47]. A key element of this mechanism is the recently confirmed expression of androgen receptors in astrocytes [48,49], but the functionality of this expression was hitherto in doubt.

In the present work, we present for the first time a direct mechanistic study of the axis androgen-astrocyte-chemokine in the context of inflammation. We tested the influence of primary androgen testosterone on CXCL1 expression and secretion, which turned out to depend strictly on the proinflammatory milieu. The use of the highly specific androgen receptor ligand flutamide, which is commonly applied as an antagonist of this nuclear receptor but has been previously shown to be able to have an agonist-like effect as well (which was also the case in our study), implicated this transcription factor in the observed phenomenon. Thus, we provide new insights on the molecular mechanism of this effect, which we found to most probably depend on the genomic action of the androgen receptor.

2. Materials and Methods

2.1. Cell Culture

Type 1 astrocyte cell line DI TNC1 was purchased from ATCC (cat. no. CRL-2005). The cells were cultured at 37 °C in a 5% CO_2 humidified atmosphere in high glucose Dulbecco's modified Eagle's medium (Mediatech, Inc., Corning subsidiary, Manassas, VA 20109, USA, cat. no. 10-013-CV) supplemented with 10% (v/v) heat-inactivated fetal bovine serum (FBS) (Mediatech, Inc., Corning subsidiary, Woodland, CA 95776, USA, cat. no. 35-016-CV), 100 units/mL penicillin, and 100 µg/mL streptomycin (Mediatech, Inc., Corning subsidiary, Manassas, VA 20109, USA, cat. no. 30-002-CI).

2.2. Viability Assay

To verify the cytotoxic effect of lysophosphatidylcholine (LPC) treatment, the integrity of the cell plasma membrane was verified by staining cells with propidium iodide (cell impermeable) and Hoechst 33342 (cell permeable). Cells were seeded into a 96-well plate at a density of 1.0×10^4 cells per well and treated with increasing concentrations of LPC (0−200 µg/mL) for 24 h. Following the incubation, cells were treated with 5 µM Hoecht33342 and 20 µM propidium iodide for 15 min at 37 °C. Subsequently, cells were washed once with phosphate-buffered saline (PBS, pH = 7.4) and fixed with 4% formaldehyde in PBS prepared freshly from paraformaldehyde. Cell viability was assessed with an automated fluorescence microscope, ArrayScan® VTI (Thermo Fisher Scientific, Waltham, MA, USA), by comparing the number of cell nuclei stained with membrane-impermeable (propidium iodide) and permeable (Hoechst 33342) dye.

2.3. Gene Expression Assay

The gene expression level was determined by quantitative real-time RT-PCR. The aliquots of 2.6×10^5 DI TNC1 cells were cultured for 24 h in 24-well plates in the presence or absence of 150 µg/mL LPC or with various concentrations of testosterone added from a stock solution prepared in ethanol. All cells, including control ones, were treated with the same amount of ethanol (0.2%). Following incubation, cells were washed once with PBS, pH = 7.4, and total cellular RNA was isolated using the InviTrap® Spin Cell RNA Mini Kit (Stratec, Birkenfeld, Germany) according to the manufacturer's protocol. Complementary DNA (cDNA) was transcribed from mRNA using the Maxima First Strand cDNA Synthesis Kit (Thermo Fisher Scientific, Waltham, MA, USA) and used for real-time PCR amplification with GoTaq® qPCR 2x master mix (Promega Corporation, Madison, WI, USA) according to the manufacturer's protocol. Each 16 µL reaction volume contained ca. 3 ng of cDNA and 0.25 µM of forward and reverse primers (for primer sequences, see Table 1). *Ywhaz*, *Ubc*, and *B2m* were used as reference genes. PCR reactions were performed in 96-well microplates using the CFX96 Real-Time PCR Detection System (Bio-Rad Laboratories, Hercules, CA, USA). The expression level of assayed genes was calculated using the ΔΔCt method and expressed as the number of mRNA copies per respective number of copies of geometric-averaged mRNA for reference genes.

Table 1. Sequences of primers used in this study.

Gene	Forward and Reverse Sequences (5′-3′)	Source
Ywhaz	Fw: AACTTGACATTGTGGACATCGG Rv: AAAGGTTGGAAGGCCGGTTA	this study
Ubc	Fw: ACACCAAGAAGGTCAAACAGGA Rv: CACCTCCCCATCAAACCCAA	[50]
B2m	Fw: GTCACCTGGGACCGAGACAT Rv: AGAAGATGGTGTGCTCATTGC	[51]
Ar	Fw: CTTATGGGGACATGCGTTTGG Rv: GCTCCGTAGTGACAACCAGA	this study
Fdps	Fw: GCAGACTCTCGACCTCATCACA Rv: CCCATCAATTCCAGCCATG	[52]
Camkk2	Fw: AGAACTGCACACTGGTCGAG Rv: CCGGCTACCTTCAAATGGGT	[53]
Cxcl1	Fw: GCCACACTCAAGAATGGTCG Rv: TGGGGACACCCTTTAGCATC	[54]
Tnfa	Fw: GACCCTCACACTCAGATCATCTTCT Rv: TGCTACGACGTGGGCTACG	[55]

2.4. Quantification of CXCL1 Secreted to the Medium by Astrocytes

At 72 h prior to medium collection, cells were seeded in 24-well plates at a concentration of 1.5×10^5 cells per well. Cells were treated for 24 h with 150 µg/mL LPC and/or various concentrations of testosterone and/or flutamide prepared in fresh medium. Control cells were incubated with an equal concentration of ethanol (0.2%) that was used as a solvent for the respective treatments. At the time of medium collection, cells reached ca. 90% confluence and were counted to calculate the amount of CXCL1 secreted relative to 1.0×10^5 of cells. Measurements were made with an enzyme-linked immunosorbent assay (ELISA) according to the manufacturer's protocol (Rat CXCL1/CINC-1 DuoSet ELISA—R&D, cat. no. DY515). Cell-free medium was bound for 24 h to 96-well plates pre-coated with the capture antibody. After 2 h of incubation, the unbound material was washed off and a detection antibody was added for another 2 h incubation. Finally, the amount of bound antibody was detected colorimetrically, and the amount of CXCL1 was calculated from the calibration curve prepared for the recombinant protein included in the kit.

2.5. Statistical Analysis

The N values reported in the study refer to independent biological replicates. The Shapiro-Wilk test was used to evaluate whether the data follow a gaussian distribution. The effects of testosterone and flutamide on CXCL1 production by astrocytes were evaluated using three three-way ANOVA and, subsequently, Tukey's post-hoc test to demonstrate the significance of differences between individual values. The evaluation of the effects of different doses of testosterone and flutamide was performed using the U Mann-Whitney test. Results of gene expression assays at the mRNA level were analyzed by the one-way ANOVA and, subsequently, Tukey's post-hoc test to demonstrate the significance of differences between individual values and the control.

3. Results

3.1. Lysophosphatidylcholine Is Not Toxic to DI TNC1 Astrocytes but Exerts a Pro-Inflammatory Effect at the Signaling Level

Since incubation with the known in vivo inflammation stimulant lysophosphatidycholine (LPC) can change the composition of cell plasma membrane, leading to cytotoxicity, we verified the cytotoxic effect of LPC on DI TNC1 astrocytes. Cells were incubated with increasing concentrations of LPC, namely 0, 50, 100, 150, and 200 µg/mL, and the integrity of their cellular membrane was assessed after 24 h by comparing the amounts of cell nuclei stained with cell membrane permeable (Hoechst 33342) and impermeable (propidium iodide) dye. At all LPC concentrations, cell membrane integrity was preserved, since the number of cell nuclei stained by propidium iodide was less than 1% of those stained with Hoechst 33342.

Next, we tested if 24-h treatment with 150 μg/mL LPC has a pro-inflammatory effect on DI TNC1 astrocytes. At the mRNA level, the expression of the *Tnfa* gene increased by 360% (Figure 1A). At the same time, LPC treatment induced the expression of the *Cxcl1* gene by 13%, providing a mechanistic explanation for the increased secretion of this chemokine by cells incubated with LPC (Figure 1B).

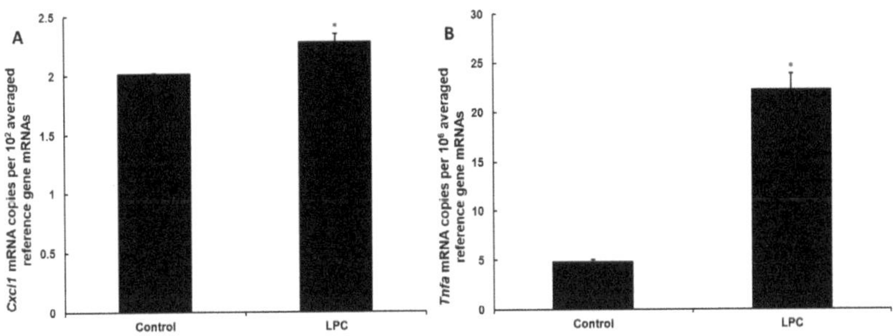

Figure 1. Incubation with LPC induces expression of proinflammatory genes in rat astrocytes. DI TNC1 cells were incubated for 24 h without (control) or in the presence of LPC (150 μg/mL). Subsequently, the expression of *Cxcl1* (**A**) and *Tnfa* (**B**) genes was quantified at mRNA level by real-time PCR, and expression level was expressed relative to a validated set of reference (housekeeping) genes. Significance of overall differences was tested by one-way ANOVA ($p < 0.05$). Significance of differences between treated samples and control was tested by Tukey's post-hoc test (* $p < 0.05$).

3.2. DI TNC1 Astrocytes Produce an Increased Amount of CXCL1 When Treated with Lysophosphatidylcholine

We have quantified the amount of CXCL1 that type I rat astrocytes (DI TNC1 cells) secreted into culture medium when incubated for 24 h with LPC (150 μg/mL) or in control conditions (cells treated with ethanol in equal volume used as a solvent for LPC). The level of CXCL1 in the culture medium was significantly increased in the group treated with LPC (Figure 2). The average concentration of CXCL1 in the culture medium was equal to 0.94 ± 0.03 ng/mL per 100,000 DI NTC1 cells. When stimulated with LPC, astrocytes produced 1.27 ± 0.03 ng/mL of CXCL1 per 100,000 DI NTC1 cells.

3.3. Testosterone Affects the Production of CXCL1 but Only in Cells Stimulated with Lysophosphatidylcholine

Considering that incubation with LPC exerted a pro-inflammatory effect on DI TNC1 astrocytes and stimulated them to produce increased amounts of CXCL1, we were interested in verifying how testosterone affects this phenomenon. The amounts of CXCL1 secreted into culture medium by DI TNC1 astrocytes were quantified after 24 h of incubation with and without LPC and in the presence and absence of 60 μM testosterone (Figure 2). Testosterone antagonized the induction of CXCL1 stimulated by LPC treatment while having no effect on the basal level of secretion of this chemokine. Cells stimulated with LPC in the presence of testosterone and cells treated only with testosterone secreted CXCL1 in the same quantity as non-stimulated, control cells. Subsequently, we have set out to explore if this effect is dose-dependent. We have stimulated DI TNC1 astrocytes for 24 h with 150 μg/mL LPC in the presence of increasing concentrations of testosterone (0–80 μM). The concentration of secreted CXCL1 decreased gradually with an increasing dose of testosterone, reaching values similar to those secreted by the cells unstimulated with LPC (Figure 3). This observation confirms that testosterone mitigates the excess secretion of CXCL1 by binding to specific effectors (receptor-like effect), whose effectiveness is dependent on its concentration.

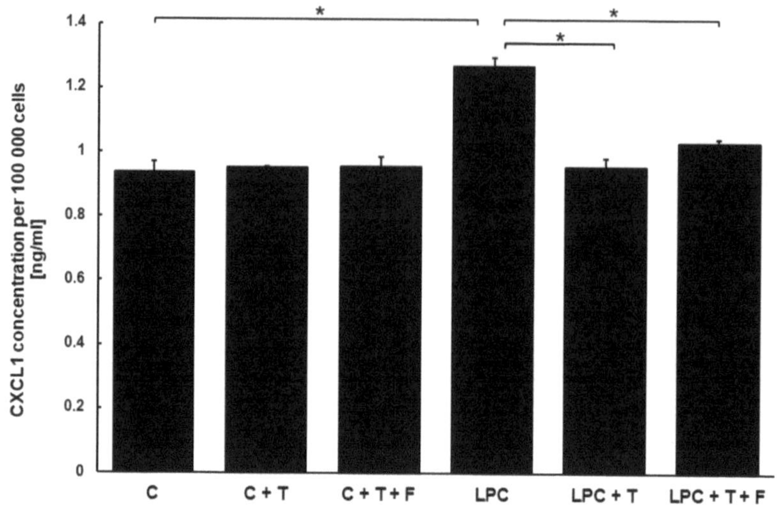

Figure 2. Quantification of CXCL1 secreted to culture medium by rat astrocytes. DI TNC1 cells were incubated for 24 h without (control, C), in the presence of LPC (150 µg/mL), in the presence of 60 µM testosterone (T), or in the presence of 60 µM testosterone and 60 µM flutamide (T + F). Subsequently, the amount of CXCL1 secreted by the cells was quantified in culture media by ELISA and it is presented as a value ± SEM per 100,000 cells. Significance of overall differences was tested by one-way ANOVA ($p < 0.05$). Significance of differences between treated samples and the control was tested by Tukey's post-hoc test (* $p < 0.001$), N = 4.

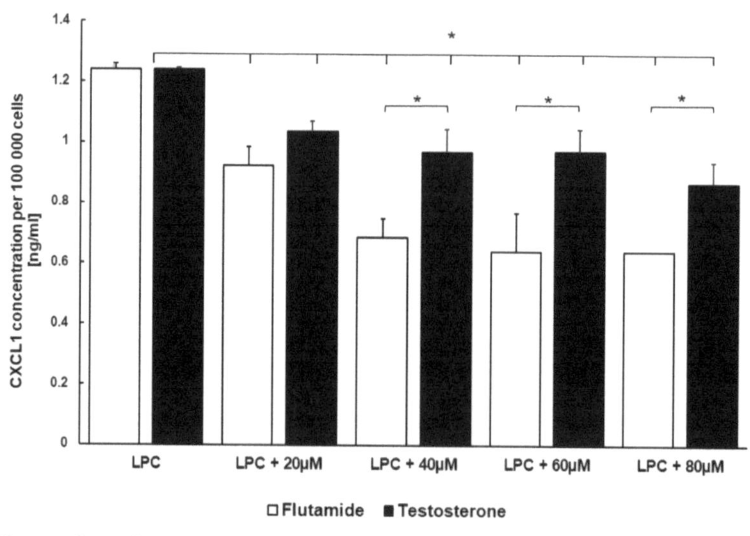

Figure 3. Quantification of CXCL1 secreted to culture medium by rat astrocytes in the presence of testosterone or flutamide. DI TNC1 cells were incubated for 24 h in the presence of LPC (150 µg/mL) and in the presence of increasing concentrations of either testosterone or flutamide. Subsequently, the amount of CXCL1 secreted by the cells was quantified in culture media by ELISA, and it is presented as a value ± SEM per 100,000 cells. * $p < 0.05$, N = 4.

3.4. DI TNC1 Cells Express Functional Androgen Receptor

Subsequently, we have verified whether DI TNC1 cells are expressing functional androgen receptor (AR), which could be the target of action of testosterone in the studied phenomenon. First, we quantified the expression of the *Ar* gene in this cell line at the mRNA level by performing quantitative real-time PCR. We measured that the androgen receptor is expressed in DI TNC1 cells, and its expression was not affected by incubation with testosterone (data shown in Supplementary Materials—Tables S1–S4, Figure S1).

To assess if the effect of testosterone is mediated through the androgen receptor, we measured the expression of known AR-dependent marker genes: *Fdps* and *Camkk2* [52] upon stimulation with testosterone (Figure 4). Both 20 μM and 60 μM concentrations of testosterone enhanced the expression of the *Fdps* gene (by 21% and 27%, respectively) and the *Camkk2* gene (by around 10% at both concentrations), showing that the androgen receptor is stimulated by testosterone in DI TNC1 cells and implying that the effects of testosterone on CXCL1 secretion may be mediated through AR.

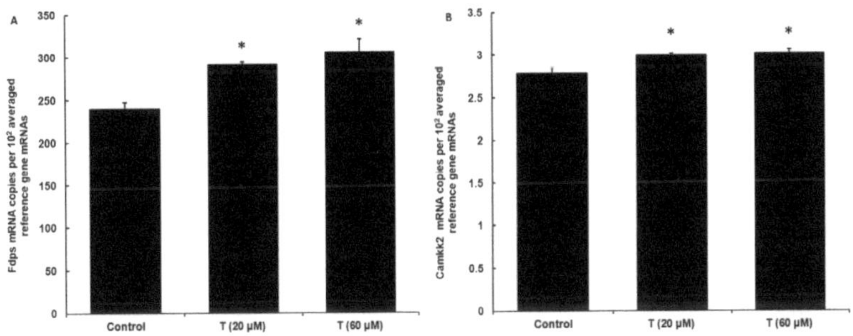

Figure 4. Incubation with testosterone induces expression of marker genes of androgen receptor in rat astrocytes. DI TNC1 cells were incubated for 24 h without (control) or in the presence of 20 μM or 60 μM testosterone. Subsequently, the expression of *Fdps* (**A**) and *Camkk2* (**B**) genes was quantified at mRNA level by real-time PCR, and expression level was expressed relative to a validated set of reference (housekeeping) genes. Significance of overall differences was tested by one-way ANOVA ($p < 0.05$). Significance of differences between treated samples, and control was tested by Tukey's post-hoc test (* $p < 0.05$).

3.5. Flutamide Similarly to Testosterone Reduces the Pro-Inflammatory Stimulus of LPC on CXCL1 Secretion

To determine if the effect of testosterone on the secretion of CXCL1 is mediated by the androgen receptor, we incubated DI TNC1 cells for 24 h with testosterone and flutamide, which is usually used as an antagonist of testosterone's effect on AR, in equal concentrations (60 μM). We tested its effects in the presence and absence of pro-inflammatory milieu (150 μg/mL of LPC). Cells unstimulated with LPC and incubated with both compounds secreted similar basal levels of CXCL1 (0.95 ± 0.03 ng/mL per 100,000 cells). Surprisingly, we observed that flutamide co-incubated with testosterone in the presence of LPC does not show antagonistic properties (Figure 2). Similar to cells treated with testosterone alone, the cells incubated with LPC in the presence of testosterone and flutamide produced almost the same amount of CXCL1 (1.03 ± 0.01 ng/mL per 100,000 cells).

To further corroborate this result, we investigated how different concentrations of flutamide (0–80 μM) affected the astrocytes in the presence of LPC (Figure 3). We observed the dose-dependent reduction of CXCL1 secretion by flutamide, but this effect was even more pronounced than the one observed with the same concentrations of testosterone, confirming that flutamide in this case probably exerts an agonistic effect on androgen receptors like testosterone, but even stronger.

4. Discussion

Inflammatory processes in the central and peripheral nervous systems, which accompany a variety of pathological states, are extremely complex phenomena that contribute to the etiology of clinically important neurological syndromes such as demyelinating and neurodegenerative diseases. To elucidate their mechanism, it is crucial to study the interplay and cross-communication between cells of the immune system and resident elements of the neural tissue, as both of these cell groups contribute to the distinctive elements of the inflammatory state. Chemokines play a pivotal role as messenger molecules. They can be secreted by non-specialized cells in order to signal specific immune cell populations to induce (or, in some situations, inhibit) their migration. They also have other properties, including activation, stimulation of the production of cytokines and other mediators, and specialized immune-related functions. There is a significant knowledge gap with regard to the involvement of individual cell types in producing the chemokine repertoire observed in neuroinflammation, for example concerning CXCL1, one of the most important chemokines with somewhat contradictory effects in the regulation of pathological inflammation. Research in this direction is needed, as this may be a potential therapeutic approach utilizing natural inhibitory mechanisms to counteract unwanted inflammation, which has deleterious consequences.

There is overwhelming evidence from animal models of neuroinflammation that CXCL1 production and secretion in the neural tissue are strictly regulated. It significantly impacts both the cellular and systemic presentation of pathological symptoms. Specifically, in some mouse models, the overexpression of CXCL1 under the glial fibrillary acidic protein (GFAP) promoter in astrocytes leads to a reduction in lesion load and enhances repair mechanisms in relapsing and remitting encephalomyelitis models [56]. Moreover, the chemokine receptor CXCR2 and its ligands CXCL1 and CXCL2 were shown to be upregulated during viral-induced demyelination, where CXCR2 signaling in oligodendrocytes seemed to play a role in their protection and the restriction of the demyelination process [57]. On the other hand, it has been shown that the rise in the expression of CXCL1 in astrocytes is associated with an increased severity of experimental autoimmune encephalomyelitis (EAE) due to the increased recruitment of neutrophils [58]. CXCL1 was reported to be upregulated during the acute phase of EAE, both in the brain and the spinal cord [8]. It has also been reported that CXCL1 was upregulated in mouse dorsal root ganglion (DRG) neurons during the asymptomatic phase of neuroinflammation. Neutrophils accumulated in the DRG produce neutrophil elastase, which is able to sensitize DRG neurons, leading to the induction of mechanical allodynia; therefore, gene silencing of CXCL1 attenuated neutrophil accumulation in the DRG and consequent mechanical allodynia [59]. Inhibition of CXCL1 signaling through CXCR2 by the use of anti-CXCR2 antibodies or pharmacological antagonists had beneficial effects for in vivo models of demyelination and encephalomyelitis, such as reduced size of lesions, increased OPC differentiation, functional improvement, enhanced myelination, and reduced lesion load. This was attributed to reduced infiltration and activation of macrophage/microglial cells under CXCR2 inhibition [60].

There are numerous natural mechanisms counteracting neuroinflammation at the level of cellular communication. Their potential therapeutic utilization is a hot topic in clinical studies, especially for demyelinating diseases. Among these, hormonal effects are very promising, including an emerging body of data on the favorable action of androgens in several in vivo models, which tie in, e.g., with epidemiological data on the penetration of demyelinating diseases in different sexes [38,61–65]. In the presence of testosterone, areas of LPC-induced focal demyelination in the spinal cord were repopulated with astrocytes to a much larger extent than in the absence of the hormone. The androgen-activated astrocytes promoted axonal remyelination through oligodendrocytes, whereas in control (untreated) lesions, Schwann cells were the main myelin-producing cell type [66]. This, along with other accumulated evidence for the anti-inflammatory action of testosterone in the CNS, is convincing at the physiological level in animal models; however, the specific molecular mechanisms at the cellular level and participating immune mediators need to be elucidated in direct biochemical experiments on isolated in vitro models, which is a prerequisite to understanding the feasibility of proposed modes of action. Therefore, the experiments presented in this paper fulfill an important role in providing basic data on how androgens can potentially counteract neuroinflammation. Our research demonstrates that they can directly (most probably via their nuclear receptor AR) suppress the stimulation of CXCL1 production in astrocytes by pro-inflammatory agents. Since CXCL1 is strongly implicated in enhancing the detrimental pro-inflammatory feedback loop by recruiting and activating neutrophils and/or macrophages, this suppression is one of the possible mechanisms explaining the moderating influence of testosterone on clinical manifestations of neuroinflammation.

While LPC is widely used in vivo as a demyelinating agent, it is also known to act as a bona fide proinflammatory mediator produced in the neural tissue itself [67,68]. It has been shown that LPC increases the production of pro-inflammatory cytokines and chemokines by immune cells [69,70]. In addition, LPC can also induce glial cell activation via the Rho-kinase pathway [71]. Enhanced expression of MCP-1 and CCR2 has been observed in activated microglia in response to LPC produced in astrocytes and neurons [72]. It has been observed that astrocytes and immature oligodendrocytes are sensitive to LPC-induced injury in vivo [68,73].

Our experimental model was composed of physiologically relevant elements, which enhanced the credibility of the proposed mechanism. Treatment with LPC mimics natural pro-inflammatory steps observed in demyelinating disease development pathways. We were able to further confirm this in our experiments showing the ability of LPC to induce the expression of another pro-inflammatory mediator, TNF-alpha. The DI TNC1 astrocyte cell line was derived from the same species and strain (Sprague-Dawley rats) and has been used in studies on experimental inflammatory demyelination, including those that identified astrocytes as potential mediators of androgen action. Our experimental approach involves measuring not only CXCL1 expression but, more importantly, its secretion to the outside environment, a central feature of the detrimental role of astrocytes in pro-inflammatory cell recruitment. Thus, the mechanism of action of the androgen-astrocyte-chemokine regulatory axis that emerges from our study can be directly applicable to in vivo models of neuroinflammation.

Taken together, our data points to a coherent mechanistic explanation of this regulatory phenomenon: Under the conditions of pro-inflammatory signaling (and only under these conditions), testosterone acts on the androgen receptor in astrocytes, preventing the signal-induced increase of CXCL1 secretion. In human monocytes exposed to parasitic (amoebal) antigens, CXCL1 secretion increased after androgen pre-treatment, which also points to the potential for androgen receptor-mediated modulation of the expression of this gene [74]. It is important to note that astrocytes produce and secrete a significant amount of CXCL1 in the resting state as well, and the molecular mechanisms responsible for this baseline level are not affected by testosterone. Identification of the exact elements (transcription factors) involved in CXCL1 expression in physiological and pathological conditions will require more profound exploration by molecular genetic techniques and is beyond the scope of the present study. However, the role of AR in the action of testosterone on astrocytes is strongly suggested by our experimental approach: we demonstrate that it is functionally expressed in the investigated cells (by showing the induction of known marker genes by testosterone [75]); testosterone acts in a dose-dependent (rather than threshold) manner on CXCL1 expression; and finally, and most convincingly, flutamide (which was applied as a presumptive antagonist of testosterone action) fortuitously turned out to have an analogous effect to testosterone in repressing CXCL1 induction. The latter argument points convincingly towards AR as the mediator of this effect, since there is a body of literature that identifies flutamide (or its metabolite, hydroxyflutamide) as a possible agonist of AR in several cell types [76–78]. This similarity between testosterone and flutamide is a powerful argument for the direct involvement of AR because there is no other known effector common to both of these chemically dissimilar ligands. It is, however, important to keep in mind that testosterone itself may indeed have other ways of inhibiting CXCL1 production in astrocytes, and therefore the effect of testosterone is potentially at least partially non-AR-dependent. One possible additional mechanism involves conversion to 17-beta-estradiol by aromatase expressed in these cells [79], with subsequent interference with the function of transcription factor AP-1, with which it is able to interact [80], and which is involved in CXCL1 induction during inflammatory signaling [81]. Importantly, estrogens have also been reported to increase CXCL-1 expression via estrogen receptor β (ERβ) [82]. Therefore, the conversion of testosterone to estrogen by aromatase could lead to a reduction of the original effect of testosterone, which could explain why flutamide alone demonstrated a stronger effect on CXCL1 level reduction than testosterone. In contrast, it has also been reported that estradiol at high concentrations down-regulates epithelial expression of CXCL1 [83]. In our study, we observed that the inhibitory effect of testosterone on CXCL1 production, while weaker at low doses, increases at the highest applied dose of 80 μM. This may be caused specifically by the shift in the effect of aromatase-produced estrogen at this concentration no longer counteracting the inhibitory effect of testosterone but enhancing it. Confirmation of the actual conversion of testosterone to estrogen occurring in astrocytes would help provide further proof for this postulate. Thus, further investigation of this mechanism is required to fully elucidate the mechanisms underlying the above effect. While we are certain that the AR-mediated pathway is involved in testosterone effects, further experiments are needed to quantify the extent of this involvement, e.g., using other AR antagonists or gene silencing.

The identification of a potential beneficial molecular mechanism of action of androgens in a model of neuroinflammation, with astrocytes as the novel site of action, is an important step in studies on hormonal regulation of CNS pathology. We demonstrate that (as was previously suggested on the basis of phenomenological in vivo data) testosterone and other androgens may indeed work via resident cells of the CNS which are not directly involved in immune activity and that astrocytes, which are already an important target in clinical studies on demyelinating and neurodegenerative diseases, acquire an even broader array of upstream regulators. This is also one of the first demonstrations of functional AR activity in astrocytic cells, while at the same time it adds to the increasing number of studies that encourage caution in the uncritical application of receptor antagonists as investigative and/or therapeutic tools since some of them (in this case flutamide) may also cause the opposite (agonistic) effect on some cell types. In general, the demonstration that pro-inflammatory chemokine secretion is an important function of astrocytes and that it can be modulated pharmacologically adds to our understanding of the complexity of neuroinflammation.

From a practical point of view, it is important to note that weak AR agonists, like testosterone and (hydroxy)flutamide, which may have beneficial effects in diseases that involve neuroinflammation, also have therapeutically favorable pharmacokinetics, being able to reach the CNS through the blood-brain and blood-cerebrospinal fluid barrier. Since CXCL1 has been implicated in many neuroinflammatory disorders and their models, such as EAE, MS, other demyelinating diseases, neurodegeneration, and infection, being able to modulate its secretion at one of its sources may be a common solution to seemingly unrelated pathologies. Of course, we do not suggest that this is the only chemokine that astrocytes use to influence the inflammatory milieu, nor do we suggest that androgens (or even AR itself) exert their documented beneficial physiological effects exclusively via the mechanism that we identified, but the fact that this signaling axis is theoretically possible in vivo is important for the interpretation of physiological phenomena such as sex differences in disease penetration or hormonal effects in MS. From the clinical point of view, another important corollary is the possibility of side effects of hormonal treatments in the CNS. However, the potentially most important therapeutic implication of our results is the indication that astrocytes are a viable target for AR-mediated adjuvant treatment of demyelinating diseases by alleviating the pathologically increased production of at least some pro-inflammatory mediators.

In the future, it will be important to verify whether AR binds directly to the CXCL1 promoter or whether its action is indirect. We also plan to work on identifying the physiologically important cellular targets of astrocyte-derived CXCL1 (resident vs. hematogenous cells) and optimizing the agonistic function of androgens in animal models.

In conclusion, the probable direct involvement of AR in the effects of androgen on the pro-inflammatory activity of astrocytes is a newly identified mechanism of hormonal regulation of neuroinflammation. This mechanism involves the inhibition of CXCL1 release, underlining the central role this chemokine plays in regulatory loops between glial and immune cells in the CNS.

Supplementary Materials: The following supporting information can be downloaded at: https://www.mdpi.com/article/10.3390/cimb46030135/s1. Tables S1–S4: Analysis of expression of the *Ar* gene in DI TNC1 cell line using quantitative real-time PCR. Figure S1: The expression of *Ar* gene in DI TNC1 cell line.

Author Contributions: Conceptualization: M.T.-K., B.B. and C.M.; methodology: M.T.-K., B.B., M.S., K.S. and L.P.; conducting the experiments: M.T.-K., M.S. and P.K., statistical analysis: P.S.; writing—original draft preparation: M.T.-K., M.S. and P.K.; writing—review and editing: B.B., L.P. and C.M.; supervision: B.B. and L.P. All authors have read and agreed to the published version of the manuscript.

Funding: This research was funded by MEDICAL UNIVERSITY OF LODZ from the research task number 501/5-062-01/201-81-134, 502-03/5-062-01/502-54-181, 502-03/5-062-01/502-54-182 and 503/1-062-01/503-51-001-19-00.

Institutional Review Board Statement: Not applicable.

Informed Consent Statement: Not applicable.

Data Availability Statement: The original contributions presented in the study are included in the article/Supplementary Materials, further inquiries can be directed to the corresponding author/s.

Conflicts of Interest: Author Claudia Mattern was employed by the company M et P Pharma. The remaining authors declare that the research was conducted in the absence of any commercial or financial relationships that could be construed as a potential conflict of interest.

References

1. Choi, S.S.; Lee, H.J.; Lim, I.; Satoch, J.; Kim, S.U. Human astrocytes: Secretome profiles of cytokines and chemokines. *PLoS ONE* **2014**, *9*, e92325. [CrossRef]
2. Stalder, A.K.; Pagenstecher, A.; Yu, N.C.; Kincaid, C.; Chiang, C.S.; Hobbs, M.V.; Bloom, F.E.; Campbell, I.L. Lipopolysaccharide-induced IL-12 expression in the central nervous system and cultured astrocytes and microglia. *J. Immunol.* **1997**, *159*, 1344–1351. [CrossRef]
3. Van Wagoner, N.J.; Oh, J.W.; Repovic, P.; Benveniste, E.N. Interleukin-6 (IL-6) production by astrocytes: Autocrine regulation by IL-6 and the soluble IL-6 receptor. *J. Neurosci.* **1999**, *19*, 5236–5244. [CrossRef]
4. Sénécal, V.; Deblois, G.; Beauseigle, D.; Schneider, R.; Brandenburg, J.; Newcombe, J.; Moore, C.S.; Prat, A.; Mantel, J.; Arbour, N. Production of IL-27 in multiple sclerosis lesions by astrocytes and myeloid cells: Modulation of local immune responses. *Glia* **2016**, *64*, 553–569. [CrossRef]
5. Wu, Z.; Zhang, J.; Nakanishi, H. Leptomeningeal cells activate microglia and astrocytes to induce IL-10 production by releasing pro-inflammatory cytokines during systemic inflammation. *J. Neuroimmunol.* **2005**, *167*, 90–98. [CrossRef]
6. Cooley, I.D.; Chauhan, V.S.; Donneyz, M.A.; Marriott, I. Astrocytes produce IL-19 in response to bacterial challenge and are sensitive to the immunosuppressive effects of this IL-10 family member. *Glia* **2014**, *62*, 818–828. [CrossRef]
7. Rubio, N.; Sanz-Rodriguez, F.; Lipton, H.L. Theiler's virus induces the MIP-2 chemokine (CXCL2) in astrocytes from genetically susceptible but not from resistant mouse strains. *Cell Immunol.* **2006**, *239*, 31–40. [CrossRef] [PubMed]
8. Glabinski, A.R.; Tuhoy, V.K.; Ransohoff, R.M. Expression of chemokines RANTES, MIP-1alpha and GRO-alpha correlates with inflammation in acute experimental autoimmune encephalomyelitis. *Neuroimmunomodulation* **1998**, *5*, 166–171. [CrossRef] [PubMed]
9. Blaževski, J.; Petković, F.; Momcilovic, M.; Jevtic, B.; Mostarica-Stojković, M.; Miljkovic, D. Tumor necrosis factor stimulates expression of CXCL12 in astrocytes. *Immunobiology* **2015**, *220*, 845–850. [CrossRef] [PubMed]
10. Sanmarco, L.M.; Polonio, C.M.; Wheeler, M.A.; Quintana, F.J. Functional immune cell-astrocyte interactions. *J. Exp. Med.* **2021**, *218*, e20202715. [CrossRef] [PubMed]

11. Eddleston, M.; Mucke, L. Molecular profile of reactive astrocytes–implications for their role in neurologic disease. *Neuroscience* **1993**, *54*, 15–36. [CrossRef]
12. Verkhratsky, A.; Parpura, V. Recent advances in (patho)physiology of astroglia. *Acta Pharmacol. Sin.* **2010**, *31*, 1044–1054. [CrossRef]
13. Haskill, S.; Peace, A.; Sporn, S.A.; Anisowicz, A.; Lee, S.W.; Smith, T.; Martin, G.; Ralph, P.; Cases, R. Identification of three related human GRO genes encoding cytokine functions. *Proc. Natl. Acad. Sci. USA* **1990**, *87*, 7732–7736. [CrossRef]
14. Iida, N.; Grotendorst, G.R. Cloning and sequencing of a new gro transcript from activated human monocytes: Expression in leukocytes and wound tissue. *Mol. Cell. Biol.* **1990**, *10*, 5596–5599.
15. Becker, S.; Quay, J.; Koren, H.S.; Haskill, J.S. Constitutive and stimulated MCP-1, GRO alpha, beta, and gamma expression in human airway epithelium and bronchoalveolar macrophages. *Am. J. Physiol.* **1994**, *266 Pt 1*, L278–L286. [CrossRef]
16. Omari, K.M.; John, G.; Lango, R.; Raine, C.S. Role for CXCR2 and CXCL1 on glia in multiple sclerosis. *Glia* **2006**, *53*, 24–31. [CrossRef]
17. Katancik, J.A.; Sharma, A.; de Nardin, E. Interleukin 8, neutrophil-activating peptide-2 and GRO-alpha bind to and elicit cell activation via specific and different amino acid residues of CXCR2. *Cytokine* **2000**, *12*, 1480–1488. [CrossRef]
18. Sawant, K.V.; Poluri, K.M.; Dutta, A.K.; Sepuru, K.M.; Troshkina, A.; Garofalo, R.P.; Rajarathnam, K. Chemokine CXCL1 mediated neutrophil recruitment: Role of glycosaminoglycan interactions. *Sci. Rep.* **2016**, *6*, 33123. [CrossRef]
19. Schumacher, C.; Clark-Lewis, I.; Baggiolini, M.; Moser, B. High- and low-affinity binding of GRO alpha and neutrophil-activating peptide 2 to interleukin 8 receptors on human neutrophils. *Proc. Natl. Acad. Sci. USA* **1992**, *89*, 10542–10546. [CrossRef] [PubMed]
20. Serdar, M.; Kempe, K.; Herrmann, R.; Picard, D.; Remke, M.; Herz, J.; Bendix, I.; Felderhoff-Müser, U.; Sabir, H. Involvement of CXCL1/CXCR2 During Microglia Activation Following Inflammation-Sensitized Hypoxic-Ischemic Brain Injury in Neonatal Rats. *Front. Neurol.* **2020**, *11*, 540878. [CrossRef] [PubMed]
21. Robinson, S.; Tani, M.; Strieter, R.M.; Ransohoff, R.M.; Miller, R.H. The chemokine growth-regulated oncogene-alpha promotes spinal cord oligodendrocyte precursor proliferation. *J. Neurosci.* **1998**, *18*, 10457–10463. [CrossRef]
22. Kadi, L.; Selvaraju, R.; de Lys, P.; Proudfoot, A.E.I.; Wells, T.N.C.; Boschert, U. Differential effects of chemokines on oligodendrocyte precursor proliferation and myelin formation in vitro. *J. Neuroimmunol.* **2006**, *174*, 133–146. [CrossRef]
23. Omari, K.M.; John, G.R.; Sealfon, S.C.; Raine, C.S. CXC chemokine receptors on human oligodendrocytes: Implications for multiple sclerosis. *Brain* **2005**, *128 Pt 5*, 1003–1015. [CrossRef]
24. Filipovic, R.; Zecevic, N. The effect of CXCL1 on human fetal oligodendrocyte progenitor cells. *Glia* **2008**, *56*, 1–15. [CrossRef]
25. Wang, L.; Yang, H.; Zang, C.; Dong, Y.; Shang, J.; Chen, J.; Wang, Y.; Liu, H.; Zhang, Z.; Xu, H.; et al. CXCR2 antagonism promotes oligodendrocyte precursor cell differentiation and enhances remyelination in a mouse model of multiple sclerosis. *Neurobiol. Dis.* **2020**, *134*, 104630. [CrossRef]
26. Müller-Ladner, U.; Jones, J.L.; Wetsel, R.A.; Gay, S.; Raine, C.S.; Barnum, S.R. Enhanced expression of chemotactic receptors in multiple sclerosis lesions. *J. Neurol. Sci.* **1996**, *144*, 135–141. [CrossRef]
27. Lustig, R.H. Sex hormone modulation of neural development in vitro. *Horm. Behav.* **1994**, *28*, 383–395. [CrossRef]
28. Zung, A.; Phillip, M.; Chalew, S.A.; Palese, T.; Kowarski, A.A.; Zadik, Z. Testosterone effect on growth and growth mediators of the GH-IGF-I axis in the liver and epiphyseal growth plate of juvenile rats. *J. Mol. Endocrinol.* **1999**, *23*, 209–221. [CrossRef]
29. Chin, K.Y.; Ima-Nirwana, S. The effects of orchidectomy and supraphysiological testosterone administration on trabecular bone structure and gene expression in rats. *Aging Male* **2015**, *18*, 60–66. [CrossRef]
30. Zhang, Y.; Champagne, N.; Beitel, L.K.; Goodyer, C.G.; Trifiro, M.; LeBlanc, A. Estrogen and androgen protection of human neurons against intracellular amyloid beta1-42 toxicity through heat shock protein 70. *J. Neurosci.* **2004**, *24*, 5315–5321. [CrossRef]
31. Białek, M.; Zaremba, P.; Borowicz, K.K.; Czuczwar, S.J. Neuroprotective role of testosterone in the nervous system. *Pol. J. Pharmacol.* **2004**, *56*, 509–518.
32. Ogata, T.; Nakamura, Y.; Tsuji, K.; Shibata, T.; Kataoka, K. Steroid hormones protect spinal cord neurons from glutamate toxicity. *Neuroscience* **1993**, *55*, 445–449. [CrossRef]
33. Asgari, N. Epidemiological, clinical and immunological aspects of neuromyelitis optica (NMO). *Dan. Med. J.* **2013**, *60*, B4730.
34. Wingerchuk, D.M. Neuromyelitis optica: Effect of gender. *J. Neurol. Sci.* **2009**, *286*, 18–23. [CrossRef]
35. Tintoré, M.; Arrambide, G. Early onset multiple sclerosis: The role of gender. *J. Neurol. Sci.* **2009**, *286*, 31–34. [CrossRef]
36. Voumvourakis, K.I.; Tsiodras, S.; Kitsos, D.K.; Stamboulis, E. Gender hormones: Role in the pathogenesis of central nervous system disease and demyelination. *Curr. Neurovasc. Res.* **2008**, *5*, 224–235. [CrossRef]
37. Pugliatti, M.; Rosati, G.; Carton, H.; Riise, T.; Drulovic, J.; Vécsei, L.; Milanov, I. The epidemiology of multiple sclerosis in Europe. *Eur. J. Neurol.* **2006**, *13*, 700–722. [CrossRef]
38. Harbo, H.F.; Gold, R.; Tintoré, M. Sex and gender issues in multiple sclerosis. *Ther. Adv. Neurol. Disord.* **2013**, *6*, 237–248. [CrossRef]
39. Disanto, G.; Ramagopalan, S.V. On the sex ratio of multiple sclerosis. *Mult. Scler. J.* **2013**, *19*, 3–4. [CrossRef]
40. Ribbons, K.A.; McElduff, P.; Boz, C.; Trojano, M.; Izquierdo, G.; Duquette, P.; Girard, M.; Grand'Maison, F.; Hupperts, R.; Grammond, P.; et al. Male Sex Is Independently Associated with Faster Disability Accumulation in Relapse-Onset MS but Not in Primary Progressive MS. *PLoS ONE* **2015**, *10*, e0122686. [CrossRef]
41. Pakpoor, J.; Goldacre, R.; Schmierer, K.; Giovannoni, G.; Goldacre, M.J. Testicular hypofunction and multiple sclerosis risk: A record-linkage study. *Ann. Neurol.* **2014**, *76*, 625–628. [CrossRef]

42. Gold, S.M.; Chalifoux, S.; Giesser, B.S.; Voskuhl, R.R. Immune modulation and increased neurotrophic factor production in multiple sclerosis patients treated with testosterone. *J. Neuroinflamm.* **2008**, *5*, 32. [CrossRef]
43. Bebo, B.F.; Schuster, J.C.; Vandenbark, A.A.; Offner, H. Androgens alter the cytokine profile and reduce encephalitogenicity of myelin-reactive T cells. *J. Immunol.* **1999**, *162*, 35–40. [CrossRef]
44. Liva, S.M.; Voskuhl, R.R. Testosterone acts directly on CD4+ T lymphocytes to increase IL-10 production. *J. Immunol.* **2001**, *167*, 2060–2067. [CrossRef]
45. Johnson, R.T.; Schneider, A.; DonCarlos, L.L.; Breedlove, S.M.; Jordan, C.L. Astrocytes in the rat medial amygdala are responsive to adult androgens. *J. Comp. Neurol.* **2012**, *520*, 2531–2544. [CrossRef]
46. Satriotomo, I.; Miki, T.; Gonzalez, D.; Matsumoto, Y.; Li, H.P.; Gu, H.; Takeuchi, Y. Excessive testosterone treatment and castration induce reactive astrocytes and fos immunoreactivity in suprachiasmatic nucleus of mice. *Brain Res.* **2004**, *1020*, 130–139. [CrossRef]
47. Gu, F.; Hata, R.; Toku, K.; Yang, L.; Ma, Y.J.; Maeda, N.; Sakanaka, M.; Tanaka, J. Testosterone up-regulates aquaporin-4 expression in cultured astrocytes. *J. Neurosci. Res.* **2003**, *72*, 709–715. [CrossRef]
48. Lorenz, B.; Garcia-Segura, L.M.; DonCarlos, L.L. Cellular phenotype of androgen receptor-immunoreactive nuclei in the developing and adult rat brain. *J. Comp. Neurol.* **2005**, *492*, 456–468. [CrossRef]
49. Mhaouty-Kodja, S. Role of the androgen receptor in the central nervous system. *Mol. Cell. Endocrinol.* **2018**, *465*, 103–112. [CrossRef]
50. Sygnecka, K.; Hein, C.; Scherf, N.; Fasold, M.; Binder, H.; Scheller, C.; Franke, H. Nimodipine enhances neurite outgrowth in dopaminergic brain slice co-cultures. *Int. J. Dev. Neurosci.* **2015**, *40*, 1–11. [CrossRef]
51. Klimas, J.; Olvedy, M.; Ochodnicka-Mackovicova, K.; Kruzliak, P.; Cacanyiova, S.; Kristek, F.; Krenek, P.; Ochodnicky, P. Perinatally administered losartan augments renal ACE2 expression but not cardiac or renal Mas receptor in spontaneously hypertensive rats. *J. Cell. Mol. Med.* **2015**, *19*, 1965–1974. [CrossRef]
52. Chen, Z.; Chintagari, N.R.; Guo, Y.; Bhaskaran, M.; Chen, J.; Gao, L.; Jin, N.; Weng, T.; Liu, L. Gene expression of rat alveolar type II cells during hyperoxia exposure and early recovery. *Free Radic. Biol. Med.* **2007**, *43*, 628–642. [CrossRef]
53. Yu, S.; Li, Y.; Zhao, H.; Wang, Q.; Chen, P. The Histone Demethylase JMJD1C Regulates CAMKK2-AMPK Signaling to Participate in Cardiac Hypertrophy. *Front. Physiol.* **2020**, *11*, 539. [CrossRef]
54. Schludi, B.; Moin, A.S.M.; Montemurro, C.; Gurlo, T.; Matveyenko, A.V.; Kirakossian, D.; Dawson, D.W.; Dry, S.M.; Butler, P.C.; Butler, A.E. Islet inflammation and ductal proliferation may be linked to increased pancreatitis risk in type 2 diabetes. *JCI Insight* **2017**, *2*, 5499368. [CrossRef]
55. Gujral, J.S.; Liu, J.; Farhood, A.; Jaeschke, H. Reduced oncotic necrosis in Fas receptor-deficient C57BL/6J-lpr mice after bile duct ligation. *Hepatology* **2004**, *40*, 998–1007. [CrossRef]
56. Omari, K.M.; Lutz, S.E.; Santambrogio, L.; Lira, S.A.; Raine, C.S. Neuroprotection and remyelination after autoimmune demyelination in mice that inducibly overexpress CXCL1. *Am. J. Pathol.* **2009**, *174*, 164–176. [CrossRef]
57. Hosking, M.P.; Tirotta, E.; Ransohoff, R.M.; Lane, T.E. CXCR2 signaling protects oligodendrocytes and restricts demyelination in a mouse model of viral-induced demyelination. *PLoS ONE* **2010**, *5*, e11340. [CrossRef]
58. Grist, J.J.; Marro, B.S.; Skinner, D.D.; Syage, A.R.; Worne, C.; Doty, D.J.; Fujinami, R.S.; Lane, T.E. Induced CNS expression of CXCL1 augments neurologic disease in a murine model of multiple sclerosis via enhanced neutrophil recruitment. *Eur. J. Immunol.* **2018**, *48*, 1199–1210. [CrossRef]
59. Zhang, J.; Harada, Y.; Hayashi, Y. A TLR-CXCL1 pathway in DRG neurons induces neutrophil accumulation in the DRG and mechanical allodynia in EAE mice. *Sci. Rep.* **2019**, *9*, 12003. [CrossRef]
60. Kerstetter, A.E.; Padovani-Claudio, D.A.; Bai, L.; Miller, R.H. Inhibition of CXCR2 signaling promotes recovery in models of multiple sclerosis. *Exp. Neurol.* **2009**, *220*, 44–56. [CrossRef]
61. Kalincik, T.; Vivek, V.; Jokubaitis, V.; Lechner-Scott, J.; Trojano, M.; Izquierdo, G.; Lugaresi, A.; Grand'Maison, F.; Hupperts, R.; Oreja-Guevara, C.; et al. Sex as a determinant of relapse incidence and progressive course of multiple sclerosis. *Brain* **2013**, *136 Pt 12*, 3609–3617. [CrossRef]
62. Pozzilli, C.; Tomassini, V.; Marinelli, F.; Paolillo, A.; Gasperini, C.; Bastianello, S. 'Gender gap' in multiple sclerosis: Magnetic resonance imaging evidence. *Eur. J. Neurol.* **2003**, *10*, 95–97. [CrossRef]
63. Khalid, R. Contributing factors in multiple sclerosis and the female sex bias. *Immunol. Lett.* **2014**, *162 Pt A*, 223–232. [CrossRef]
64. Fazekas, F.; Enzinger, C.; Wallner-Blazek, M.; Ropele, S.; Pluta-Fuerst, A.; Fox, S. Gender differences in MRI studies on multiple sclerosis. *J. Neurol. Sci.* **2009**, *286*, 28–30. [CrossRef]
65. Bove, R.M.; Healy, B.; Augustine, A.; Musallam, A.; Gholipour, T.; Chitnis, T. Effect of gender on late-onset multiple sclerosis. *Mult. Scler. J.* **2012**, *18*, 1472–1479. [CrossRef]
66. Bielecki, B.; Matters, C.; Ghoumari, A.M.; Javaid, S.; Smietanka, K.; Abi Ghanem, C.; Mhaouty-Kodja, S.; Ghandour, M.S.; Baulieu, E.E.; Franklin, R.J.M.; et al. Unexpected central role of the androgen receptor in the spontaneous regeneration of myelin. *Proc. Natl. Acad. Sci. USA* **2016**, *113*, 14829–14834. [CrossRef]
67. Ghasemlou, N.; Jeong, S.Y.; Lacroix, S.; David, S. T cells contribute to lysophosphatidylcholine-induced macrophage activation and demyelination in the CNS. *Glia* **2007**, *55*, 294–302. [CrossRef]
68. Plemel, J.R.; Michaels, N.J.; Weishaupt, N.; Caprariello, A.V.; Keough, M.B.; Rogers, J.A.; Yukseloglu, A.; Lim, J.; Patel, V.V.; Rawji, K.S.; et al. Mechanisms of lysophosphatidylcholine-induced demyelination: A primary lipid disrupting myelinopathy. *Glia* **2018**, *66*, 327–347. [CrossRef]

69. Hung, N.D.; Sok, D.E.; Kim, M.R. Prevention of 1-palmitoyl lysophosphatidylcholine-induced inflammation by polyunsaturated acyl lysophosphatidylcholine. *Inflamm. Res.* **2012**, *61*, 473–483. [CrossRef]
70. Bach, G.; Perrin-Cocon, L.; Gerossier, E.; Guironnet-Paquet, A.; Lotteau, V.; Inchauspé, G.; Fournillier, A. Singlelysophosphatidylcholine components exhibit adjuvant activities in vitro and in vivo. *Clin. Vaccine Immunol.* **2010**, *17*, 429–438. [CrossRef]
71. Sheikh, A.M.; Nagai, A.; Ryu, J.K.; McLarnon, J.G.; Kim, S.U.; Masuda, J. Lysophosphatidylcholine induces glial cell activation: Role of rho kinase. *Glia* **2009**, *57*, 898–907. [CrossRef]
72. Inose, Y.; Kato, Y.; Kitagawa, K.; Uchiyama, S.; Shibata, N. Activated microglia in ischemic stroke penumbra upregulate MCP-1 and CCR2 expression in response to lysophosphatidylcholine derived from adjacent neurons and astrocytes. *Neuropathology* **2015**, *35*, 209–223. [CrossRef]
73. Hussain, R.; Ghoumari, A.M.; Bielecki, B.; Steibel, J.; Bohem, N.; Liere, P.; Macklin, W.B.; Kumar, N.; Habert, R.; Mhaouty-Kodja, S.; et al. The neural androgen receptor: A therapeutic target for myelin repair in chronic demyelination. *Brain* **2013**, *136 Pt 1*, 132–146. [CrossRef]
74. Sellau, J.; Groneberg, M.; Fehling, H.; Thye, T.; Hoenow, S.; Marggraff, C.; Weskamm, M.; Hansen, C.; Stanelle-Bertram, S.; Kuhl, S.; et al. Androgens predispose males to monocyte-mediated immunopathology by inducing the expression of leukocyte recruitment factor CXCL1. *Nat. Commun.* **2020**, *11*, 3459. [CrossRef]
75. Itoh, N.; Itoh, Y.; Tassoni, A.; Ren, E.; Kaito, M.; Ohno, A.; Ao, Y.; Farkhondeh, V.; Johnsonbaugh, H.; Burda, J.; et al. Cell-specific and region-specific transcriptomics in the multiple sclerosis model: Focus on astrocytes. *Proc. Natl. Acad. Sci. USA* **2018**, *115*, E302–E309. [CrossRef]
76. Masiello, D.; Cheng, S.; Bubley, G.J.; Lu, M.L.; Balk, S.P. Bicalutamide functions as an androgen receptor antagonist by assembly of a transcriptionally inactive receptor. *J. Biol. Chem.* **2002**, *277*, 26321–26326. [CrossRef]
77. Nguyen, T.V.; Yao, M.; Pike, C.J. Flutamide and cyproterone acetate exert agonist effects: Induction of androgen receptor-dependent neuroprotection. *Endocrinology* **2007**, *148*, 2936–2943. [CrossRef]
78. Prekovic, S.; van Royen, M.E.; Voet, A.R.D.; Geverts, B.; Houtman, R.; Melchers, D.; Zhang, K.Y.J.; Van den Broeck, T.; Smeets, E.; Spans, L.; et al. The Effect of F877L and T878A Mutations on Androgen Receptor Response to Enzalutamide. *Mol. Cancer Ther.* **2016**, *15*, 1702–1712. [CrossRef]
79. Kata, D.; Gróf, I.; Hoyk, Z.; Ducza, E.; Deli, M.A.; Zupkó, I.; Földesi, I. Immunofluorescent Evidence for Nuclear Localization of Aromatase in Astrocytes in the Rat Central Nervous System. *Int. J. Mol. Sci.* **2022**, *23*, 8946. [CrossRef]
80. Thiel, G.; Welck, J.; Wissenbach, U.; Rössler, O.G. Dihydrotestosterone activates AP-1 in LNCaP prostate cancer cells. *Int. J. Biochem.* **2019**, *110*, 9–20. [CrossRef]
81. Shieh, J.-M.; Tsai, Y.-J.; Tsou, C.-J.; Wu, W.-B. CXCL1 Regulation in Human Pulmonary Epithelial Cells by Tumor Necrosis Factor. *Cell. Physiol. Biochem.* **2014**, *34*, 1373–1384. [CrossRef]
82. Karim, H.; Kim, S.H.; Lapato, A.S.; Yasui, N.; Katzenellenbogen, J.A.; Tiwari-Woodruff, S.K. Increase in chemokine CXCL1 by ERβ ligand treatment is a key mediator in promoting axon myelination. *Proc. Natl. Acad. Sci. USA* **2018**, *115*, 6291–6296. [CrossRef] [PubMed]
83. Salinas-Muñoz, L.; Campos-Fernández, R.; Olivera-Valle, I.; Mercader, E.; Fernandez-Pacheco, C.; Lasarte, S.; Pérez-Martín, L.; Navarro-González, M.T.; Sánchez-Mateos, P.; Samaniego, R.; et al. Estradiol impairs epithelial CXCL1 gradient in the cervix to delay neutrophil transepithelial migration during insemination. *J. Reprod. Immunol.* **2019**, *132*, 9–15. [CrossRef] [PubMed]

MDPI AG
Grosspeteranlage 5
4052 Basel
Switzerland
Tel.: +41 61 683 77 34

Current Issues in Molecular Biology Editorial Office
E-mail: cimb@mdpi.com
www.mdpi.com/journal/cimb

www.ingramcontent.com/pod-product-compliance
Lightning Source LLC
Chambersburg PA
CBHW041407210926
51850CB00013B/3201
9783725842759